Tommy McClanahan

Farm Animal Health and Disease Control

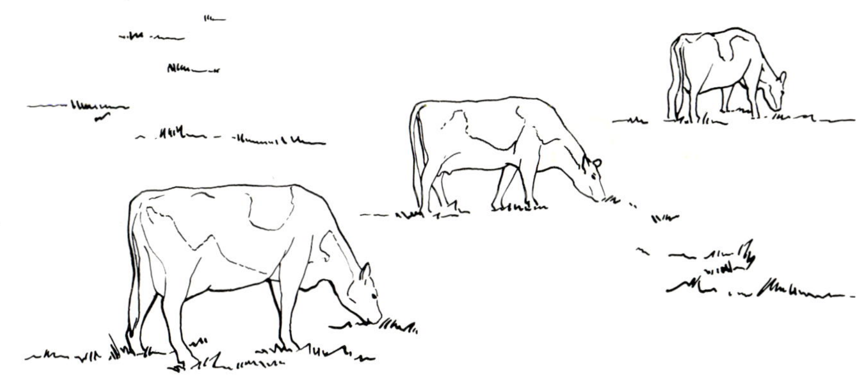

Farm Animal Health and Disease Control

JOSEPH H. GALLOWAY, B.V.Sc., M.R.C.V.S.

Director of the Vivarium and Assistant Professor of Physiology and Biophysics, Georgetown University School of Medicine, Washington, D.C.

LEA & FEBIGER PHILADELPHIA

Reprinted, 1974

ISBN 0-8121-0310-6

Library of Congress Catalog Card Number: 77-123420

Printed in the United States of America

Preface

THIS BOOK has been written for agriculture students.

For the past five years, I have been teaching a course in livestock diseases and sanitation, and have seen the need for a short introductory text outlining the principles of preventive veterinary medicine and disease control. There are many good texts concerning the diseases of a particular species of domestic animal, and there are many farmers' veterinary encyclopedias. However, a book seemed needed for a one-semester course where the coverage must, of necessity, be broad.

In planning this text, I have had no thought of encouraging the agriculture students to assume the role of veterinarians, for which of course they lack training, but rather I hope to acquaint them with the causes and the methods of eradication, prevention and control of infectious diseases of economic importance to the livestock industry.

The matter of treatment has been purposely avoided, since it is felt that treatment belongs in the hands of skilled veterinarians. The prevention of disease by proper management has been emphasized, since here the farmer has the primary responsibility.

The book is divided into seven parts. The first part deals with the agencies concerned with the eradication of diseases of economic or public-health importance, and with the methods and procedures by which eradication and control may be accomplished.

The second part of the book is concerned with specific diseases of economic importance. It is hoped that in this way the text may serve the student as a reference volume in the future. Only those diseases and conditions preventable by prophylactic means are covered. Part 3 is concerned with a few selected diseases best controlled by tactical measures. Part 4 deals with exotic diseases that can pose a threat to the livestock industry of this country, and Part 5 points out the dangers of poisonous substances. Because of the economic importance of parasites to the livestock industry, Part 6 of the book deals with the internal and external parasites most often encountered in veterinary practice.

In the preparation of this book, free use has been made of current literature. However, unless specifically noted, acknowledgments have been kept to a minimum and a list of selected references is given in Part 7 for those wishing to obtain further details. In choosing the specific diseases to be presented in this text, liberal use was made of the National Report of Animal Diseases prepared by the United States Department of Agriculture.

Washington, D.C. JOSEPH H. GALLOWAY

Contents

PART 1
General Principles

1
Introduction

PREVENTIVE medicine for farm animals is important both for human public health and livestock production. Animal diseases directly transmissable to man can cause varying types of ill-health. In addition to this direct effect, human health and well-being may be affected through the loss of animals, or their products, from animal diseases or mismanagement.

In a recent analysis of the livestock industry, it was pointed out that, because of our rapidly expanding population, the nation will need 50 percent more meat by 1975. This will be accomplished only by thorough planning and increased attention to the health of our livestock. No single sickness, injury or death can be shrugged off as uncontrollable, impractical to treat, or unavoidable. The livestock industry is big business, and like any other business must concern itself with making a profit. Poor planning or lack of attention to seemingly small problems, especially concerning herd health, can make serious inroads into profits.

In the economic production of livestock, every female should produce living offspring and raise them to market weight. Every animal dying before reaching market weight due to abortion or disease, every animal retarded due to mismanagement, represents the loss of a sizable sum of money to the producer. Therefore, the least number of losses from conception to consignment is the goal of the efficient operator.

The most desirable production practices are those that prevent losses of marketable animals. However, many factors make these problems far from easy to control. Factors to be considered, either singly or in combination, include infectious and contagious diseases, vitamin and mineral deficiencies, genetic abnormalities, nutritional deficiencies, plant, mineral and insecticide toxicities, and internal and external parasites.

The objective of a breeding program is to produce the largest number of offspring with the highest weaning weights at a minimum cost. Therefore, the primary considerations in producing a profitable crop must be vigorous healthy parents, adequate nutritious feedstuffs, and an effective barrier to diseases.

All animals should be examined thoroughly before breeding. The procedure for examination rests with each producer, but it is recommended that the services of a veterinarian be utilized to examine animals for breeding abnormalities and diseases.

During gestation, dams should be observed from time to time for signs of abnormality. If at all possible, they should be examined for pregnancy periodically after being put with the male, and, if open, the cause should be determined. Although it may be difficult to examine for pregnancy on many large spreads, the efficient rancher or farmer does control his herd by determining the open females. For maximum efficiency of the operation, barren females should be detected early and sold or replaced.

The following organisms may cause abortion if proper preventive measures are not exercised: *Trichomonas foetus, Vibrio fetus, Leptospira pomona, Brucella abortus.* Epizootic bovine abortion, and other conditions such as nutritional deficiencies, injuries, heat stroke, fatigue, undue handling and stress, and internal and external parasites can also result in heavy losses.

Control and treatment of diseases of farm animals must be predicated on well-planned programs of preventive medicine and efficient management. Therefore, let us examine some preventive health measures and divide them into two categories, i.e., strategic and tactical. Strategic preventive measures are based upon a knowledge of seasonal occurrence of infections, stress and weather conditions. Tactical measures, on the other hand, are aimed at preventing increased infestations or infections and treating unusual stresses or other conditions brought about by weather, transportation, or accident. Strategic measures are worked out well in advance and put into operation on a planned schedule. Tactical measures, although planned in advance, are not usually put into operation until actually needed.

Phase One

For the purpose of this discussion, let us presuppose that a cattle ranch in operation for some time is making a concerted effort to map out a strategic and tactical approach to preventive herd health for the next year. Only healthy cows and bulls have been selected, and "D-day" is the breeding season. Strategic plans will insure that the bulls are healthy, fertile, vigorous, and free from any leg or foot condition. The cows will be in good condition, free from vaginal discharges, and with no history of retained placenta, prolapse, or previous difficult calving. About four months after joining the cows with the bulls, all cows should be examined for pregnancy; any found to be open should be removed from the herd and examined by a veterinarian. The same general criteria may be applied to all breeding operations, regardless of species being produced.

Phase Two

Phase two of our strategic planning must be concerned with the calving period. In general, this is the most important time of the whole operation and a breakdown in schedule would be disastrous. Every ranch has a different set of circumstances to contend with at this time, but generally speaking calving time is frequently mismanaged. Oftentimes not much can be done to alleviate the most objectionable features. However, if at all possible, calves should not be crowded into small lots with older cattle, nor crowded in muddy lots that have been used year after year, nor kept in damp, drafty sheds or barns. Every calf should be given an injection of vitamin A and selenium if in a deficient area. The veterinarian will suggest appropriate bacterins to guard against calf scours, pneumonia, and blackleg.

Phase Three

Phase three of the strategic plan is concerned with weaning time. Prior to weaning, all female calves should be vaccinated with Strain 19 to prevent brucellosis, bull calves should be castrated, and all calves should receive Leptospira bacterin to prevent leptospirosis. Due to the stress of weaning they should also be vaccinated for shipping fever and revaccinated for blackleg and malignant edema. Creep feeding should be started weeks before weaning to reduce weaning stress.

Tactical Measures

Tactical measures associated with Phase One include: providing extra bulls in case of accident or injury to the first joined, prompt care of feet, especially in wet weather, to insure against loss of production due to foot rot, examination and treatment for pinkeye or other abnormal conditions of the eye, and replacement of cows found to be barren when checked for pregnancy. Many of these measures may be carried out during the other phases if the need arises.

Control of Parasites

The most insidious inroads into the cattle producer's profit are made by internal and external parasites. Here again strategic and tactical procedures are useful in cutting the losses caused by these organisms. Strategic treatments are based upon the knowledge of the seasonal occurrence of parasites, while tactical treatments are aimed at preventing increased infestations following climatic conditions favorable to the parasites.

A recent survey showed that as many as 8 percent of calves may be lost through parasitic worm infestations and that the mortality may be much higher in regions of high rainfall. However, the greatest monetary loss from parasites in cattle—as well as other livestock—results not from death but from the failure of young stock to prosper and grow at an optimum rate. Roundworms and flukes are very important in high-rainfall areas and, although climatic factors do not favor these worms in drier, less verdant areas, they cannot be ruled out as important agents of losses in those areas where pastures are irrigated.

Under normal conditions it is impossible to maintain grazing animals entirely free from worms. Indeed, this would be undesirable as the young would then not develop immunity. Immunity is important and advantage should be taken of it in planning for control. Strategic measures involve rotating of pastures, spelling each field at least six weeks to eliminate most of the larvae, avoiding overstocking and overcrowding, discing pastures at frequent intervals to disperse fecal matter, maintaining a high level of nutrition, routinely examining all stock twice a year for parasites and drenching when necessary. It is especially important to check for parasites early in the winter and in the summer.

Tactical measures to combat worm parasites include keeping pens and yards as clean as possible, and drenching all grazing animals three weeks following a good rain after a prolonged dry spell. Larvae of most species require about four weeks to develop to the adult stage in animals; therefore, at three weeks they are at the susceptible stage and can be killed before they lay eggs.

External parasites are also vulnerable to strategic and tactical measures of control. With the advent of systemic insecticides the days of the cattle grub may be numbered. Depending upon the region, the activity of the heel fly may vary, but in general the application of organophosphate spray late in the fall will kill the minute larvae in situ and will provide a measure of control against ticks and lice as well. Among the ectoparasites, lice and mites are most active in the winter months. It is advantageous to dip or spray all stock, including the very young animals, in the fall and again in the spring. The fall treatment will hold down an otherwise disastrous infestation and the spring treatment will catch those developing during the winter. Tactical sprayings and dippings may be done at any time when scabies or mange becomes a problem.

Knowledge of the life cycle of parasites and of periods of stress can be of great value in planning efficient and effective strategic and tactical measures to protect the health of herds and consequently profits.

Responsibility for Disease Control

Veterinary preventive medicine has a wide field of influence but its practice cannot be the responsibility of the veterinarian alone. The veterinarian by his training is in a unique position to understand epidemiology and to advise on the control of animal diseases, but he must collaborate with the producer on matters of management, feeding, and breeding. Disease control involves the practice of both clinical and preventive veterinary medicine, and, although we may think of clinical medicine as concerned mainly with individual animals, it is usually preliminary to the prevention and control of diseases in flocks or herds. The veterinarian must encourage livestock owners or managers to prevent animal diseases by promoting positive animal health programs. He must encourage the owners to believe that positive animal health and maximum productivity are his main objectives, because preventive veterinary medicine can be efficiently practiced only with the full cooperation of the animal owner or manager. *Steps taken to keep animals healthy will cost less in the long run than restoring them to health and productivity after they become sick.*

2
Disease Control Methods

IF OUR methods of preventing disease were no better today than they were one hundred years ago, we might now be spending tremendous amounts of money to fight against the elemental problems of malnutrition and hunger instead of being the best-fed nation in the world. During recent years science has been moving relentlessly forward against the scourge of transmissible diseases.

A major accomplishment was proving that living organisms cause disease and that microorganisms always originate from some other organisms, be they plant or animal. In 1863 a French scientist demonstrated that anthrax organisms could be shown in the blood of sheep that died of that disease, and that the organisms would multiply if kept under suitable conditions. Later, in 1876, the noted German bacteriologist Koch showed conclusively that the organisms demonstrated by the Frenchman could be grown on artificial media and were, therefore, the cause of anthrax in animals and people. From the early work of Koch, scientists now know how to grow microorganisms, how to produce disease with them, and how to make them into protective vaccines. However, that was only the beginning of the programs to protect animals from transmissible diseases.

Research workers had to learn how to produce each disease they studied in order to have sick animals with which to work. This in itself was a tremendous task. Some of the questions they sought were: How do microorganisms cause death? Where do they grow in sick animals? How do they escape from such sick animals? How long will they live outside the animal's body? What substances would kill the microorganisms? The bacteria causing brucellosis in cattle multiply in the pregnant uterus and in the udder. Brucella organisms escape with the calf at the time of birth, from the discharge from the uterus a few days or weeks after abortion or birth, and in the milk of the dam. Anthrax organisms may escape from infected animals in discharges from the nose, in the urine, and in feces. It has been found that anthrax spores can live for fifty years or more in soil even when exposed to bright sunlight and dry air.

Brucella organisms, on the other hand, are usually destroyed in a few days if exposed to direct sunlight or dry air.

It has been learned that animals may appear healthy and yet spread microorganisms causing such diseases as tuberculosis, brucellosis, glanders and coccidiosis. This discovery clarifies the disappointing results that had followed attempts to eradicate diseases from infected herds by removing all animals showing symptoms. The carrier animals were not removed, and they continued to spread infection.

Much work has been done to find methods of detecting symptom-free carrier animals. Governmental agencies have been instrumental in developing reporting procedures which will make it possible to control many diseases by preventing exposure. The basic principles concerned in accomplishing this task can be divided into two parts: (1) the determination of an endemic infection, and (2) the prevention of direct or indirect contact between disease-free animals and infected animals, or contaminated premises, equipment, feed, or vehicles.

By a system of reporting, state and federal veterinarians in various parts of the country learn where infection may be endemic. This may be done by making careful and repeated examinations of suspected animals, by examining animals passing through public stockyards, by requiring health certificates for all animals moving through interstate transportation systems, and by requiring veterinarians in the field to make reports of important infectious and contagious diseases. When a particular infectious disease has been reported, trained men will then examine the herds or flocks from which it has been reported to determine the extent of the disease, and, if necessary, will establish a quarantine. Sometimes a combination of physical examination and diagnostic test is the standard procedure. If suspicious cases are found, the veterinarian may collect material and send it to a laboratory for tests. Sometimes, however, symptoms and lesions are so typical that the diagnosis is made without laboratory confirmation.

For some diseases the veterinarian relies almost entirely on diagnostic tools—the tuberculin test for tuberculosis, the johnin tests for Johne's disease, the anaplasmosis agglutination test, the pullorum agglutination test, and many others.

Preventing contact between diseased and healthy animals often is difficult. The easiest and most economical way to accomplish this is to separate all diseased and exposed animals from healthy animals. The suspect animals are then given curative treatment and held in isolation until they are free of infection. At the same time, all contaminated premises are cleaned and disinfected. This procedure will eradicate disease by destroying the infectious agent at its source. To remove sick animals while leaving healthy animals in a contaminated area really means to continue the possibility of infection and the spread of disease organisms into an otherwise clean and uncontaminated area. Therefore, apparently healthy animals *should* be removed from the contaminated focus to a clean area and kept under observation. Depending upon the type of disease, infected animals may be held in isolation and quarantined on the same premises with little danger. However, sometimes such procedures are unsafe; for instance, any attempt to hold animals infected with foot-and-mouth disease on premises with other susceptible animals would probably be disastrous.

Infected animals (including man) are the source of all infections. They are always potentially dangerous. Slaughter of infected farm animals is usually the best procedure for actually preventing exposure and spread of easily transmitted diseases, which may be so infectious that it is well-nigh impossible to prevent their spread if sick and healthy animals are kept on the same premises. Slaughter is also the method of choice in handling diseases of a chronic nature from which animals do not recover. Some animals may live for months or years with these diseases, during which time they discharge large numbers of the organisms on the pastures or into barns.

Because of the danger of carrier animals, it has been the procedure in the United States to slaughter all animals affected with certain serious diseases such as tuberculosis. The government usually pays indemnities for slaughtered animals if the owners agree to follow programs of disease prevention prescribed by state and federal offices of disease control.

The causative agents of some diseases may be found in all parts of the carcasses of animals dying from those diseases. Therefore, carcasses should be disposed of as quickly and thoroughly as possible, by burning, sterilizing with heat, or burying deeply to prevent feral animals from disturbing the carcasses and further spreading the disease.

Premises contaminated with the disease-producing agents are potentially dangerous. Thorough cleaning and disinfection of barns, stables, and sheds exposed to disease-producing agents are necessary. Contaminated pastures present special problems. Spores of anthrax or blackleg organisms may live indefinitely in the soil. Viruses, on the other hand, may disappear from pastures in a relatively short time. Eggs, larvae, and immature arthropod and nematode organisms may infest pastures for a number of years. The plowing of pastures increases the danger of spores coming to the surface but lessens the danger from parasitic infestations; it decreases bacteria and viruses by exposing them to drying in direct sunlight.

Protection from exposure becomes increasingly easier as the amount of infection decreases. However, care should be taken to prevent unusual movement of animals from infected premises into premises clean and free from disease. The most common way to expose and infect animals in disease-free herds is to introduce infected animals into the healthy herds. If a farmer or rancher needs to add animals to a disease-free herd or flock, he should insist on official health certificates covering both the animals to be added and the herds from which they originate. The animals he buys should not be exposed in transit to infected animals or to contaminated trucks, cars, or pens. It is a wise precaution to hold newly purchased animals in separate quarters for three weeks or longer, as healthy-appearing animals may be harboring an infectious or contagious disease; they may pass all diagnostic tests, and still transmit the disease to other unexposed animals.

Increased resistance is becoming a more and more important factor in preventing transmissible diseases. It should be possible to increase resistance to some diseases by selective breeding. However, breeding farm animals for disease resistance is a long-term, costly operation. By natural selection, several breeds in different parts of the world have become somewhat resistant to diseases endemic in those areas; likewise, economic as well as environmental methods may have played a part in this natural selection.

Vaccination has been a practical method of protection against transmissible disease since Pasteur developed vaccines against some of the common diseases of that time. Vaccines give good protection against many of the transmissible diseases of livestock and poultry, among them some of the diseases which are most important today. No vaccine is absolutely safe or completely effective all the time; however, the practical value of vaccines has been demonstrated in many millions of protected animals.

Some vaccines give immediate and long-lasting protection. Some give immediate but short-lived protection. Some do not give satisfactory protection until 10 to 20 days after they are used. Some vaccines protect against only one type of disease, while others are polyvalent and protect against closely related microorganisms causing diseases with different manifestations.

The use of vaccines is the most effective method for protecting animals against acute infectious diseases when epizootics appear in countries with ineffective quarantine laws and few veterinarians or regulatory officials.

Countries with better laws and better control methods may attack such epizootics more vigorously with quarantine and eradication programs. However, the use of vaccines alone does not usually result in the complete eradication of disease. By the same token, the combination of quarantine and elimination of infected animals—to prevent exposure of disease-free animals—and vaccination has been successful in eliminating some diseases and protecting the animal population against them. This combination of eradicating infected animals and vaccinating susceptible exposed animals has brought about the elimination of several devastating diseases in the United States which are still prevalent in other countries of the world: foot-and-mouth disease, rinderpest, contagious bovine pleuropneumonia, Texas fever, glanders, and dourine are examples of such exotic diseases.

Protection against transmissible diseases is as important to the livestock producer as are good breeding and good feeding practices. Accepted protective measures should be included in the day-to-day operation of the livestock farm just as good feeding, good management, and the selection of good breeding stock. This is primarily the responsibility of the livestock producer. Veterinarians, livestock sanitary officials and research workers with animal diseases perform important functions in this area. However, the programs they recommend cannot succeed without the whole-hearted cooperation of the producer in carrying out these procedures. The ultimate objective is complete freedom from the transmissible diseases by which herds and flocks may be decimated.

3
Definitions

IT IS much easier to control a disease that is understood than an unknown malady. No longer do serious infectious diseases occur in devastating epidemics in this country, or in many parts of the world. This great achievement is the result of cooperative efforts by the entire agriculture health team in attacking the weak points in the disease cycles. Much of this success has been due to years of patient work and research in working out the reservoirs of these diseases, in isolating the causative agents, in identifying the vectors and studying their life histories, and in understanding the complex host-parasite interrelationships resulting in disease, inapparent infection, or in immunity. Livestock producers and veterinarians must have an appreciation of all these factors, often called the natural history or epidemiology of disease, in order to apply control measures intelligently. Therefore, we will begin this study by listing definitions of pertinent phrases.

The host-parasite and host-vector relationship is a complex of several primary factors, namely, parasite or causative agent of disease, vector, and host, which results in disease or inapparent infection and in immunity.

Infection: the presence of microorganisms in the body. The entry and development of or multiplication of infectious agents in the body.

Disease: an illness due to a specific agent or its toxic product arising through transmission and multiplication of that agent or its products from reservoir to susceptible host. Disease may further be defined as any change from the normal.

There can be infection without disease, but no disease without infection. Infection is not synonymous with infectious disease; there may be inapparent infection or manifest disease. Normally healthy individuals live in equilibrium, a state of truce with a variety of pathogens some of which can cause disease as changes occur in nutrition, weather and other factors. Apparently healthy people may harbor Demodex mites in the pores of the nose, tubercule bacilli in the lungs, enteric bacteria and protozoa in the alimentary tract, malarial parasites in the liver or reticuloendothelial system, filarial worms in the lymph nodes, and the fungi of athlete's foot between the toes. One wonders if apparently healthy people are ever really completely free from some of these microorganisms. The same applies to domestic animals.

Reservoir: the sum of all natural habitats of the microorganism. Microorganisms may be found in arthropods such as ticks, chiggers, mites, or any vector in which there is transovarian transmission of the pathogen from parent to offspring. Birds, vertebrates, rodents, and other species of animals may harbor a multitude of transmissible pathogens. The major problem in vector-borne disease control lies in the fact that it is impossible to kill or control all animals acting as reservoirs of a disease. Likewise, soil contaminated with bacteria and viruses causing diarrhea, dysentery, and other bacterial or viral diseases, some of which are due to spore-forming organisms which exist for considerable lengths of time in the free-living state, remains the primary focus for infecting reservoir animals.

In an epidemic, the moderate, severe and fatal cases are often easily located and reported. On the other hand, the mild, the atypical and abortive cases are the important ones because they are sources of infection for new cases; they keep the epidemic smoldering. In virus diseases such as foot-and-mouth disease and rinderpest, the virus is circulating in the peripheral blood and thus is available to infect additional vectors during the first few days of the disease. Virulent diseases have been introduced repeatedly into the United States and other areas of the world by carriers in which the virus was incubating but before clinical signs of disease were evident. It has been observed many times that an epidemic has resulted when nutrition declined, environmental sanitation broke down, and crowding and stress due to shifting populations increased. Under such conditions, a typical or mild case of a disease becomes moderately severe to severe, and severe cases terminate fatally.

Microorganism: a small organism living in or on, or at the expense of, a larger one. Microorganisms which may transmit disease-causing pathogens, or which are disease-causing pathogens in themselves, are viruses, rickettsia, bacteria, spirochetes, protozoa, helminths, and arthropods. The number of microorganisms necessary to initiate disease varies with the virulence of the organism and the resistance of the host. In general, the larger the number of microorganisms, the greater the chance of infection. For example, a bite of one infected mosquito may introduce enough protozoan parasites to initiate a clinical attack of malaria. On the other hand, it may require bites of thousands of mosquitoes and the injection of great many filarial worm larvae to bring about a clinical case of filariasis.

Virulence: a complex property which combines infectivity, invasiveness and pathogenicity.

Infectivity: the ability to initiate and maintain an infection in the host. This depends on the ability of the parasite to establish an initial beachhead in the host by evading or overcoming local defense mechanisms such as skin barriers, phagocytes, or antibodies.

Invasiveness: the power to progress from the initial infection further into the host. Microorganisms may grow in superficial tissues, in deep tissues, in the lymph; others may invade the bloodstream causing viremia, bacteremia, rickettsemia, and septicemia. After microorganisms have entered the bloodstream they may be carried to other organs, such as the liver, spleen, and bone marrow.

Pathogenicity: the ability to injure the host, once an infection is established. The principal cause of pathogenicity in most microorganisms is toxicity. Many toxins liberated by bacteria affect nervous tissue, heart muscle or kidney tissue. Strains of parasites vary from highly virulent to avirulent.

Host: one who receives and entertains another, that is, any living animal affording subsistence and lodging to microorganisms. There is a host-parasite relationship between the microorganism and the animal it has invaded. When a microorganism invades a host, one of several reactions may occur: (1) the microorganism may die quickly; (2) the parasite may survive but without causing any obvious symptoms of disease, that is, its presence may cause a reaction which may prevent reinfection or superinfection or there may be an inapparent infection; (3) the microorganisms may survive and cause disease with or without a host reaction which may or may not cure the disease, prevent reinfection or superinfection; and (4) the microorganisms may kill the host.

Susceptible host: a host not possessing resistance against a particular pathogenic agent and for that reason liable to contract the disease if exposed to the specific microorganism.

Resistance: the sum total of body mechanisms which impede the progress of invasion of microorganisms. There are two main aspects of such resistance, nonspecific and specific. Nonspecific resistance is directed, not against any particular disease, but against infection in general. There are genetic aspects to nonspecific resistance, in other words, species or racial resistance; secondly, there are physical and chemical barriers to infection. Skin rids itself of surface bacteria by the sloughing of scales from the skin. The acetic acid in perspiration is toxic to many bacteria. Tears not only contain a bactericidal substance but wash invading organisms through the tear ducts into the nasal cavities. The nose is lined with ciliated epithelial cells which urge microorganisms toward the pharynx. Sticky mucous membranes trap microorganisms, which are either coughed up or swallowed. In the mouth, suction and drainage sweep microorganisms into the stomach. Most bacteria and other organisms are destroyed by the strong, acid digestive juices.

A third means of nonspecific resistance is demonstrated by antimicrobial activities of blood cells, in particular the leukocytes of the circulating blood. A fourth mechanism is phagocytosis by leukocytes and the reticuloendothelial system. Microorganisms may be destroyed by white cells flowing in the blood. In addition special white cells, phagocytes, macrophages, or histiocytes, are built into the lining of blood vessels, particularly in the liver, spleen and bone marrow. They are part of the reticuloendothelial system which functions in part to destroy pathogens and dead cells by a process known as phagocytosis. In many infections the white cells try to dispose of foreign particles by ingesting and destroying them, or by giving off enzymes that will kill, destroy or digest them. The white cells may themselves be killed in the process.

Attacks by microorganisms are frequently countered by the development of antibodies and antitoxins. The humoral theory stated by many scientists, for our purposes, proposes that to each action of the microorganism there is a reaction by the host. The microorganism itself, or its products, contains antigen, a substance which when injected into mammalian tissues or bloodstream stimulates the formation of antibodies that react specifically when mixed with antigen. Antibodies are substances appearing in the blood or body fluids as the result of stimulation by an antigen and which react specifically with the antigen. Antibodies are modified fractions of gamma globulin.

There is a time sequence in the appearance and disappearance of antibodies. Complement-fixing antibodies appear early following infection but do not last; neutralizing antibodies appear later but may last for years.

4
Management of Health

EFFICIENT and economical animal husbandry demands healthy livestock. Poor health lowers production while fatal disease stops production entirely. Disease is the main limiting factor in the poor efficiency of animal husbandry in many countries; it is a burden which can be greatly lessened, even if it cannot be entirely avoided. It has been conservatively estimated that rinderpest, a disease widespread in the tropics, causes the death of two million animals each year. In Pakistan alone, it has been calculated that foot-and-mouth disease, a comparatively mild complaint, causes an annual loss of several millions of dollars, while in Europe it is even more costly. It is believed that in some parts of Africa the loss from parasitic diseases is over a hundred million dollars per year. Worldwide losses due to animal diseases and parasites account for the largest economic drain on the livestock industry.

Although the waves of epizootics which have swept with deplorable regularity over many parts of the world have to an appreciable extent been averted, subdued, or dissipated by the application of strict veterinary sanitary measures in North America, they are still within the experience of many farmers and ranchers and are part and parcel of their business awareness. Other factors probably have an equally devastating effect on the economy of animal husbandry: the state of impaired health which follows the failure of the body completely to suppress some causal agent of disease that devitalizes its victim and reduces or entirely stops productivity; the morbidity caused by an inadequate intake and sometimes by an excess of food, or the chronic state of susceptibility which arises from malnutrition; the inefficiency caused by heavier burdens of parasites than the body can successfully resist; and the loss of use of vast areas of fertile territory to parasites and poisonous plants fatal to animals. The average farmer or rancher cannot be an expert veterinarian nor is it necessary that he should be; however, he ought to know those diseases which, by their widespread effect, cause morbidity and mortality in his livestock, and he should have some idea of the action he can take to counteract them. Government veterinary services are organized to help animal husbandmen to maintain the health of their livestock because it is in the public interest that the animal wealth of the country is protected. The treatment of individual animals, provided their sickness entails no danger to the community, is the business of the owner, and even to him, from the purely economic point of view, is of secondary importance. It is impractical that every sick animal have the attention of an expert or veterinarian, and so the responsibility of protecting his own and his neighbors' livestock falls on each farmer or rancher. It is his duty to recognize immediately any abnormality in his livestock and to be aware of the possibility of its infectious or contagious nature. He should immediately contact his veterinarian for assistance should he suspect a disease of economic importance.

In most countries contagious or infectious diseases are reportable to public authorities, who may place quarantines upon flocks or herds with diseases of economic importance.

Prevalence of a certain disease may be estimated by the study of government morbidity reports of diseases of animals. Unfortunately, it is often difficult to ascertain the causes of poor health and unthriftiness. If the condition is well known, the cause may be understood and the cure at hand. If it is localized, the veterinarian on examination may be able to identify it or advise how it can be identified, but in many cases it is through the initiative of the owner that the condition is eliminated. He must not expect abnormalities to correct themselves.

Contagious and infectious diseases are caused through the invasion of the body by microorganisms. These are single-celled creatures which multiply by the simple process of division; however, in adverse circumstances some may form spores which are capable of withstanding conditions which would be fatal in the vegetative stage. Microorganisms range in structure and size from the invisible, or ultramicroscopic, viruses to the simple bacteria seen through a microscope under fairly high magnification to the more complex, comparatively large microorganisms such as protozoa which are visible under fairly low magnification. Many microorganisms elaborate toxins, the poisonous effect of which may damage the tissues, destroy the body defenses and cause death.

The body is invaded most frequently through the natural orifices (the mouth, the nose, the genital organs, etc.) or through broken or damaged skin. Some disease agents gain admission through external vectors such as ticks or biting flies. These vectors become infected when ingesting the blood of a diseased animal and transmit the microorganisms when they move to feed on another, the infective agent being introduced by the mouth parts of the insect. For a time after introduction the microorganisms apparently have no harmful affect on their host, but they nevertheless multiply at as great a rate as defensive mechanisms of the host will allow. Their presence stimulates the host to produce antibodies to combat the microorganisms. The defense may be so effective that the invader is overcome immediately or, if not, is unable to multiply quickly enough to harm the host, in which case the animal may become a carrier. With an effective defense, the animal is immune to a particular microorganism. A state of immunity may be a breed characteristic, that is, genetic in nature, or more commonly it may be the acquired protection afforded by a reservoir of antibodies built up by a former invasion of the same type of microorganism or the passive immunity provided by colostrum. If the infective agent is not checked, it may multiply within an organ or throughout the whole body and ultimately will give rise to the symptoms characterizing a specific disease. Symptoms are not present in the early, incubative stage, while the initial multiplication is proceeding, but appear after the microorganisms have overcome the body's defenses and are the signs of the damage done by the microorganisms.

The newborn animal receives many of the

antibodies possessed by its dam in the colostrum, so that it starts life protected to a certain extent against the common diseases in its environment. The newborn is soon exposed to a host of pathogenic microorganisms and with the help conferred by its dam overcomes the infection, if not too virulent, until it begins to make its own antibodies. Once the young animal's own protective mechanism begins to function, at each fresh exposure its immunity increases. In this respect indigenous livestock are superior to livestock without the same disease experience. A slightly troublesome or even unimportant disease to the former may be fatal to the latter when first exposed to a contaminated farm or area. Thus, all new importations should be held in quarantine on the periphery of a farm or ranch until they have been gradually exposed to local conditions.

The ability of the body to react to invasion is the basis of the protection offered by vaccines and other biological products. These products take one of several forms: (1) the infective agent is attenuated to such a state of impotence that when injected into the body it merely stimulates the tissues to react to produce antibodies; (2) the dead infective agent, or its modified toxins, in solution, provokes the body to produce antibodies or antitoxins; (3) antibodies elaborated in the serum or colostrum of some animals are extracted for use in other animals. By the first two products, an animal is encouraged to develop its own protective mechanism and to *acquire* immunity before danger arises, but with the last the immunity of another is *passively* conferred upon the animal. The *acquired* immunity needs time to develop so that it will be ready to counteract infection when it occurs. If attempts are made to produce it after infection has taken place, these are either without effect or possibly harmful. Once immunity has been acquired, it remains effective for some considerable time, sometimes for life. The *passive* immunity, on the other hand, is conferred immediately by the introduction of antibodies into the body. This usefully augments the animal's own disease protection mechanism, and passive immunity can be successfully induced either immediately before or after infection; it has no permanency and is lost comparatively quickly. A particular type of passive immunity is the immunity of the newborn acquired through intake of colostrum (see page 23).

The outcome of infection is dependent upon two factors, the invading microorganism and the animal host. The microorganism may be of such virulence that death quickly follows infection, or it may have become attenuated by unfavorable circumstances so that it has lost its strength and is easily dealt with by the host. The virulence of the microorganism may have been increased by animal passage to such an extent that it overpowers the host. On the other hand, however, it may be so attenuated by passage that symptoms are mild and easily overlooked.

Animals vary in relation to susceptibility. An animal may be weakened by inadequate feeding, poor housing, overwork, or concur-

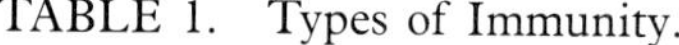
TABLE 1. Types of Immunity.

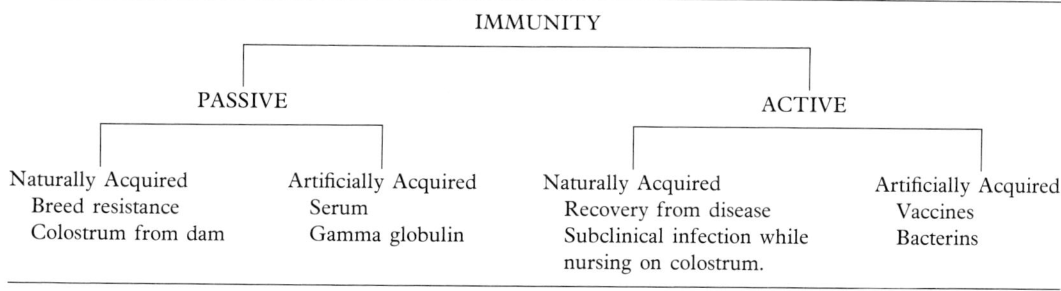

rent disease so that an otherwise mild infection, thus facilitated, becomes disastrous. On the other hand, the vitality associated with proper management, good feeding, and the absence of stress may minimize either the infection or its effects, as the natural defenses of the body are quickly brought into action, the antibodies elaborated and immunity acquired.

Biological products, of one kind or another, have been designed to give some degree of protection against many of the common contagious diseases. Some are more effective than others. Those used against the virus diseases are generally the most efficacious, as is the immunity acquired against these diseases under natural conditions. The bacterial diseases can be countered by the same means, but the immunity resulting from the natural bacterial infection is often not strong or lasting; it has to be repeated periodically if immunity is to be maintained.

All forms of medication, both biological and chemical, should be considered the last line of defense rather than the first or only one. In any case, their efficiency can be increased greatly by good management aimed at reducing the chances, the intensity, and the spread of infection.

It is unwise to expose susceptible livestock to disease, and even the most thoughtless farmer or rancher appreciates the danger of direct contact when disease is apparent. The difficulty is that the disease is not always obvious, and infection can be disseminated widely either by a carrier animal—which is apparently not affected—or by arthropod vectors. Further, the contact may be indirect and the infection passed by either inanimate objects or mechanical agencies. If one has some idea of the nature of the causal organism, a fair guess can be made regarding the manner by which it is spread.

The viruses are generalized in distribution and thus all parts of the body, and its excretions, are a source of danger. Viruses are either passed by direct contact or picked up from contaminated material. They are easily carried in food or water, or may be inhaled after they have become airborne on droplets of moisture or dust. Arthropod vectors are important reservoirs and transmitters of virus diseases to livestock.

Bacterial diseases are, with some notable exceptions, usually more confined in their distribution within the host body but they are equally as virulent as the viruses. Those infecting the respiratory organs are distributed quite widely by coughing and sneezing. Others are spread by direct or indirect contact with the diseased animal or its excretions. Once again, food and water can be easily contaminated and are common sources of infection; the causal microorganisms are found in blood, pus, or other discharges from the body, and can be easily deposited on feed bins, in water troughs, or other sources of feed and water.

A few years ago there were only a half dozen vaccines for animal diseases. Today, there are over 200 different vaccines, antisera, antitoxins, and similar products, and the list is increasing all the time.

Years of research and testing have given us more and better biological weapons against livestock diseases, but one feature about them has remained the same: they must be used with utmost care. They are made from disease-producing organisms or their products.

Precautions and guides for handling, storage, and use of veterinary biologicals licensed by the U.S. Department of Agriculture will be found on the label or container containing the product. Success with these products hinges on properly timed and skillful administration of a dosage prescribed for a specific disease. Failure to observe important precautions could endanger thousands of animals.

To help assure that veterinary biologicals are safe and effective, the U.S. Department of Agriculture Biologics Division licenses manufacturers and evaluates biologicals for safety and potency. Products of approved manufacturers can be identified by the U.S. license number appearing on the label of each container.

Modern biologicals and good husbandry practices not only prevent heavy disease losses in individual herds or flocks but also are key factors in stemming widespread outbreaks of infectious or contagious disease. A veterinarian or livestock extension agent in a particular area can provide information about when to vaccinate and against what diseases to protect livestock. Vaccines and other biologicals, however, should not be considered as substitutes for good sanitation, good feeding, and other management practices promoting good animal health.

It is poor management to wait until a disease has occurred before initiating a vaccination program. Animals need one to two weeks after vaccination to acquire active immunity. Since the occurrence of disease may vary by origin, by region, by year, and by season, it is wise to plan a program well in advance of diseases expected in any area. Further, federal or state requirements for vaccination may have to be satisfied in order to carry out plans for marketing livestock.

How Animals Fight Disease

Animals may inherit immunity to disease or they may acquire this immunity. The power to resist disease can be acquired in two ways: (1) as the result of successfully overcoming a natural infection or (2) as a result of administration of a biological such as vaccine or bacterin.

The immunization of livestock dates from Pasteur's development of effective vaccines against anthrax and rabies. Immunization is invaluable in protecting against a variety of viral, bacterial and even parasitic diseases. The immunization method has been used with varying success for the control of many diseases and now is considered as basic to some branches of animal husbandry as good feeding and management. Research is constantly adding to the list of diseases that can be controlled by preventive immunization.

Vaccination is an important tool in protecting individual animals from contagious diseases such as hog cholera which occur year after year in the same areas. It is a more dramatic curb of epizootics, protecting both uninfected herds in a contaminated area and susceptible livestock in disease-free areas. Federal and state programs are often initiated to bring diseases under control through a combination of quarantine, vaccination in each new area of infection, and disposal of infected animals.

Vaccination may produce active and continuing immunity to a disease. No vaccine, however, can provide 100 percent protection for all animals, because animals differ in their response to vaccination and the amount of resistance they develop. Proper vaccination usually provides an animal with enough protection to withstand exposure to a disease that would have been fatal without vaccination. Many vaccines expose animals to mild attacks by specific disease microorganisms, or the products of disease-producing microorganisms may be contained in the biological. This stimulates the animal's built-in system of defense against invading microorganisms. Antibodies are nature's way of fighting disease microorganisms. Therefore, when a microorganism enters the body, the animal's cells form antibodies to combat the invasive microorganism. Even after overcoming the mild infection caused by a vaccine, the animal's body continues to produce protective antibodies. Within one or two weeks, enough antibodies are present to fight off future attacks by the same microorganisms and active immunity is therefore established.

Antisera give passive immunity to disease microorganisms and toxins. This form of immunity is immediate but short-lived, usually lasting from 2 to 4 weeks. Protection is provided by the antibodies contained in an antiserum produced in another host. When the supply of antibodies is exhausted, protection ceases. Administration of an antiserum does not stimulate an animal's body to produce antibodies of its own. Currently, there are more than 200 types of veterinary biologicals used to fight animal diseases, and vaccines account for more than 90 percent of the biologicals produced in the United States. The remainder are products used in treatment or diagnosis of animal diseases. Some biologicals are sold for use only by veterinarians; however, many may be purchased and used by livestock producers.

Testing

Serological Testing

The fact that a disease antigen will cause antibodies to be produced and will react with them is the basis for several diagnostic tests. Such tests are called serological tests because they are accomplished with the use of serum. It is possible to use a known antigen to identify its antibody in an animal's blood serum, or to use known antibodies to identify their specific antigens.

When the antigen and antibody are homologous, the cells bearing the antigen become linked with the antibody and show such characteristics as precipitation or agglutination. These reactions are specific evidence of the disease, since antibodies would not be produced if the animal had not been exposed to the antigenic pathogen.

Fluorescent Testing Technique

While many tests give clear-cut results, and perhaps most do so under given conditions, some test reactions occur obscurely and require skillful interpretation. A new technique coming into wide use simplifies the interpretation of such tests by making reaction products fluoresce.

To use the method, a test serum containing a known antibody can be treated with a fluorescent chemical which adheres to the antibody protein. When the tagged antibody encounters its antigen counterpart, the fluorescent antibody concentrates around the antigen and fluoresces brightly in the presence of ultraviolet light. A positive reaction can be observed easily in tissues under a microscope, although it might be difficult without the fluorescent tag. This method, with some variations, has been used with encouraging results in the past few years, and may greatly extend the scope of serological diagnosis.

Hypersensitivity

Animals as well as man are subject to distressing hypersensitivity to certain proteins and chemicals. The allergic condition develops locally in cells where the stimulus occurs and is properly a phase of cell chemistry.

The individual's response may be a typical immune reaction or may resemble one. The typical antigen-antibody mechanism is involved in the former but not in the latter. Unlike an infectious organism, the excitant in these cases is not immediately and directly harmful. The antigen does not cause a reaction at first, but preconditions the cell for a strong reaction on the next or later contact. Susceptible individuals react excessively. The antigen is not toxic in itself, but the immune reaction sometimes yields toxic by-products that are harmful, sometimes fatal.

Typical immune-type hypersensitivity reactions may be caused by certain foods, drugs, or other chemicals, pollens, dusts, danders, poison, poison ivy, antibiotics, and injections of immunizing serum from a different species. Antibodies are formed and react with sensitizing substances. Toxic products seem to cause the hypersensitivity, but spasm of the smooth muscle causes the distress. Itching, sneezing, excessive secretions, swelling of tissues and distressing symptoms develop. Sensitivity occurs immediately on the second or later contact of the irritant with the cells, increases with each subsequent exposure, and may cause shock or even death. Cells are not destroyed, and the condition is generally short-lived. Hypersensitivity is an individual matter, and any animal can experience an immune type of hypersensitivity to a variety of substances. The condition is best known in humans, but some investigators think that immune hypersensitivity may play a part in explaining unthriftiness in livestock.

Immunity

Internal Parasites

Throughout most of the history of immunological science, veterinarians were chiefly concerned with microorganisms which produce and respond to immune effects in higher animals and with blood antigens which also cause immune reactions. Then inanimate substances came under investigation. In recent years, attention has been given to immune effects involving larger parasites, that is, the nematodes, and insect larvae infesting the organs and internal tracts of livestock. Many researchers have noted that animals are generally infected when young, less so in adulthood.

It has been demonstrated that cattle surviving lungworm infections often become immune. Recently, a vaccine has been prepared by exposing a larval stage of the cattle lungworm to X-rays. The irradiated larvae undergo only partial development in the host and produce a solid immunity without causing the clinical disease. Antigens present in various organs and tissues and in the secretions and excretions of many-celled parasites are being studied for their ability to act as "vaccines." Antigens believed to be important in immunity to certain cattle nematodes have been found in molting fluid secreted to facilitate each change in the life cycle of the parasite. Antigens have been extracted from various organs and tissues of the swine kidney worm, principally the excretory glands, intestines and esophagus. These substances precipitate on contact with antibodies present in the serum of swine infected with this nematode, and are being studied as experimental vaccines for pigs.

The cultivation of helminth parasites in glass tubes is a recent development which may have important applications in the field of immunology. Certain nematodes grown by this technique have been shown to produce antigens which may be identical to those normally produced by parasites within the host. In the near future large numbers of parasites for immunological studies may be easily harvested from cultures instead of from experimental animals.

Man has learned to use the forces of immunology in the natural state, to his own betterment. He can use them deliberately for the improvement of livestock production and the general benefit of man. Scientists learned long ago that they can apply the principles of immunology to the alleviation of suffering in man and animals, producing better vaccines and producing them more efficiently, and have used this to great advantage in furthering the cause of livestock health.

Vaccines

Vaccines are used to provide relatively long-lasting immunity against many diseases. They are prepared from virulent, attenuated, weakened, or dead viruses and bacteria. The term *vaccine* formerly meant any microorganism in a biological product. However, in modern usage, it is restricted to viruses only.

Live Virus Vaccine

Live virus vaccine is produced by inoculation of live virus into a medium such as chick embryo; the virus is permitted to grow, and the vaccine is prepared from the infected fluids and tissues of the embryo. Care should be used in the administration of live virus vaccine as the vaccine itself may serve as a means of spreading the disease to susceptible animals.

Modified Live Virus Vaccine

Modified live virus vaccine is prepared by processing the disease-causing virus in such a way that it no longer causes disease but stimulates immunity.

Desiccated Vaccine

Desiccated vaccine is freeze-dried vaccine that before use must be reconstituted to a liquid state by addition of a diluent, usually distilled water.

Monovalent Vaccine and Monovalent Bacterin

Monovalent vaccine and monovalent bacterin are biological products used to stimulate immunity to a single-disease organism.

Polyvalent Vaccine and Polyvalent Bacterin

Polyvalent vaccine and polyvalent bacterin are biological products which stimulate immunity to two or more disease organisms.

Antiserum

Antiserum is used for quick protection against a disease. It contains sufficient antibodies to provide protection for two to four weeks. More lasting immunity is obtained against some diseases by using a vaccine simultaneously with antiserum. Large doses of an antiserum may have some curative value and may be used in treating diseases refractory to other types of treatment.

Antitoxin

Antitoxin is injected to neutralize poisons or toxins caused by an invading disease microorganism and to produce short-lived immunity similar to that produced by antiserum. Antitoxins contain large numbers of antibodies.

Bacterin

Bacterin is used to stimulate immunity against bacterial diseases. It contains a standardized number of killed bacteria. Upon injection, a bacterin causes an animal to produce antibodies that will fight future invasions of the same type of bacteria.

Mixed bacterin contains standardized numbers of four or more bacterial species and is used to prevent conditions attributable to the microorganisms used in making the product.

Diagnostic Agents

Diagnostic agents and diagnostic antigens are biologicals used to detect and diagnose disease, either by causing a typical reaction following injection into an animal (diagnostic agent) or producing standards in laboratory blood tests (diagnostic antigen).

Administration of Biologicals

Biologicals should be administered by a veterinarian whenever possible. Only a person with knowledge of animal diseases and experienced in the use of biologicals should attempt immunization of animals, as one inept in this procedure could endanger an entire herd.

Vaccinate only healthy animals. Immunization will be adversely affected by anything that lowers resistance or causes stress to the animal. This includes overwork, exposure to cold, lack of proper feed, shipment over long distance—especially in cold and stormy weather—and chronic infections or presence of parasites.

To increase chances for successful immunization, eliminate as many adverse conditions as possible, free animals of parasites, treat chronic respiratory infections, eliminate deficiencies in diets, and protect animals from cold and dampness.

Age is also a factor in immunization. Neither the very young nor very old animals respond as well to vaccination as those between these extremes. In the very young, a passive immunity should be employed as the antibody-producing system has not yet developed. In the very old, the antibody-producing system may be overworked and, therefore, a passive immunity is to be desired.

Role of Colostrum

Since all animals are highly susceptible to disease after birth, nature has provided a means of transmitting immunity from mother to offspring. This resistance is provided, primarily, by antibodies developed in the dam following exposure to infections. Newborn animals are born without protective antibodies, but they begin to be protected a few minutes after their first meal of colostrum. As the newborns grow, they develop their own protection and rely less on their mother's immunity.

Antibodies are concentrated primarily in the gamma globulin serum protein in the blood. Young animals are born with practically none of this vital protein. Gamma globulin of colostrum is absorbed intact by the cells lining the intestinal tract and is transferred immediately to the bloodstream. Within minutes after nursing, antibodies are found in the blood. The cells continue to absorb whole particles of gamma globulin until they are completely filled with this protein. If gamma globulin is not present in sufficient quantities, other soluble proteins are absorbed in an apparent attempt to meet the emergency; if the cells become filled, they cannot use gamma globulin which may become available later. Normally, a dam will provide a quantity of colostrum gamma globulin during the first 24 hours equivalent to that contained in her entire bloodstream. Nearly one-half of this quantity is secreted by the dam and ingested by the offspring during the first nursing period. The first colostrum has a protein content of 14 to 20 percent and is 5 to 6 times higher in gamma globulin than serum.

The absolute amount of gamma globulin absorbed by the various species is different; however, one-half of the gamma globulin ingested during the first nursing period is found in the bloodstream of the pig when peak levels are reached 6 to 12 hours later. At this time gamma globulin levels are 2 to 3 levels higher than in adult hogs. After 24 to 48 hours gamma globulin levels fall rapidly for 7 to 10 days, decrease more slowly for an additional 2 weeks, stabilize for 3 to 4 weeks, and then gradually rise. The same general pattern applies to all species of livestock.

At first glance it would appear that newborn animals are provided with an excess of antibodies contained in gamma globulin. Under ideal conditions this is the case. There is little need for production of antibodies, and all protein can be used for body building or growth. Ideally, between one and two weeks of age the young animals begin to adjust to environmental disease agents and produce their own active antibodies for additional protection. In the event that a young animal is unable to obtain colostrum from the dam, the animal husbandman would be well advised to draw a sample of blood from the dam, allow the sample to clot, and draw off the serum (which has a high gamma globulin content, although not as high as colostrum itself). This substitute colostrum can be given by mouth to the young animal with assurance that it will protect him in the same manner as the colostrum.

The longer the period following birth before a high gamma-globulin level is reached in the bloodstream of the newborn, the greater the chance for infection to become established. The antibody-producing mechanism of young animals is called upon to produce excessive amounts of gamma globulin in competition against protein for growth; thus growth rate is reduced. This is always the case even though disease may not be apparent.

Any condition which tends to decrease the colostrum flow of the dam immediately after birth has a detrimental and long-lasting effect on newborn animals. Factors such as difficult parturition, digestive upsets, metritis and mastitis are easily recognized. Mental anxiety or distress of the mother, a major, complicated, and frequently unrecognized problem, often is an underlying factor in any of the above conditions.

Transmission of immunity from the dam to the newborn is a unique phenomenon, without peer in the prevention of infectious diseases under the primitive, natural conditions in which it is involved. The frequency of infections in young animals indicates that it will not prevent disease under ordinary management conditions. Therefore, the following suggestions are made in this light: (1) Expect dams to transfer only immunity which they possess. Even though a nursery area may look clean, it represents a different environment from the gestation area and may harbor many agents from previous breeding periods in spite of conscientious sanitation. (2) Recognize that many chronic infections induce poor immunity; therefore, little protection is transmitted to young animals. Eradication should be practiced wherever possible. Isolate young animals which sicken to prevent seeding to other young animals. (3) Practice recognized vaccination for disease which may be prevented, thus maintaining a high level of immunity by artificial means. (4) Handle dams as easily and quietly as possible prior to and at parturition. Parturition is surrounded by varying degrees of emotionalism in all species of animals. (5) Provide comfortable quarters for all dams with newborns in a draft-free, warm, protected area.

5 Sanitation Procedures

Natural Agencies

Protection against infectious animal diseases lies primarily in avoiding contact with the infected animal or with infected material. The best way to do this is to keep stock segregated to the extent that they do not mix with other animals, share facilities of feeding and watering, or use ground or accommodations upon which infection may still linger. Such isolation can seldom be followed completely. Under the most careful management, occasions arise when a calculated risk must be taken; more often, a slip is made by the farmer or rancher, his employee, or some other person who does not heed signs and warnings. One of the most common mistakes is to introduce new animals into a healthy herd without taking adequate quarantine precautions. Another common mistake is to accept, without quarantine, the return of an animal to the herd after it has been exposed to the chance of infection, for instance through its presence at a market or fair or auction yard, its transport in a truck that has not been properly cleaned, a cattle chute or crush, or some other place where animals are congregated.

As the possibilities of infection are seldom absent, it is therefore necessary to design management so that if disease is contracted it may be controlled with the least cost. For that purpose the stock should be divided into as many independent units as economically permissable, and crowding within the units should be avoided. Each unit should consist of animals of the same sex and same age group. It is important that animals of varying age groups not be mixed at any one place, because a latent infection can be passed on to susceptible animals.

Effective protection against disease lies in timely vaccination when possible, local segregation, division of the stock into manageable units, adequate nutrition, proper housing, and efficient supervision. One of the first duties of the farmer or rancher, to himself and to his neighbors, is to detect immediately

3

the abnormality in his animals as the first sign of disease appears and to understand the possibility of its contagious nature. It is of the utmost importance that contagious diseases are detected early, and so, if local conditions cause an owner to suspect the presence of a disease, or if he finds his suspicions are justified, he should immediately seek the help of his veterinarian.

An infected animal is an incubator for the microorganisms of the disease it harbors and can pass them on to all susceptible animals. The healthy animals should, therefore, be removed from close proximity to the disease without delay. This usually means that the sick are allowed to stay on the infected ground and the healthy are removed to uncontaminated areas. This is not always convenient if only one or a few animals are sick, but if the premises are a source of infection the obviously healthy must be removed; to move the sick is, after all, only increasing the extent of the infected area. It may not be so important to follow that rule when a disease transmitted by an insect vector is suspected, as removing the sick removes the reservoir from which the vector becomes infected and tends to increase the area over which the infective microorganisms may be transmitted.

The second important step is to segregate the apparently healthy animals which have been in contact with the sick, and to keep them in quarantine over the maximum incubating period. Under certain circumstances, particularly when the disease is an especially virulent one, it may be expedient to slaughter the sick and, in the case of contagious diseases, those animals that have been in contact with them. However, it is advisable to do so only on the advice of a veterinarian. It is risky, often dangerous, to try to hide the presence of contagious disease by slaughter and disposal of the carcasses.

Much can be done to stop spread of infection by using chemicals which kill microorganisms or their spores. Some chemicals are more potent against one class of microorganisms than others and, if proper use is to be made of such material, some judgment is required in the selection of the best for any particular occasion. However, none is of much use if its application is not thorough. Chemicals should be particularly directed against known concentrations of microorganisms, that is, the blood from the carcass of an animal that has recently died, pus and vaginal discharges, or the feces of an animal suffering from dysentery or scours.

All disease-producing microorganisms are adversely affected, and most are quickly killed, by direct exposure to strong sunlight and dry currents of hot air; on the other hand, moist warm air may favor their multiplication. Infective material should therefore be exposed, where possible, to direct sunlight so that complete desiccation is facilitated. Other agencies of physical disinfection contributing to the destruction of microorganisms are heat, cold, desiccation and agitation. Sunlight is the most potent, and its powers of destruction are enormous. Its efficacy is entirely due to the ultraviolet range of the spectrum and it is at its greatest wavelengths between 2800 and 2400 Angstrom units. Unfortunately, these ultraviolet rays have little penetrating power; they cannot pass through glass or translucent sheets or through clouds and industrial haze. The value of sunlight in animal buildings is thus unreliable. Desiccation from fresh air and wind will contribute to the destruction of microorganisms, especially if they have become exposed by thorough cleaning of a building or agitation of the soil. High temperatures will also accelerate the destruction of exposed microorganisms, but cold, particularly freezing temperatures, may actually preserve them. Another process is antibiosis: many bacteria and fungi produce substances antagonistic to other microorganisms. Penicillin and streptomycin are agents of this nature, with well-known antibacterial action. In the soil, pathogenic microorganisms can be acted upon by antibiotics produced by nonpathogenic organisms normally inhabiting the soil. Warm, moist conditions will assist the action of these saprophytic agents.

Fire is the most effective method of destroying microorganisms and the material they contaminate, and should be the first choice as a disinfectant whenever practical. For ordinary farm disinfection, dry heat applied by any other means is not so reliable, merely because of the difficulty of application. For many years, moist steam under pressure has been successfully used in sterilization and disinfection. The most resistant disease-producing agents are the spores of anthrax, but even they can be killed if boiled or exposed to live steam for a sufficient length of time. The momentary application of boiling water is ineffective, but prolonged boiling of any contaminated article will sterilize it with certainty.

Dry heat is not as effective as moist heat, and may be dangerous to wooden buildings if safety measures are not exercised. Among the nonspore-forming bacteria the thermal death time ranges from a few hours at 116 F to 60 minutes at 140 F or 5 minutes at 158 F. The most susceptible bacterial spores will succumb, though some may be extremely resistant. For example, *Bacillus anthracis* may survive 90 minutes at 320 F, and *Clostridium tetani* 15 minutes at 284 F. Some spores may even survive heating at 572 F for 10 minutes. The transitory heating from a flame thrower must therefore be at a very high temperature to achieve disinfection. Likewise, under moist heat, *Bacillus anthracis* may survive up to 15 minutes, and clostridial spores up to 300 minutes, at 200 F. The uncertainty of steaming is thus apparent. While it is clearly a useful cleansing agent, it cannot be considered a reliable disinfectant when used in buildings where the microorganisms may be protected in cracks and crevices. Steam is more useful on equipment, but its powers are greatly increased by incorporating a detergent and disinfectant with the steam or hot water. It is again important to point out that the presence of organic matter will interfere with disinfection by heat.

Modern Methods of Manure Disposal

Any method of animal husbandry requiring that farm livestock live in close proximity to their own bodily excreta is dangerous, preconditioning to disease. Intestinal and urinary discharges of livestock are seldom devoid of disease-producing microorganisms. In areas where animals are crowded into poorly drained enclosures and where there is no sunshine to dry the excrement, feed and water facilities are often contaminated with fecal material. Such a practice is detrimental to the health of livestock, and is considered as chronic mismanagement from the standpoint of disease prevention.

No single step is so important to the health of livestock, especially those kept in small, closed spaces, as the frequent removal of excrement in the surrounding area. If there is any difference in the degree of importance of this step, greatest care should be given to the surroundings of those animals that naturally prefer to take their food from the ground, such as swine.

Experience seems to indicate that in the loose housing barn, in which manure is compacted by the trampling of the livestock, there are advantages that must be weighed against daily removal of the excreta. There seems to be foundation for the belief that, in these almost dry, compacted manures, heat production and chemical changes exert a deleterious action on the microorganisms contained in the droppings.

Storage and final disposal of liquid and solid manure is a matter of considerable sanitary importance. These substances have a rich intermixture of parasites and their ova, and at times the specific microorganisms of many well-known diseases. These pathogenic invaders may live for a considerable length of time in unsanitary surroundings. If animals are kept continuously in contact with excreta under crowded conditions, it means that they will be exposed to unbroken life cycles of many generations of pathogenic microorganisms.

Older methods for the storage of manure required the use of pits or storage areas. It was expected that such areas would be far enough away from buildings that the danger of contamination of the immediate surroundings of the animals was reduced to a minimum. Manure pits or sheds were floored to control seepage, covered and screened to keep the animals away and to control flies. It was considered important to provide a fly-proof enclosure around such pits or sheds, although in some instances it was impractical to provide such sophisticated protection. Parasiticides were often sprayed on manure piles, but this procedure was not entirely satisfactory in controlling the development of fly larvae. Spraying also was questionable from the viewpoint of producing resistance in the developing larvae. When this happened, larvae developed into adult flies resistant to subsequent attacks by the chemical.

One of the most practical methods of assuring a degree of fly control was the rapid drying of fecal material so that the fly eggs would not develop into larvae, or maggots, and subsequently into adult flies.

In yards for animals kept under crowded conditions, hard surfacing, especially with concrete and with appropriate drainage, is undoubtedly a most sanitary method. First, the ground is sloped so that drainage will be toward one side of the yard, where a tile drain is placed to conduct the fecal material and urine away from the animal enclosure into an irrigation ditch or other place of removal; the accumulated animal waste will be carried either directly in irrigation water to adjacent fields or into a sewage lagoon where it will be fermented in time, as in any sewage disposal plant. Sewage lagoons have only recently been developed. They serve a useful purpose in preventing undue pollution of adjacent streams with raw feces and urine from large animal feedlots or even from small barns and enclosures on individual farms.

Recommended lagoon design is intended to provide for disposal of waste at a minimum of cost without creating health hazards or public nuisances, especially from objectionable odors. Recent research has shown that the worst odors emanate from confined animal enclosures, and the least objectionable come from enclosures with partially slotted floors over a channel flushed daily into a lagoon. Therefore, where animals are kept in close confinement, it is suggested that an automatic flushing system under slotted floors, with drainage into a sewage lagoon, is most efficient.

The raising and feeding of livestock on raised floors, through which the manure falls, is not a new concept. Poultry have been raised on wire floors for many years, and in recent times swine have been reared and fattened on slotted floors over storage pits, or pits that drain into lagoons.

The keeping of cattle on slotted floors has aroused some interest in this country. At least two steel fabricators offer steel members for the construction of such floors, usually in conjunction with complete steel buildings.

The interest in feeding cattle on concrete or slotted floors is an extension of the confinement feeding currently practiced, although feeding on concrete floors has been done in parts of Europe for some time. The current interest in concrete or slotted floors is coupled with interest in increased cattle density, as shown by recent experimental procedures.

Slotted floors appear to have some advantages over concrete floors since they are self-cleaning, the animals walking the manure through the slots. The manure thus forced through the slots may drop onto a floor for eventual mechanical cleaning or into storage pits from which it may be pumped out with a sledge pump into a lagoon. This latter method appears to be the most desirable from the standpoint of flies and odor control. A properly maintained lagoon gives off very little odor and provides no breeding place for flies. Animals tightly confined on concrete must be kept clean and probably should be bedded down in shavings, straw, or some other similar material.

One of the advantages of slotted floors, or

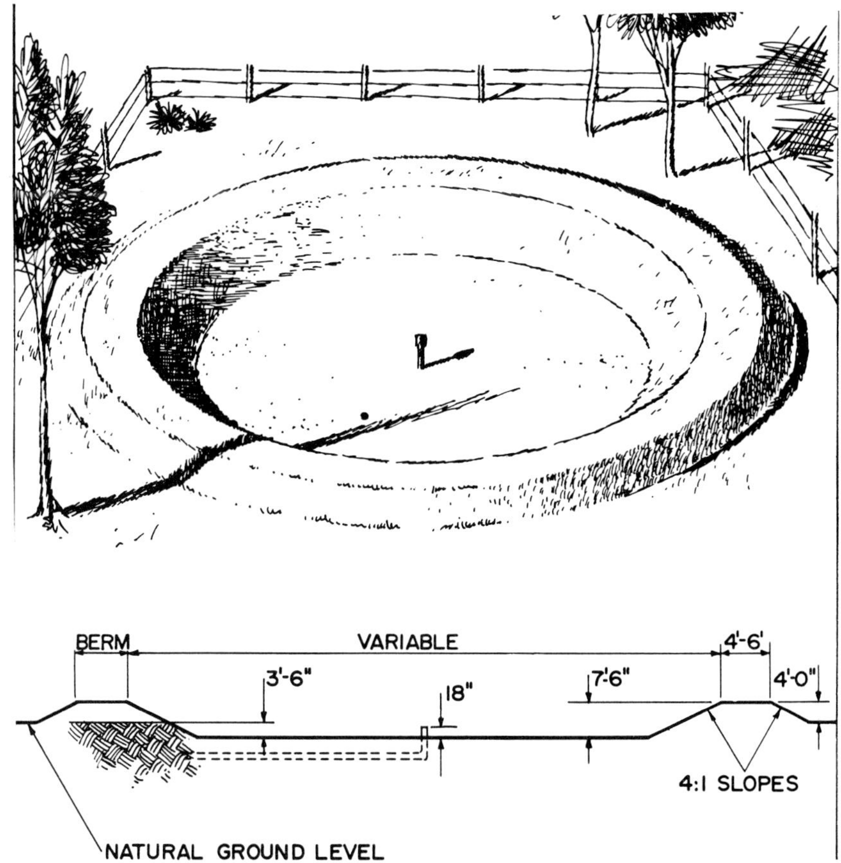

FIG. 1. Farm waste lagoon. (From National Hog Farmer Bulletin F19.)

other means of intensive confinement, is the ease with which they fit the idea of complete housing where climate dictates. The geographical areas where the use of slotted floors is currently greatest are those where climate control appears desirable, especially winter control.

Animals fed in close confinement are generally quiet and do not expend energy in play, as in traditional feedlots. Several investigations of the value of intensive confinement on both slotted and concrete floors under western conditions have favored the slotted floors. In eastern states, both sheep and swine are being reared on slotted floors with good results.

Slotted and concrete floors appear to have much to offer. However, as in other management innovations, patience is a virtue and time spent on proper evaluation may be money saved. It is difficult to look at the results achieved in other countries and apply them immediately to local conditions. In the western part of the United States, it has been

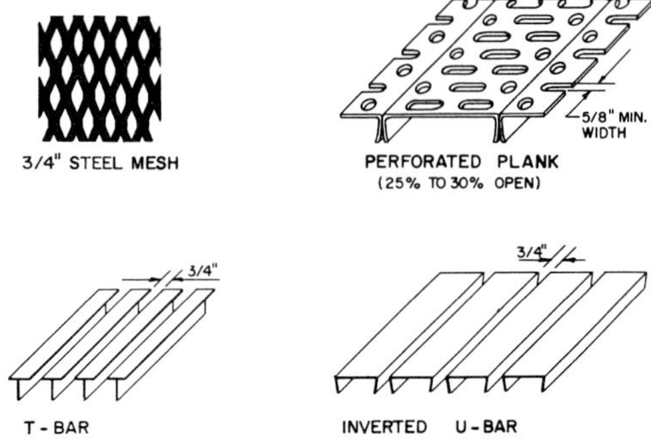

FIG. 2. Steel shapes for slotted floors. (From National Hog Farmer Bulletin F12.)

accepted that concrete slabs, with an elevation to provide drainage into irrigation ditches, adequately meet local conditions. However, this sort of manure removal is of little value in those areas of the midwest and east where animals must be confined during the colder months of the year.

Sanitation is one of the most effective and still one of the cheapest ways to prevent disease. In fact, the livestock producer is often the real cause of disease, because the only effective insurance against disease losses is a prevention program. Disease is spread primarily in three ways: by physical contact, by contaminated feed and water, and by air movement. Physical contact is probably most important because it assures direct transfer of a virulent infective agent from one animal to another. "Head-to-tail" contact is important in the transmission of many infectious bacterial and viral diseases, as well as some of the parasitic diseases which gain entrance to the body through the digestive tract. Nose-to-nose contact will transfer any pathogen capable of invading the body either through the lungs and respiratory tract or through the digestive tract. Body-to-body contact will spread external parasites and, occasionally, such skin diseases as ringworm.

Management stresses can be important when they involve comfort and sanitation. Cattle and swine are expected to live and gain rapidly under many diverse conditions which may vary widely from those under which they were raised. First, there is crowding. Instead of having acres per animal, as on the range,

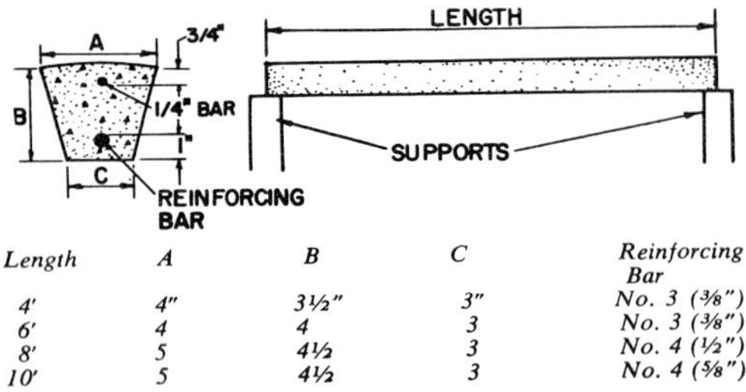

Length	*A*	*B*	*C*	*Reinforcing Bar*
4′	4″	3½″	3″	No. 3 (⅜″)
6′	4	4	3	No. 3 (⅜″)
8′	5	4½	3	No. 4 (½″)
10′	5	4½	3	No. 4 (⅝″)

FIG. 3. Concrete beam design. (From National Hog Farmer Bulletin F12.)

feeder cattle, swine, and lambs are crowded with many other animals into small areas. This leads to the establishment of a social order—a graduation from the animal which always gets to the feed bunk or water trough first to the one which gets what is left after all the others have had their fill. The cleanliness of the bunks and troughs is also important; the cleaner they are, the more each animal will eat and drink to assure maximum growth.

Modern methods of manure disposal, when fully accepted by livestock producers, will provide several advantages both profitable for the producer and beneficial for the livestock. These are: (1) a saving in labor, (2) a possible increased production because of greater efficiency, (3) a practical solution to the problems of odor control and manure handling, (4) saving of bedding costs, (5) saving of feeding costs, (6) less chance for livestock to come into contact with pathogenic microorganisms.

Sterilization and Disinfection

Most chemical disinfectants do all that is claimed for them by reliable manufacturers, but they must be applied as their makers direct. Even the most efficient and effective chemical needs time to kill; the sprinkling of a disinfectant over a contaminated floor, for example, is generally futile, while soaking the floor with disinfectant could rightly be expected to be effective. It must not be forgotten that simple mechanical methods of cleaning, brushing, scraping, or flushing are often essential preliminaries to the application of disinfectant. Gross dirt cannot be treated effectively except by burning or deep burial.

Disinfection is generally affected by chemical agents. The lethal effects of disinfectants are due, in the main, to their ability to react with the protein and, in particular, the essential enzymes of microorganisms. Any agent that will coagulate, precipitate, or otherwise denature proteins will act as a general disinfectant. Among these agents are phenols, alcohols, acids, salts of heavy metals and hypochlorides as well as heat in certain radiations.

Physical conditions, such as heat and radiation, and chemical substances which destroy microorganisms are the two broad groups of agencies used for sterilization or disinfection. The classical meanings of the words *disinfection* and *sterility* are still valid, but new terms have been introduced and the old terms are sometimes used with modified meaning. Thus the terms *antiseptic, disinfectant,* and *sterilant* are used for similar substances, and *disinfection,* and *sterilization* for similar processes. The term *disinfectant* usually implies a germicide with little irritant effect on the tissues, while the term *sterilant* is coming into use possibly because *disinfectant* often implies a strong-smelling phenolic substance.

Sterility means *incapable of reproduction,* and so, in the hygienic sense, the complete absence of any form of life. The word is sometimes used more loosely to indicate absence of pathogens, ignoring the small number of harmless microorganisms which may not be destroyed. The word *sterility* should always be used in its strict sense.

In practice, the destruction of pathogens is often sufficient to control infection; the term *disinfection* is then used, particularly with reference to the surface of equipment, the interior of a room or building, or a large area. *Antisepsis* refers to the destruction of pathogens on the surface of a living organism or tissue.

A disinfectant is an agent that can achieve this end, usually a chemical agent. In the general context of disinfection, other terms are used that need accurate definition. A disinfectant is by custom applied to inanimate objects. In contrast, an antiseptic is an agent eliminating infection on living tissues, but it may also sometimes be used to signify agents used in a weaker concentration than a disinfectant to render harmful microorganisms innocuous either by killing them or by preventing their growth. A sanitizer is an agent reducing the number of contaminants to a level judged safe by public-health requirements. In disinfection an absolute elimination of microorganisms is generally required, so that sanitizers are not effective. They are used, however, in the partial aerosol cleaning of the atmosphere in populated buildings, an increasingly common practice.

A germicide is an agent that kills all microorganisms, and the term may therefore be considered synonymous with disinfectant; it is, however, sometimes taken to include the destruction of bacterial spores, and therefore a germicide may be less potent than a disinfectant.

The disinfection of a building can be accomplished by natural processes or by artificial means. Before discussing these in detail it should be emphasized that cleaning is an essential preliminary to disinfection, since organic matter will considerably reduce the power of disinfectants.

Cleaning

Cleaning is of the greatest importance in all aspects of sterilization. Cleaning may be defined as the complete removal of all extraneous material, and especially organic matter, which may harbor microorganisms. The modern fashion of chemical disinfection has tended to reduce the significance of cleaning. Heat may in time penetrate a film of dried organic material and kill microorganisms, but such a film may protect organisms indefinitely against all types of chemical sterilants or radiation. Aside from this, efficient cleaning removes about 99 percent of the bacteria on a filthy object and is, therefore, an integral part of the sterilizing processes. Organisms which survive are almost invariably spores or resistant cocci of no pathogenic importance. Spore-forming pathogens are the unfortunate exception, however. When destruction of these microorganisms becomes necessary, more drastic methods must be employed.

Factors Influencing Chemical Disinfectant Activity

Three basic phenomena are of importance for disinfection by chemical means: (1) absorption of the compound by the cell wall; (2) penetration into the cell cytoplasm; (3) reaction of the compound with one or more of the cell constituents. The properties of absorption and penetration in relation to the cell are not exclusive to the substance itself; they can be influenced by other constituents in the immediate environment, for instance those affecting surface tensions, and other physical-chemical properties. An example is the effect of aqueous solutions of phenol produced by sodium chloride, which enhances the activity of the phenol. The most important factor is, however, the chemical constitution of the disinfectant. Thus, the activities of alcohols and phenols in homologous series increase proportionately with their molecular weights to the limit of their solubilities.

Chemical disinfectants can more readily attack the cell of the aqueous phase natural to the organism. Conversely, any solvent reducing the concentration of the disinfectant in the aqueous phase has the consequent effect of reducing the activity of the product. Oils, fats and alcohols have this affect on phenol; its activity with these solvents is depressed. Emulsification of phenols in soap solutions appreciably enhances their activity. This characteristic is exploited in preparations such as Lysol and various disinfectant fluids, which for this reason are more efficiently absorbed by the microorganism. Various inorganic salts also increase the power of disinfectants; for example, the absorption of phenol by the microorganism is greatly increased in this way.

The actions of osmosis and surface tension are also of importance. Some microorganisms are highly vulnerable to changes in tension. Reduction of surface tension will generally increase the activity of a disinfectant; this is the case with phenol, resorcinol and hexoresorcinol, where disinfecting ability is directly related to lowering of surface tension. The same is true with the quaternaries, in which there is cytolitic damage resulting in leakage of growth material from the cell.

Many disinfectants have a selective action for different microorganisms. Microorganisms respond to changes in pH value and, as every protein has its own characteristic isoelectric point, each responds individually and will be influenced by the acidity or alkalinity of the disinfectant.

Complete disinfection is not an instantaneous matter; it takes place gradually. However, more microorganisms are killed at the beginning of the process than at the end. There is an initial lag period before activity commences. An examination of the number of microorganisms surviving at different stages during disinfection shows that the number of cells killed in unit time bears a constant relationship to the number of surviving microorganisms. Thus, after the lag phase, destruction of the cells is rapid at first but tends to slow up, so that eventual destruction of all microorganisms takes considerable time.

The activities of most disinfectants increase with temperature, but there are a few exceptions. The so-called temperature coefficient time is the measure of the change in velocity of disinfection per degree of rise in temperature. The coefficient is an exponential factor as well as a dilution coefficient. The effect of dilution, however, varies widely among disinfectants.

Almost invariably, when disinfection is carried out on the farm, organic matter is present. It can be said that organic matter always interferes with action of the disinfectant. It may do so in the following ways: (1) the organic matter may protect the cell by forming a coating on it and preventing the ready access of the disinfectant; (2) the disinfectant may react chemically with the organic matter, resulting in a noneffective product; (3) the disinfectant may form an insoluble compound with the organic matter, and destroy its potential activity; (4) particulate and colloidal matter in suspension may absorb the disinfecting agent so that it is potentially removed from the solution; and (5) fats and oils may inactivate the disinfectant.

Bactericides and Bacteriostats

The generally accepted definitions are that a bactericide kills bacteria, whereas a bacteriostat merely prevents growth or proliferation of bacteria. In general, the suffix *-cide* applies to any agent that kills microorganisms, while *-stat* applies to one that merely prevents their growth; thus bacteriostat is a term occasionally used but having little relevance to the critical needs for sanitation. In practice this distinction may be difficult to justify, as vegetative cells of the bacteria which cannot grow usually die, although sometimes very slowly. The difference in effect, therefore, may be a matter of time, concentration and temperature. For practical purposes we may assume that, if living cells cannot be recovered by cultural methods after removal of the chemical, the reaction is bactericidal. If living cells are recovered, then the action is bacteriostatic. It is often difficult to decide when a cell is dead, and this is only one of many reasons why laboratory tests may be unreliable as a guide to the efficiency of a germicide.

Most pathogenic microorganisms perish rapidly once outside the animal body, but, unfortunately, enough may survive to cause renewed infection. Vegetative bacteria and viruses can live several months if protected with organic matter, while the spores of bacteria—for example *Clostridium tetani* and *Bacillus anthracis*—can live almost indefinitely in the soil or in the cracks and crevices of buildings. Even the coccidial oocyst may survive for years in infected quarters.

Commonly Used Disinfectants

Hypochlorites

Chlorine or hypochlorite has many advantages. It is cheap, convenient to use, powerful, and has a wide antibacterial spectrum. Its greatest disadvantages are corrosiveness, strong odor, and neutralization by organic material. The former may be minimized by using in cold solutions at a pH of 9 or higher; however, the solution becomes more bactericidal as the pH approaches the neutral point. Commercial preparations usually contain 9 to 12 percent and domestic preparations about 1 percent of the available chlorine.

Quaternary Ammonium Compounds

Next to hypochlorite the quaternary ammonium compounds have hitherto been the most popular. They are convenient to use, of very low toxicity to animals, without appreciable odor or taste, and noncorrosive, but relatively expensive. They are powerful agents against gram-positive organisms but are less efficient against gram-negative organisms. This is their greatest disadvantage. They are incompatible with soaps and ionic detergents, but can be used with alkalis and nonionic detergents. Alkalinity increases their bactericidal power, but they are weak detergents.

Working concentrations vary from 1 : 1000 to 1 : 20,000 according to the particular quaternary ammonium used, the temperature, the time, the alkalinity and the percentage kill desired. Weight for weight, they are less effective than chlorine, but their other advantages far outweigh this fact.

Alkalis

Although generally regarded as detergents, caustic alkalis have a strong germicidal activity. Bactericidal activity falls rapidly with decreasing pH and is influenced by the nature of the anion. Hot caustic soda solutions at 1 to 3 percent are especially useful for killing spores, one of the main advantages of the use of alkalis.

Iodine

Although useful as an antiseptic, iodine has certain disadvantages as a sterilant. It has a very powerful odor, stains badly, is not very soluble in water, and is expensive. It is readily soluble in iodide solutions and alcohol, but this method increases its cost and may produce a solution irritating to skin.

Iodophors

Although of recent introduction, iodophors are growing in popularity. They are prepared by the reaction of iodine on nonionic detergent, in acid solution, and they have both detergent and sterilizing properties. It is claimed that the soluble iodine in this form has the same killing power as the available chlorine in hypochlorites.

Chloro-compounds

The usefulness of the chloro-phenols and related compounds has been established, but they are odorous and may be irritating. Chloramine-T does not suffer from these disadvantages, but is mild in action. Among interesting new compounds are dichlorocyanuric acid and dichlorodimethylhydantoin. These are of low toxicity and nonirritating. Dichlorophene is more effective against gram-positive organisms and fungi than hexachloraphene. Both have been popular as antiseptics. The latter has a phenol coefficient of about 40 against *Staphylococcus aureus* and of about 15 against *Salmonella typhi.*

Strong claims have been made for the efficiency and general suitability of chlorhexydene diasatate and the chloroxolenols as antiseptics. The odor of some of these substances makes them unsuitable as sterilants.

The Phenol Coefficient

The phenol coefficient of a disinfectant may be defined as the ratio of the killing power of the disinfectant to the killing power of pure phenol when determined under standard conditions. It is obvious, therefore, that the most important factors in such a determination are the conditions under which the test is made. The conditions under which phenol coefficients and other germicide tests are determined are given in publications by the U.S. Department of Agriculture.

The Action of Chemical Disinfectants

Chemicals destroy microorganisms in a variety of ways. A few of the chemicals have only one type of action, while others bring about death by a number of different types of action.

Probably the most varied of any of the chemicals are the inorganic salts. It has been observed that salts of various kinds in low concentrations are stimulating to the growth of bacteria and are important as buffers in growth media. In high concentrations, however, most salts are definitely toxic and hasten death. Salts vary in toxicity; sodium chloride is toxic only in high concentrations while mercury bichloride is toxic in low concentrations. It has been shown that the toxic action of many salts, as well as other types of disinfectants, may be increased by the addition of sodium chloride. This is due to increased dissociation and dispersion of the disinfectant, resulting in an increased effect on bacterial cells. However, the addition of sodium chloride to mercuric chloride lowers the toxicity of the latter.

Salts do not produce bacterial death by osmotic effects. Bacteria are resistant to changes in osmotic pressure and can live in distilled water as well as in rather high salt concentration. Salts do, however, exert a dehydrating effect on the media in which bacteria grow, and thereby cause inhibition of growth and eventual death. Due to the dissociation of salts, most of the germicidal action is caused by the effect of ions upon the bacterial cell. This effect may be the result of the influence upon cell permeability, the lyotropic action upon cell protoplasm altering cell metabolism, and the inactivation of enzymes on which the cells depend for the synthesis of food substance.

Oxidation is one of the most common methods by which chemicals cause death. Many salts, for example potassium permanganate and sodium perborate, are active oxidizing agents. The halogen compounds also are noted for this kind of chemical action.

Some chemicals used in sterilization are active reducing compounds. These, it is true, are not as commonly used as the oxidizing agents. The ferrous salts, sulfites, and thiosulfites are good examples of reducing compounds.

Many of the most effective chemicals form irreversible compounds with bacterial protoplasm by the coagulation of the protein. The salts of the heavy metals, that is, silver, mercury, zinc, copper and bismuth, are active in this manner. The derivatives of benzene, the coal tar products, chief among which are phenol and cresol, are used widely as the basis of many commercial disinfectants. These chemicals in their purest state, saponified or altered by the replacement of an H atom by another chemical, cause the death of bacteria by the coagulation of bacterial protein.

Miscellaneous Compounds

Alcohol, especially ethyl alcohol, is considered by many to be a most effective antiseptic, and is credited by some as a disinfectant. The efficacy of alcohol is dependent upon the concentration. Investigation and experience have shown that 70 percent alcohol is most efficient; concentrations above and below that level are ineffective. Alcohols in general are more bactericidal in the higher molecular weights. They are expensive and thus used less widely than other substances.

Isopropyl alcohol has been shown to be a more effective germicide than the more commonly used ethyl alcohol. It is used in the 98 to 99 percent pure state and is noncorrosive to instruments. The pungent odor of this alcohol is objectionable, and for that reason it is not widely used.

Formaldehyde gained great popularity as a disinfectant in the days when infected dwellings were fumigated. Its value as a disinfectant in that procedure was due to its solubility in water; it is usually sold commercially as formalin, an aqueous alcoholic solution containing approximately 40 percent formaldehyde. Formalin is an effective germicide and is used not only in the killing of animal and human pathogenic bacteria but also for treating seeds against fungi. This chemical is used as an attenuating agent for bacteria, toxins, and viruses which are to be used as immunizing agents.

Potassium permanganate was formerly used extensively in veterinary medicine as an antiseptic in drinking water for poultry, for which it seemed to have definite value. Potassium permanganate has also been used as a wound dressing and as a footbath for livestock. The stain produced by the chemical has limited its general use as an antiseptic, however. Hydrogen peroxide is not employed extensively as a disinfectant, due to the ease with which it combines with organic matter. It does have some virtue as a cleansing agent for deep wounds, but its effervescing action belies its real value, and it should not be depended upon to any great extent.

Investigations of the synthetic soaps or detergents have revealed that they have germicidal activity. Such compounds are classified as either cationic or anionic. The cationic detergents have greater germicidal activity than the anionic compounds. Cationic detergents are active in the alkaline range, while the anionic are active in the acid range. The great popularity of these compounds as detergents, wetting agents, and emulsifiers has resulted in the synthesis of over 1,000 different ones in recent years. Most are nontoxic to living tissues and are safe to use as skin disinfectants. Some have been given internally to experimental animals without toxic effect, and Zephiran has been shown to be an active germicide in a dilution of 1 to 80,000.

The Desirable Properties of a Disinfectant

There are many disinfecting agents, with variable properties. However, several properties should be found in any desirable disinfectant. Criteria for selecting an appropriate and effective agent for disinfection are as follows:

1. The disinfecting agent must be free of strong and objectionable odors.
2. The disinfecting agent must not be destructive to materials; in other words, it should not be corrosive to the material which it is designed to disinfect, nor bring about any other type of destruction.
3. A disinfectant should not remain strongly poisonous for a long time after its application. Some agents require a long period of time to become completely effective; however, the poisonous properties should not remain long after application or they themselves may cause poisoning to livestock.
4. A desirable disinfectant must not combine chemically with other chemicals so as to become inert.
5. An effective and desirable disinfectant must not be excessively irritating nor poisonous when inhaled, as this property would be undesirable from the public-health point of view.
6. A desirable disinfectant must be effective at ordinary temperatures, although warming a solution or warming the surface on which the disinfectant is to be applied enhances its killing power. Conversely, cold reduces killing power. Therefore, the desirable disinfectant must be effective at ordinary temperatures.
7. The disinfectant must be effective when diluted with water, and must readily and uniformly mix with water because it is the universal solvent. A disinfectant that does not mix with water may cause several problems.
8. The disinfectant must be in such a concentration and in such a form that it may be readily and economically transported. The best disinfectant in the world would not be efficient nor feasible if it could not be transported easily and economically to the place where it is to be used.
9. The disinfectant must be priced reasonably.

The foregoing has dealt with chemical disinfecting and the ways in which it is brought about. There are also nonchemical means of disinfection. Mechanical agencies such as cleaning and scrubbing and the physical removal of organic matter are means of nonchemical disinfection. There are also natural agencies of nonchemical disinfection, including sunlight, heat, filtration, sedimentation, and time.

The USDA, in the interests of serving the public, publishes an official list containing those cresylic disinfectants permitted for use on equipment and animals quarters. All federal employees supervising the disinfection of infected or exposed cars, trucks, boats, other vehicles, stockyard pens, chutes, alleys, premises, etc., are required to use a product permitted for that use under federal regulations. The permitted list of cresylic disinfectants issued June, 1965, follows. (All disinfectants are to be diluted in the proportions of 4 ounces to one gallon of water.)

CRESYLIC DISINFECTANTS

ACCO Cresylic Solution
Acresel
Anchor Cresylic Compound
ARCO 50% Cresylic Solution
Baird's Solution Cresol—Compound U.S.P. XIII
B&B Cresno 16-N
Belltex Farm Disinfectant
Bourbon Cresylic Disinfectant
B.P.C.O. Cresolis Compound
C-4 Brand Soluble Cresylic Disinfectant
Carbola Liquid Disinfectant
Carson's 50% Cresylic Disinfectant
Cento Discresol
Central's Liquor Cresolis Saponatus U.S.P. XIII
Columbia Cresul Fluid
Co-op Cresylic Disinfectant
Cooper's Saponified Cresyl Solution
Corn States 50% Cresylic
Cres-A-Check
Cresilin
Cresnol Cresol Compound
Cresolutol
Crespolin
Crestall Fluid
Cres-Tone 50% Cresylic
Cresylic Solution 50%
Cresyline Cresylic Compound
Crystal Cresylic Disinfectant

Curt's Cresylic Compound
Deolysin
Diamond H. Cresyl Fluid
Dixon Germ (Check) Cresylic Disinfectant
Dolge Cresylic Disinfectant
F.O. Cresylic Disinfectant
Franklin Cresolis
Germalene Cresol Compound
Germo Cresolis
G.L.F. Soluble Cresylic Disinfectant
Globe 50% Cresylic Disinfectant
Harco Saponated Cresylic Disinfectant
HVL Cresylic Disinfectant
Hy-Kresol
Imco Brand Technical Cresol Compound
Jen-Sal Cresylic Disinfectant
KaDeCo Cresylic Acid Solution 50% HMC
Kerol
Kremulso
Liquor Cresolis Saponatus U.S.P. N.F.
Midland Cresylic Disinfectant
Miller's Cresylic Disinfectant
New M.F.A. 50% Cresylic Disinfectant
NCL 50% Cresylic Solution
Palmer's Technical Cresol Compound
Purina Cre-so-fec
Quist Solution Cresol
Sanfax C61
S.O. Germite
Supersan Cresylic Compound
Tekresol
U.C. Cresolis
Val-A-Saponified Solution
Varco 50% Cresylic Solution
Varco Liquor Cresolis Saponatus XII
Warlasco 50% Cresylic Solution

6
Agencies of Disease Control

THE LIVESTOCK industry of the United States is relatively efficient compared to many areas of the world. This nation is one of the safest in which to raise livestock, although diseases, parasites, and insect pests exact a high toll each year. State and federal measures have been developed to combat diseases, but economic losses still occur. The greatest losses result not from death of animals but from the loss of meat, milk, or fiber when animals become debilitated. The livestock industry is continuously challenged to reduce these losses.

Communicable diseases of livestock can be eradicated only when diseased animals are prevented from mingling with the susceptible. However, the more animals are isolated, the less immunity they develop to common pathogens. Viruses, bacteria, and parasites are prolific, insidious, elusive, and invisible. They can strike without warning, causing untold mortality and morbidity in unprotected livestock. As animal populations increase, the standards of management must also increase; otherwise, the ravages of diseases will be frequent and costly. Although the manner of disease spread is complex, much of it is preventable if proper precautions are taken. Prevention of disease spread must be a consequence of cooperative efforts among livestock producers, state and federal agents and veterinarians.

Accredited Veterinarians

For many years, federal regulatory agencies have relied on the ability and the integrity of accredited veterinarians in the cooperative control and eradication of livestock diseases. Most state and federal regulations evidence this reliance by specifying that certain livestock movements may be made only when certified by full-time state or federal veterinarians, or by an accredited veterinarian. Accredited veterinarians are practitioners who have been examined and certified as to their competence. They are privileged to cooperate with regulatory disease-control programs not only protecting the livestock industry of the nation but adding to the well-being of mankind. This is a responsibility neither lightly given nor lightly assumed. Therefore, the accredited veterinarian is the first bulwark in the line of defense against ever-present animal disease.

Most veterinarians in large-animal practice are accredited by state and federal agencies to participate in those activities having a direct relationship to the economic diseases prevalent within a given area. As a consequence, the veterinarian accepts the responsibility of notifying government officials of the presence of reportable diseases within his area. The accredited veterinarian is obligated to report to the state and federal officials any outbreak, or any case diagnosed by him, of any of the reportable diseases and to seek additional aid and laboratory diagnosis to confirm the presence of the disease.

In addition to supplying veterinary services for the individual farm or ranch owner on a routine and emergency basis, the accredited veterinarian serves as a contract veterinarian for the state or federal government in certain eradication programs. In this respect, he is paid by the government to perform services to protect the livestock of the area. That service, therefore, is free to the livestock or ranch owner. The veterinarian serves in such programs as tuberculosis, brucellosis, hog cholera, and scabies eradication, and any other programs determined to be of economic importance. Thus, the local veterinarian serves a multiple role: (1) He is the regulatory official responsible for the testing, vaccination, quarantine, and disposal of reactor animals of economic importance. (2) He serves the public in such programs as rabies vaccination and the eradication of economic diseases. (3) He may serve in a public-health capacity by inspecting meat and milk, and supervising animal activities—primarily the movement of livestock—having a bearing on human health.

The accredited veterinarian is responsible for the examination of livestock and the issuance of health certificates when livestock are moved across boundaries of states or counties—anywhere that cattle, sheep, or hogs enter into interstate commerce.

County, District, or Area Veterinary Services

In highly developed counties in many areas of the United States, there are state, federal and county veterinary organizations participating in activities of economic importance to livestock producers and associated with programs aimed at preventing communicable diseases from spreading and from being transmitted to humans. A veterinary officer is often associated with a county board of health to handle animal conditions of public-health importance. In sparsely settled states, some counties exert a regulatory capacity not found in the more heavily populated states, namely, the control of the movement of livestock and the inspection of livestock going through local abattoirs.

State Veterinarians

The office of state veterinarian has been created in each state for the purpose of controlling communicable diseases of economic importance within that state. The state veterinarian is the senior veterinary official within the state and his responsibilities are to the governor, or to the Livestock Disease Commission, or to the Livestock Sanitary Board, or to the Department of Agriculture, depending upon the administrative structure of the state. The duties of the state veterinarian are to evaluate the disease probabilities within a state, to establish livestock disease controls, and to enforce those controls by regulations to prevent the widespread dissemination of diseases of economic importance to livestock producers. Whenever necessary, the state veterinarian may establish quarantines of a particular farm, an area, or the entire state. He establishes rules and regulations concerning the importation of animals from other states and approves the conditions of shipment into his state; the state veterinarian of one state may place a restriction on all animals emanating from any other state where a serious communicable disease may be present.

The state veterinarian is responsible for the issuance and renewal of licenses of all veterinary practitioners. He also serves as the head of the Veterinary Examining Board of the state, or as an ex-officio member of the Board. He is responsible for the initiation of legislation concerning livestock disease control, and serves as a consultant to the legislature in this area. He investigates violations of disease control regulations, cooperates with federal officials in the approval of accredited veterinarians, examines any cases in which violations of accreditation standards are suspected, and acts where the rules and regulations concerning eradication practices have been violated.

The state veterinarian is responsible for the establishment of diagnostic laboratories to investigate and confirm the diagnoses of diseases referred by local veterinarians in the field. In essence, then, he is in charge of the state diagnostic services, and it is under his direction that communicable diseases are investigated.

Federal Regulatory Agencies

The Animal Health Division of the United States Department of Agriculture is responsible, at the federal level, for the formulation and administration of cooperative federal-state programs for the control and eradication of animal diseases.

The responsibility for protecting the health of the nation's livestock includes full-scale or limited eradication programs, epidemiological, laboratory and field diagnostic services, and a continuing interest in all animal diseases, domestic or foreign, that are threats to livestock. To safeguard livestock producers in the United States from losses due to animal diseases, every possible effort must be made

to prevent the introduction of foreign animal diseases, to stamp out promptly any infection that may gain a foothold, and to employ any adequate and established measures to this end. If the microorganism of any disease normally nonexistent in this country is introduced and threatens the livestock industry, the Secretary of Agriculture has the authority to cooperate with the states concerned in drastic eradication measures, including the purchase and destruction of diseased or exposed animals and contaminated material.

Among the regulatory features of material assistance in combating animal diseases are federal and state quarantines; campaigns for disease control and eradication; record keeping to disclose the extent and distribution of various diseases; public stockyards inspection; testing livestock before interstate shipment; cleaning and disinfecting premises and vehicles; immunization of swine against hog cholera; dipping of cattle and sheep for scabies; and the enforcement of the so-called "28-hour law." Supervision over the production of biological products and control of drug remedies are also important phases of the work.

A long-term program of eradication, undertaken county by county and state by state, with active cooperation among federal and state livestock sanitary officials, livestock producers and veterinarians is commonly called a campaign.

Federal and state quarantines are of great value in the control and eradication of animal diseases. These measures are usually effected through rules and regulations based on legislation which in many instances is general but which confers on the enforcing officers ample authority to prescribe definite and detailed specifications for quarantine.

In combating most infectious diseases of livestock, control of the movement of the diseased and exposed animals is essential. This can seldom be accomplished without some kind of quarantine. The principal purpose for the establishment of quarantine is to confine the infection to the smallest possible area and to hold it there until it can be eradicated through the use of appropriate measures.

Several of the most serious communicable diseases of animals have not gained a permanent foothold in this country, primarily due to the efforts of regulatory veterinary officials at ports of embarkation. Sometimes it is possible to prevent a highly infectious disease from getting a foothold by the strict enforcement of a local quarantine. This is well demonstrated by the practice of holding animals offered for importation into the United States in quarantine at ports of entry for a period of observation. This practice in a number of instances has prevented the introduction of foreign animal diseases into this country, the most noteworthy case having been the detection of a disease of economic importance in animals from a country where the disease had not been reported to be prevalent.

When an outbreak of a serious disease occurs, it is the practice of both federal and state officials to impose drastic quarantine measures. These not only prohibit all movement from infected premises but prohibit or greatly restrict the movement within the quarantined area of livestock and materials considered likely to serve as means for the spread of the disease. Although the quarantined area covered by regulations from federal and state authorities is usually identical, in some instances the state may, as a precautionary measure, establish a more stringent quarantined area, from which a limited movement of animals and farm products is permitted only under the close observation of state veterinary officials. When diseases of economic importance have become widespread and established, local quarantines may not be adequate to control the movement of livestock and the vehicles used in their transportation. In such instances, a federal quarantine is imposed, and the interested officials cooperate by putting state quarantines into effect. To be effective, and to have the support of interested agencies and livestock producers, quarantines must be appropriate for the particular disease being combated. These procedures may range on the one hand from complete prohibition against the movement of all animals, produce, and vehicles, and even restrictions on human beings, to, on the other, physical examination and movement under proper certification or official permit: animals are subjected to prescribed observations and treatment before being allowed to enter into interstate commerce.

Since quarantine measures interfere in varying degrees with the operations of livestock producers, they should be imposed only when other means would be ineffective; they should be lifted as promptly as conditions warrant. It would be impossible, however, to control and eradicate some of the infectious diseases in this country without the authority of both state and federal agencies to impose strict quarantines.

While complete eradication is the final objective of all campaigns, two quite different principles are involved calling for correspondingly different methods of procedure. Diseases caused by, or transmitted by, external parasites may be effectively controlled by treatment of the affected animals for the destruction of the parasites or by eradication of the vector per se. On the other hand, bacterial or virus diseases are determined by diagnostic tests, and animals found to be infected are appraised and slaughtered. Owners of destroyed animals are indemnified by the state and federal governments within certain regulatory limits. Efforts toward the control and eradication of communicable animal diseases within the states are primarily the function of the respective state authorities; the direct authority of the federal government extends only to the control of the interstate movement of livestock from districts where disease is known to prevail. Authority to enforce local quarantines and to compel the destruction or the treatment of infected or exposed animals rests entirely with the states; consequently, the work of federal and state cooperative projects is done chiefly under state laws and regulations. State authorities undertake to proceed in harmony with the policies and practices agreed upon by federal and state veterinary regulatory officials.

Infected animals are the source of all infection. They are always potentially dangerous. Therefore, slaughter of infected animals is usually the best procedure for actually preventing exposure and spread of easily transmitted diseases, such as foot-and-mouth disease; this affliction is so infectious that it is almost impossible to prevent its spread if sick and healthy animals are kept on the same premises. Slaughter of all animals affected with certain infectious diseases is a standard procedure.

Philosophy of the Animal Health Division

The best economic treatment of livestock or poultry diseases is eradication. Preventing the introduction of foreign animal diseases and eradicating domestic diseases of major economic significance will ultimately eliminate the need for a continuous control program and the annual cost associated with it. This can be done effectively and efficiently through close cooperation with the states, with modern methods, and with a minimum of trade interference.

The Animal Health Division:

1. conducts nationwide state-federal cooperative programs for control and eradication of animal diseases.
2. suppresses the spread of disease through control of interstate and international movement of livestock.
3. is aware of the overall disease situation nationally and internationally, and maintains the capability of dealing with foreign animal diseases.
4. administers laws to insure humane treatment of transported livestock and certain laboratory animals.
5. collects and disseminates information on disease morbidity and mortality throughout the country.
6. provides for increased technical, managerial, and professional competence through continuous employee development and training.

The Animal Health Division is organized so that the director of the Division has under his control a group of assistant directors, one for each of the four major districts of the United States, and several national animal diagnostic laboratories. Therefore, each state belongs to a larger district. Within each state there is a federal veterinarian-in-charge, responsible for the Animal Health Division's programs. Under the veterinarian-in-charge for each state, variable numbers of veterinarians are designated as district veterinarians. They are responsible for the activities of several area veterinarians and of the accredited veterinarians in private practice within that particular area, as their activities relate to federal and state diagnostic and regulatory activities. The activities of the area veterinarians are directly related to the activities on the farms and ranches; they assist the accredited veterinarians in diagnosis and issue local quarantines where diseases of economic importance are located. If a reportable communicable disease is suspected, it is their responsibility to solicit the aid of local, state, or federal animal disease diagnostic laboratories to determine by further tests the accurate diagnosis of the condition; in the meantime, they issue a restrictive quarantine until the disease has been diagnosed as either an innocuous malady or one of economic importance.

The continued high level of the economy is due in part to the large numbers of healthy livestock in the nation. Although losses to the livestock industry in the United States due to animal diseases and parasites have been estimated to be more than two billion dollars each year, our nation is better off than most other countries in the world in terms of animal diseases. Many livestock diseases of other lands do not exist here. (Conversely, some nations have successfully eradicated diseases still widespread in this country, and for which no eradication programs have been authorized or undertaken to date.) The Animal Health Division is alert to the shifting patterns of animal diseases. Liaisons with scientists around the world have been maintained for the development of plans to cope with emergency situations should exotic diseases find their way into the nation's livestock.

Many regulations are considered by the public as a burden imposed on commerce for purposes they do not readily comprehend. However, regulations are important to the disease eradication programs. Methods of disease dissemination are thoroughly studied, and regulations are then drawn to prevent the spread of diseases. If these regulations were not enforced, programs for control would be ineffective.

Animal Quarantine Laws

The Animal Quarantine Laws are contained in the federal regulations. They are designed to prevent the spread of communicable diseases by controlling the interstate movement of livestock, including poultry, which are apparently free of diseases or exposure thereto. Special provisions permit the interstate movement of reactors to tuberculosis, brucellosis, and paratuberculosis tests, but only under certain carefully supervised conditions which insure proper handling until final disposition.

The regulations also provide for the cleaning and disinfection of all cars, boats, and other vehicles used in the interstate transportation of diseased livestock and poultry. These sanitary precautions apply likewise to stockyards, holding pens, and other premises used in connection with such shipments.

Inspections for compliance with the laws are conducted throughout the United States at highway and railroad points, stockyards, and livestock centers. Apparent violations are reported to the Department of Agriculture for further investigation and possible prosecution.

28-Hour Law

With the advent of railroads, a new epoch began in the delivery of livestock to markets. Cattle, in fact all breeds of livestock, were herded into crude, ill-equipped railway cars—some of which contained no provision for shelter, or feed, or water—and were maintained in these conveyances for great lengths of time. The overland truck was also used for transport, and with similar results. Mounting public clamor led to an act passed in June, 1906. This Act is essentially a law to prevent cruelty to animals while in interstate transit. It prohibits the confinement of animals in a car for a period longer than 28 consecutive hours without unloading them, in a humane manner, into properly equipped pens, for a period of at least five hours for rest, water, and feeding. In some instances, animals may be fed and watered without unloading, provided that adequate space is available in the railway cars for rest. In some cases, by written request, accidental causes or acts of nature, which cannot be anticipated or avoided by the exercise of due diligence and foresight, may excuse continuous confinement for 36 hours or longer. Although the law is applicable only to railroad and water transport, attempts have been made to apply its humane principles to motortruck transport as well.

Public Stockyard Law

By an Act of Congress dated May 29, 1884, the Commissioner of Agriculture was authorized to organize a Bureau of Animal Industry, to appoint a chief, and to empower him to employ personnel to initiate special investigations into certain contagious, infectious, or communicable diseases along the lines of transportation to all parts of the United States. In this general language lies legal authority for inspection of public stockyards.

For several years, Texas fever was the only disease subject to stockyard control. In 1897 inspection was extended to sheep scabies and in 1903 to cattle scabies. By 1905, activities were enlarged to embrace inspection for communicable diseases of all livestock received at public stockyards.

Since its beginning, public-stockyard inspection has been important in controlling or eradicating Texas fever in cattle, dourine and glanders in horses, scabies in sheep and cattle, foot-and-mouth disease, and vesicular exanthema.

The stockyard service proved its importance in controlling and eradicating vesicular exanthema. Since most major markets were involved, the manner in which vesicular exanthema was handled unquestionably prevented the development of additional foci of infection. On many occasions, stockyard inspection not only stopped the spread of infection but also helped to locate farm sources where the disease had not been known to exist.

The cooperation between the management of the stockyard companies and the Department of Agriculture in controlling the vesicular exanthema epidemic cannot be overemphasized. It demonstrated that in these days of rapid transport, by working with marketing interests, the USDA can effectively control the spread of livestock diseases.

Stockyard-inspection activities were enhanced when, in an effort to prevent the spread of brucellosis, provision was made in 1957 for specifically approved stockyards and slaughtering establishments to handle reactor and suspect animals. These approved establishments operate under state inspection. Cattle may move interstate to them without having to meet certain prior requirements. Subsequent movement from such markets, however, must be in compliance with federal regulations.

From an economic standpoint, no service supplies more information on the health of the livestock population than the stockyard inspection. An inspection of premises to learn which diseases exist in livestock would be an impractical and expensive procedure. A satisfactory method of making a good estimation is by inspecting the 60 to 65 million animals annually moving through 56 major marketing centers.

This service provides a means of preventing the interstate spread of communicable diseases. It also gives buyers at inspected markets the assurance that they are getting healthy livestock.

Morbidity and Mortality Reporting

In 1955, the USDA established a system for collecting and disseminating statistics on livestock diseases. Reporting will not, in itself, prevent the spread of disease, but it is an important foundation in building sound programs of livestock disease prevention, control, and eradication. In the succeeding years, most states have assumed the responsibility for collecting information within the individual states and supplying it to the Animal Health Division for the morbidity and mortality report. The purpose of the collection of statistics is to furnish continuing information enabling all regulatory agencies to estimate the prevalence of disease in livestock. The reports also alert regulatory officials to changes in disease incidence and provide a means to help them plan programs for eradication of serious diseases.

Reporting includes four basic steps: collection of information, processing, dissemination and use. To be effective, this must be a continuous cycle with each step coordinated with and supporting all other steps. Despite its laudable ambitions, however, the animal disease reporting service has several weak spots. Reports rarely show all occurrences of a given disease. It is necessary for local practitioners to participate in the service, and some fail to cooperate. Further, some reports do not include all diseases observed, while others include some diseases more consistently than they do others; some may be based on incorrect field diagnoses. Additional weaknesses are directly related to the failure of some livestock owners to consult veterinarians; thus occurrence is not reported. It is also possible that several cases occurred before an individual owner contacted his veterinarian, and that further cases will occur and will not be reported to him after he has made the original diagnosis. No reporting system can reflect all occurrences of every disease, particularly those that are common or widespread. Constant effort is needed to improve the system to keep the effects of these shortcomings at an absolute minimum.

The widest possible range of accurate informational sources is needed if the final mortality and morbidity reports are to have any real meaning. Practicing veterinarians, veterinary colleges, veterinary service departments of agricultural colleges and universities, diagnostic laboratories, inspection services at public stockyards and auction markets, ante- and postmortem inspections at slaughtering plants operating under state, federal, and municipal inspection, and inspections by other regulatory officials are all important sources for useful information. This information must be accumulated in detail to provide a meaningful survey of animal diseases within a given area.

An efficient reporting system is of inestimable use in the evaluation of research requirements. It is invaluable if control and eradication programs are to receive adequate advance planning. Systematic disease reporting by regulatory inspectors at stockyards and slaughtering establishments is of special value, since these data can be directly related to known animal numbers.

Modern disease-reporting techniques have many advantages. They are of material assistance in recognizing possible modes of dissemination among animal species, both wild and domestic; they provide indirect evidence of the effectiveness of animal disease control measures. By providing sound disease statistics on geographical and seasonal patterns, the reports serve as an additional protective measure to the entire livestock industry and therefore to human health.

Animal Inspection and Quarantine Division

International inspection and quarantine measures seek to prevent livestock diseases of foreign origin from gaining entrance into the United States as thousands of animals and millions of pounds of animal products are imported each year from all over the world.

Absolute protection against the entrance of foreign diseases through importations is impossible. The only effective measures are constant inspection and quarantine. Public understanding and support are essential if these are to be successful.

The United States is one of the few major livestock-producing countries of the world that remain free of devastating animal diseases prevalent in most countries.

State and federal laws governing the movement of livestock and their products are necessary to prevent the introduction and spread of disease. Before necessary laws were promulgated, many animal diseases were introduced. Prior to the building of our extensive system of roads and railways, diseases did not tend to spread rapidly. However, today, with our rapid system of transport, animal diseases may rapidly become widespread unless stringent methods of control are initiated whenever a disease of a reportable nature is discovered.

There are two basic ways by which this country may be protected against diseases of foreign origin. The first is the absolute prohibition of all imports. Under this system, the government prohibits the importation of all animals and commodities that might transmit disease, but then provides for an exception to this prohibition when the national benefit to be derived is greater than the potential

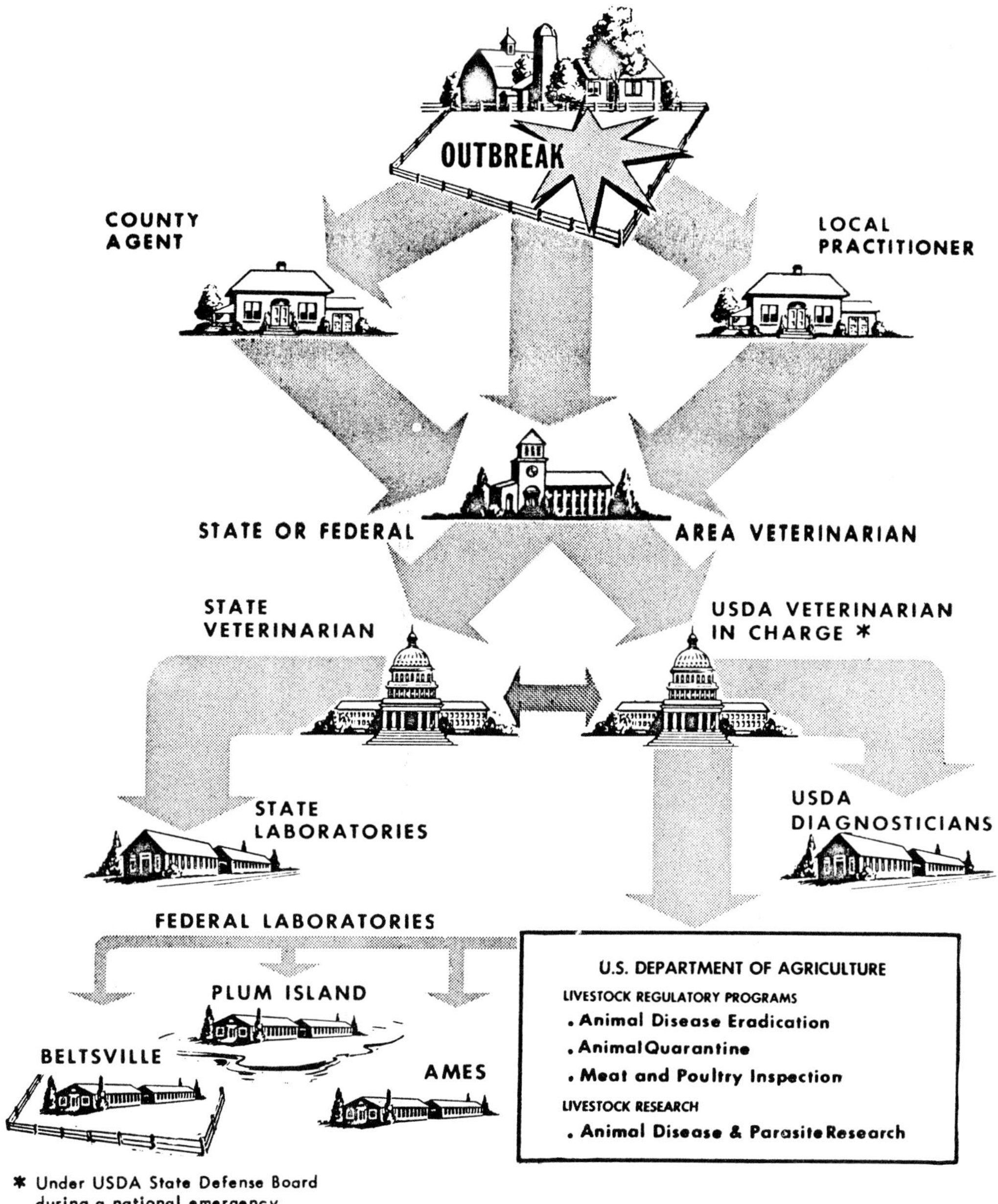

FIG. 4. Scheme for reporting outbreaks of disease.

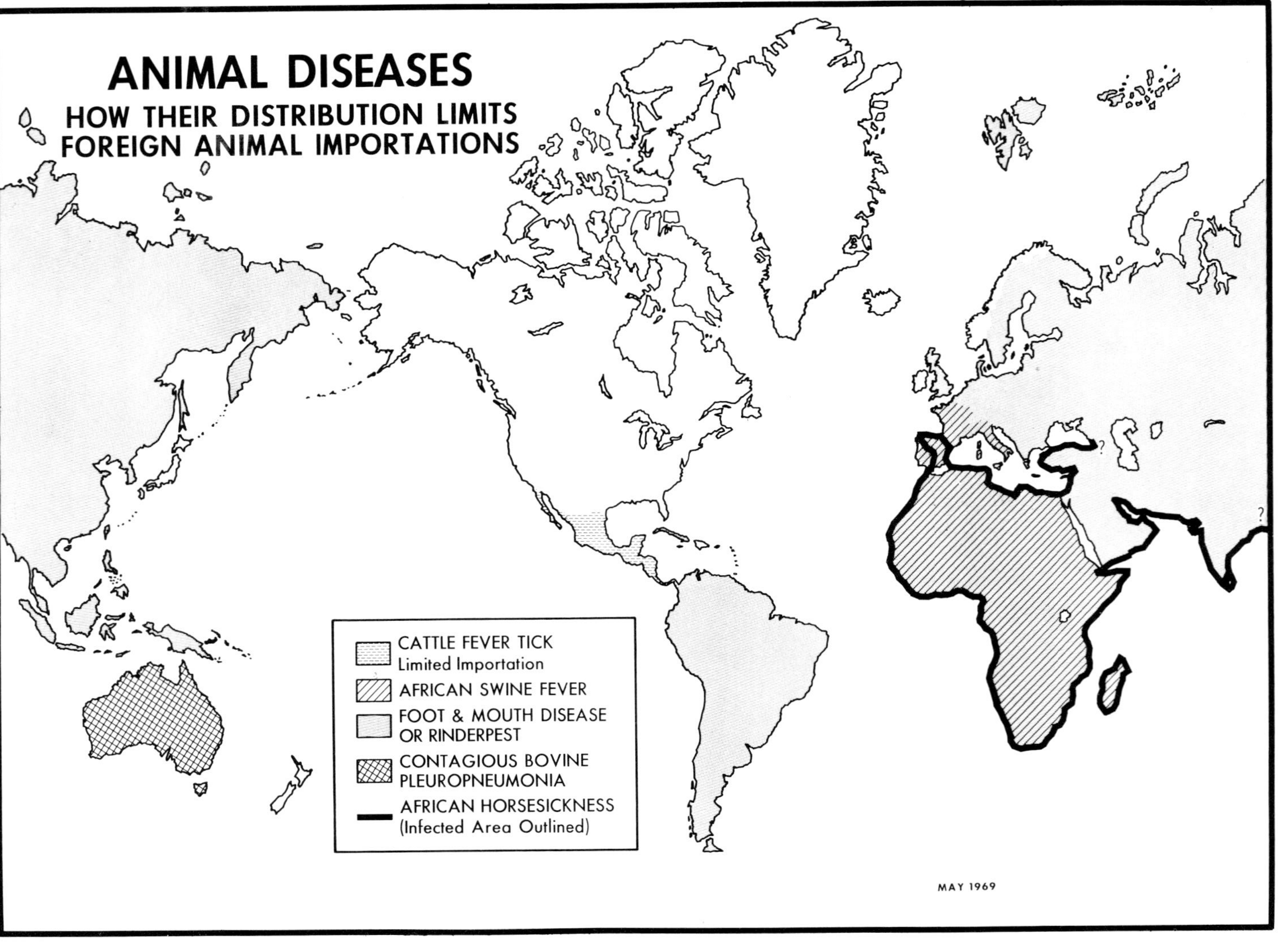

FIG. 5. World distribution of diseases.

danger from possible disease introduction. This is a relatively easy way to administer regulations, because by taking no action the officials preclude any importation that in their opinion might introduce diseases of foreign origin.

The second method involves the establishment of specific regulations governing imports. This requires the publication of detailed regulations applicable to each species of animal, product, or material that may be offered for entry into the United States. Under this system, importations can be prevented only when appropriate officials have taken action to show cause why a particular importation does not meet the applicable import regulation.

With few exceptions, animals offered for entry must be accompanied by a certificate of health issued by an official veterinarian at the point of origin showing that the animals have been in that country for at least 60 days preceding shipment, that they have been inspected and found to be free from certain communicable diseases, and that they have not been exposed to such disease.

The responsibility for protecting the United States against foreign animal diseases has been delegated to an agency of the national government from the time the first legislation was enacted until today. The responsibility was originally given to the Treasury Department, when the first legislation was passed in 1865 to prohibit certain importations of cattle. Some 20 years later, this responsibility was transferred to the Department of Agriculture. Six years later, authorization was granted for the designation of specific ports of entry to be used as animal quarantine stations. This legislation further provided for presidential authority to suspend any or all importations because of disease, when necessary.

The Act of February 2, 1903, authorized

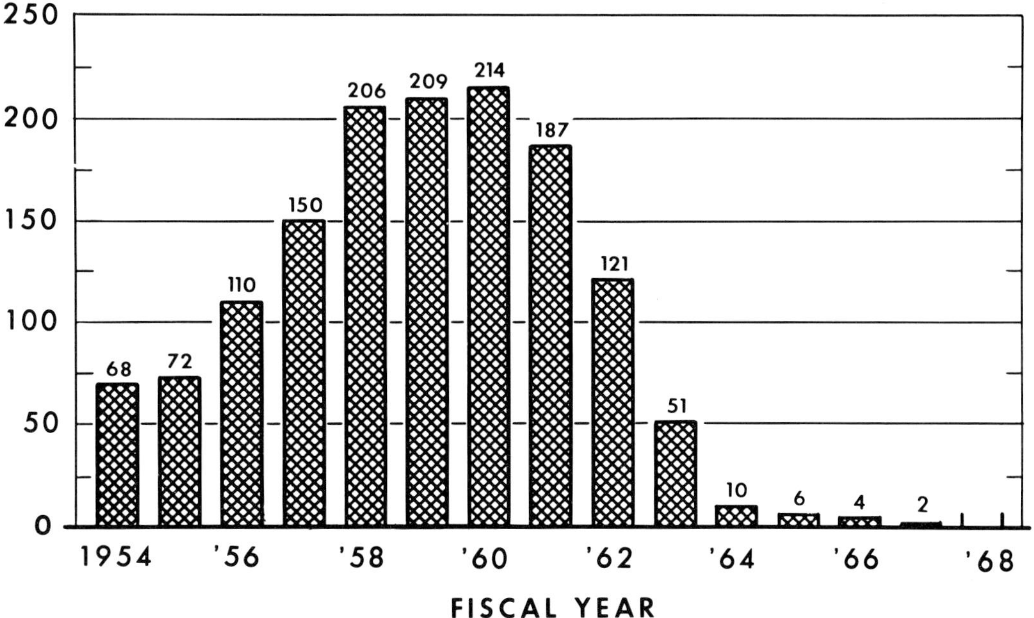

FIG. 6. Graph reflecting incidence of sheep scabies.

the Secretary of Agriculture to promulgate regulations applicable to import animals and to assume other necessary measures to protect against introduction of animal disease.

Despite passage of the laws enumerated, foot-and-mouth disease gained entry into the United States nine times between 1884 and 1929. Although each epizootic was eradicated, the economic loss to the country and to the livestock producers was staggering. Without doubt, these epizootics led to legislation in 1930 to prohibit the importation of domestic ruminants and swine, and fresh, chilled, or frozen meat from all ruminants and swine, from any country declared by the Secretary of Agriculture to be infected with foot-and-mouth disease or rinderpest. In 1958, the law was amended to include a similar prohibition against wild ruminants and swine unless imported under stringent restrictions, including permanent postentry control in USDA-approved zoological parks.

Finally, in 1962, an Act was passed which extended and better defined the authority to seize and destroy international shipments of animals being moved or held contrary to American laws.

Other statutes previously cited are usually referred to as the Animal Quarantine Laws. They provide the authority for imposing restrictions applicable to imported animals, animal products, hay, straw, and similar material that may transmit diseases of foreign origin, as long as such restrictions do not constitute an outright prohibition against such importations.

Because some imported animals may be carriers of latent infections, or may have been exposed to contagious or communicable diseases in transit, quarantine is for a sufficiently long time to insure that the animals are free from disease or exposure. Quarantine is considered the most important step in any introduction of new animals to a herd or flock. It stands as the barrier between susceptible livestock and the importation of new disease.

Control over animals intended for shipment to the United States is based primarily on a series of requirements that include:

1. inspection and certification of the animals by a veterinarian of the national government of the country of origin.
2. knowledge about the status of animal diseases in the country of origin.
3. isolation of the animals while being processed for shipment.
4. completion of preliminary tests in preparation for shipment.
5. a period of quarantine at the embarkation port to better insure against animals having been exposed to disease immediately prior to shipment.
6. completion of precautionary treatments if any are permitted or required.

In addition to the original health certificate issued by the veterinarian of the national government of the country of origin, a second document, a permit, serves to provide control over the importation of animals into the United States. This is a prior permit issued by authorities in the United States to the importer. The import permit:

1. states that no other animals may be permitted aboard the transporting carrier except those for which an import permit has been issued.
2. approves the ports of call, if any, that are permitted by the carrier, and specifically forewarns that no other stops are permitted without the permit becoming invalid.
3. designates the port of arrival at which the animals must be offered for entry into the United States.
4. provides for control over the source of hay, feed, and bedding on route in order to eliminate possible disease exposure.

At the port of entry, personnel of the Animal Quarantine and Inspection Division pass judgment on the animals being offered for entry. Control measures at the port of entry include:

1. veterinary inspection of all animals to determine that the accompanying documents are

in order and the animals appear to be free of evidence of disease or exposure thereto.

2. supervision over the cleaning and disinfection of conveyance, materials, and bedding in contact with imported animals.
3. movement of the animals from the carrier to the quarantine facilities at the port of entry, where they are supervised during their quarantine period.
4. completion of various tests required before the animals may be released from quarantine.
5. precautionary treatments that may be required while in quarantine.
6. consignment of the animals to approved destinations when appropriate.
7. supervision of disposition of animals if rejected for entry.

The restrictions on animals being offered for entry into the United States are believed by some importers and others to constitute a superabundance of precautionary measures and an unnecessary duplication of effort with respect to many of the handling procedures. Nevertheless, each step is considered to be useful and necessary to insure that the United States is not devastated by the introduction and dissemination of animal diseases of foreign origin.

The problem of disease introduction with respect to animal products is considered by some scientists to be greater than that for the animals themselves. At present, the possibility of performing definitive diagnostic tests is greater for animals than for most animal products. Further, each animal in a shipment must be qualified with respect to tests and precautionary treatments or inspection, whereas final determination regarding imported animal products is generally, but not always, completed on a sampling basis. The import volume and complexity of both animals and products are increasing, and the advent of advanced jet-powered aircraft compounds the problems beyond any previously experienced.

The ultimate goal should be definitive tests for detecting all infected, carrier, and exposed animals, and any contaminated animal products and related materials. Only slightly less important would be adequate and safe means for destroying microorganisms without destroying the animal or product involved.

With increased world trade and commerce, and now with space travel upon us, the general field of preventive veterinary medicine must be emphasized. In the final analysis, the main losses from animal diseases are in the important producing areas and the toll is greatest among young animals, many of which never reach market. The practical course by which a livestock owner may reduce losses is: to make a careful study of the probable local danger from each disease, and to obtain publications containing directions for dealing effectively with the danger; to establish a high degree of farm sanitation; and to consult a veterinarian for further methods of prevention, diagnosis, and control, including the use of biological products.

PART 2
Strategic Diseases

7
Anaplasmosis

ANAPLASMOSIS is an infectious and transmissible disease of cattle, of prime concern to the beef and dairy industries over the past fifty years. In bovine species, erythrocytes are invaded and destroyed by the causative agents, *Anaplasma marginale* and *Anaplasma centrale,* protozoa-like microorganisms. This invasion manifests itself biologically by rapidly progressive anemia and jaundice in adult animals and anemia of lesser extent in calves. In recognition of this anemic condition, a new and more specific designation of *bovine infectious anemia* has been recorded in some veterinary literature.

Historically, the major breakthrough in identifying anaplasmosis as a separate entity occurred in 1883 when workers (Smith and Kilborne) dealing primarily with babesiosis (Texas fever) discovered a new inclusion of the peripheral cytoplasm of erythrocytes. Their findings were published in Bulletin No. 1, Bureau of Animal Industries, United States Department of Agriculture. Further research led to the realization that anaplasmosis was due to a pathogenic protozoa-like factor, and that its invasion of erythrocytes displayed clinical symptoms similar to babesiosis. Although anaplasmosis is recognized primarily in semitropical areas, the widespread shipment of cattle, and especially commercial breeding stock, from herds of the southeastern United States has led to the increased incidence of anaplasmosis in more temperate areas of this country. Recent estimates indicate the cost of the disease to beef and dairy producers to be well over fifty million dollars annually.

Geographically, endemic areas within the United States have been designated, and correlations with semitropical climatic locations are found. Heavy morbidity and mortality losses occur in the Gulf coast states and along the Pacific coast, mainly in California. In addition, northern ranges of the Rocky Mountains are recognized as enzootic areas. Prevalence of anaplasmosis in these locales is primarily due to the large arthropod vector population, especially ticks and mites.

Etiology

The causative agent is a microorganism classified as *Anaplasma marginale.* This nomenclature is justified by the fact that microscopic study demonstrates the organism to be devoid of cytoplasm (literal translation of the term *Anaplasma* means without cytoplasm). Analyses of infected animals invariably reveal the *Anaplasma* bodies proximal to the outer cellular membrane of erythrocytes, thus the term *marginale.* This was the only form inducing disease within the United States until recently. Reports from other parts of the world, viz. Africa and Argentina, indicate that a subspecies, *A. marginale* var. *centrale* is involved in pathogenesis. This second species has now been demonstrated in the United States.

Most authors refer to *Anaplasma marginale* as a protozoa-like microorganism, although recent investigations indicate a close relationship to rickettsial organisms.

Transmission

Transmission is accomplished by biological and mechanical means. The former involves arthropod vectors, especially the blood-sucking varieties. Of prime importance are the ticks, although mites, lice, mosquitoes, and biting flies have been incriminated. These vectors feed on cattle harboring the disease and then on uninfected animals, thus transferring the pathogenic agent. A significant factor in this method is the interval between feedings. Experimental evidence indicates that the chelicera and other sucking mouth parts must be wet with blood to cause an active translocation of *Anaplasma* bodies. In most climatic areas, any disruption in feeding exceeding four minutes will lower the virulence of the agent because of coagulation of the erythrocytes. However, the ability of tick species to incorporate the microorganisms within their bodies in a virulent state must not be discounted. It has been proven experimentally that female ticks can retain *Anaplasma* for periods up to six months without lowered pathogenicity.

Recent research has disclosed the phenomenon of transovarian transfer of *A. marginale* from the maternal tick to the ova. The infective organism remains viable in the ovum and larval stages of the tick from one season to the next. In the case of the three-host tick, the infective organism may be transmitted at any blood meal. This means of transmission is apparently the way *Anaplasma* is able to over-winter in an enzootic area. The developmental stages in the life cycle of arthropods will be discussed in a later chapter.

Numerically, arthropods exhibit wide seasonal fluctuations. Relatedly then, the most critical period involving population peaks of anaplasmosis vectors occurs during the months of late summer and early fall. Statistical field studies correlate the incidence of the disease with the variation in vector populations.

Mechanical transmission involves the transfer of blood from one animal to another via various operations performed upon herds. Of prime concern are castration, dehorning, ear tagging, tattooing, vaccination, and blood samples drawn with bleeding needles. Transmission normally occurs when sanitation has been neglected.

Transmission in utero has been reported in certain bovine species. Dams free of the disease and then infected during gestation have produced calves carrying the pathogenic organism. However, this transfer mechanism is believed to occur infrequently. The animal is more likely to abort than to give birth to a full-term calf.

Factors Influencing Susceptibility

All breeds of cattle and many other ruminants are susceptible to anaplasmosis. Worldwide surveys have demonstrated the *Anaplasma* organism to have a marked specificity

TABLE 2. Principal Tick Vectors of Anaplasmosis in the United States.

Scientific name	Common name	Stages of life cycle when *Anaplasma* organism carried
Argas persicus	Fowl tick	Nymph, adult
Dermacentor variabilis	American dog tick	Larva, nymph, adult
Dermacentor andersoni	Rocky Mountain spotted fever tick	Egg, larva, nymph, adult
Dermacentor occidentalis	Pacific coast tick	Egg, larva, adult
Dermacentor albipictus	Winter tick	Larva, nymph, adult
Rhipicephalus sanguineus	Brown dog tick	Nymph, adult
Ixodes scapularis	Black-legged tick	Larva, nymph, adult

toward ruminants, especially those of the bovine species. Therefore, anaplasmosis is principally considered as a disease of cattle.

Sheep and goats appear to demonstrate some degree of susceptibility; however, in most cases the infection is a latent, mild type. In 1955, a breeding ewe flock grazing on wheat pasture in western Kansas was observed to have a "debilitating condition." The etiological agent was isolated and classified as *Anaplasma ovis.*

A significant factor in epizootic areas is the ability of wildlife, especially native deer, to harbor the pathogenic organism. Known carriers in the United States are black-tailed deer, white-tailed deer, and mule deer of western range areas. In many cases, deer do not succumb to the disease but rather serve as reservoirs, thus posing great danger as a potential source for infecting healthy beef and dairy herds, through bloodsucking vectors.

Some *Anaplasma*-like organisms of an obscure nature have been isolated in swine and poultry, but to date researchers have not elucidated the *A. marginale* relationships. *Anaplasma*-like infections in man have not been reported.

Three factors influencing susceptibility are of note: (1) age of the individual, (2) level of sanitation and health in the herd, and (3) the degree of parasite control.

The correlation of age and susceptibility has been substantiated by numerous research and field studies. Calves normally have an innate physiological ability to resist the *Anaplasma* invasions, and generally evidence a mild type of infection. Conversely, older animals do not resist infection by *Anaplasma* and readily succumb to the effects of the destruction of red blood cells. In some herds mortality in animals over one year of age has exceeded 50 percent. Further, it is recognized that animals over three years of age may have a mortality of 90 percent.

While sanitation and parasite control are not directly related to susceptibility, nevertheless they have an influence. Herds allowed to become heavily parasitized and cattle maintained in unsanitary environments demonstrate increased susceptibility.

Symptoms

Symptoms are primarily related to erythrocyte destruction and the resulting anemia. In cases of mild infection, often seen in calves, the pulse rate quickens, diarrhea or constipation may be present, respiration increases, and temperature may range from 103 to 106 F. Some important field symptoms involve changes in behavior. Calves go off feed (anorexia), become "dumpy" or dejected, remain apart from the rest of the herd, and are exhausted due to anemia. In most cases, infection in young animals is short-lived, and they rarely succumb to anaplasmosis.

Symptoms in mature animals present a different picture. The rapid destruction of erythrocytes by the *Anaplasma* organism

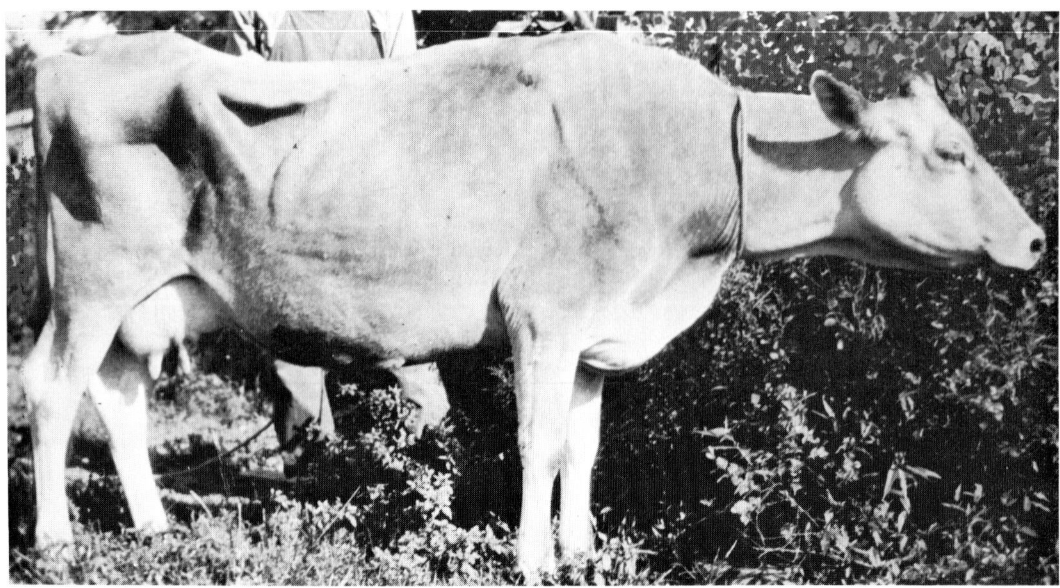

FIG. 7. A typical case of acute anaplasmosis.

places great stress upon the animal. The severity of the anemia is represented by extremely rapid or labored breathing, a pulse rate of 100 to 140, a temperature of 104 to 107 F, excessive salivation, general weakness and pallor, frequent urination, inappetence, psychotic, frequently aggressive, actions due to anoxia of the central nervous system, and abortions during all stages of pregnancy (chiefly due to the high fever).

Icterus (jaundice) is commonly observed in *Anaplasma*-infected cattle. Principally, it is caused by increased concentrations of bilirubin in the circulating plasma fluids. This results in a yellowing of epithelial tissue, especially mucous membranes of the muzzle, nasal cavity and eye. Mammary-gland tissue is also discolored, and because of this anaplasmosis has often been termed "yellow-teat disease" by stockmen.

Pathology

The incubation period occurs following transmission of the etiological agent to a susceptible animal, a state of *Anaplasma* proliferation and dissemination in the new host. It is the interval between initial exposure and microscopic detection of *Anaplasma* bodies on stained blood films, or the manifestation of clinical signs of the disease. The incubation period may last 15 to 45 days, depending on the resistance of the host and the virulence of the organism.

The clinical period is manifested by icterus and anemia with secondary symptoms. It is estimated that the parasite invades 50 to 77 percent of the circulating erythrocytes during this period. Hematological changes involve a net decrease in erythrocyte numbers. Erythropoiesis, or red blood cell production, is unable to meet the demands caused by the rapid invasion and destruction of blood cells. During this brief period, the animal will lapse into an acute or peracute condition with death rapidly occurring. If, however, antibodies can be produced during this period, the animal will probably enter a period of convalescence. The *Anaplasma* apparently acts as foreign protein (antigen), thus causing antibody formation. In young animals fetal splenic erythropoiesis coupled with antibody production accounts for suppression of the disease; removal of the spleen in calves results in exacerbation of all symptoms and death. In older animals, antibody production to combat *Anaplasma* is less efficient and increased blood formation to replace damaged cells is more difficult.

If an animal survives a mild infection, or if clinical signs improve following treatment, the *Anaplasma* may have been destroyed or the organisms may be lying dormant in the spongy portions of the long bones. The animal is classified as a carrier when microscopic blood stains reveal a decrease in *Anaplasma,* anemia and icterus subside, and the organism is lying dormant in some part of the body. During this period a delicate immunological balance exists between host and parasite. Experimentally splenectomized bovine carriers lose this equilibrium and relapse into clinical states. The gross postmortem findings are indicative of the stress imposed upon the hematopoietic system during infection. Pallor and icterus of the tissues are evident. Erythropoietic suppression is shown by a watery consistency of the blood and a lighter red color. The spleen is greatly enlarged; the liver is enlarged, with icterus and distension of the gall bladder.

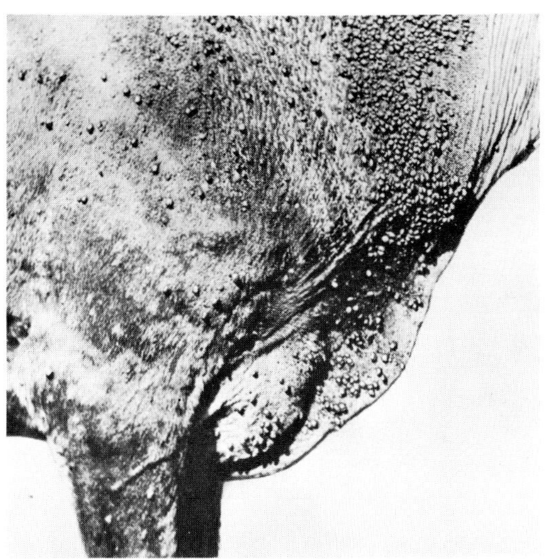

FIG. 8. Neck and shoulder of a bovine heavily infested with ticks, the vectors of anaplasmosis.

Diagnosis

Diagnosis is accomplished by observing clinical manifestations and employing laboratory tests. Infected animals exhibit anemia, icterus, rapid or labored breathing, temperature of 103 to 107 F, general weakness, irrational behavior, loss of appetite, constipation, and a decrease in milk production. Rapid death is common during the acute and peracute stages of infection. When anaplasmosis is suspected by outward symptoms, blood studies are necessary to verify a tentative diagnosis. When microscopic examinations of stained blood samples disclose *Anaplasma* bodies, diagnosis is confirmed. However, these bodies rapidly deteriorate and in many cases are not observable under a microscope. Therefore, additional methods may be necessary.

The main serological techniques used to diagnose anaplasmosis are: (1) the complement-fixation test, (2) the fluorescent-antibody technique, and (3) the antigen-antibody agglutination test.

The complement-fixation test is not only a valuable aid in diagnosing clinical cases but is 95 percent reliable in disclosing latent carriers. However, this method requires delicate procedures and is time-consuming.

The fluorescent-antibody technique subjects suspected *Anaplasma*-containing blood samples to fluorescein isothiocyanate. This precipitates an antigen-antibody-dye complex which under ultraviolet light fluoresces a yellow green, denoting infection.

The antigen-antibody agglutination test is extremely accurate in diagnosing the carrier state. A commercial test kit is currently being produced by Diamond Laboratories of Des Moines, Iowa. It employs a capillary tube in which a mixture of serum and a prepared antigen is incubated for 24 hours. Macroscopic aggregates in the tube indicate an infected animal, while absence of the aggregates is evidence of a negative test. A new field test for anaplasmosis has been developed by scientists at the National Animal Disease Labo-

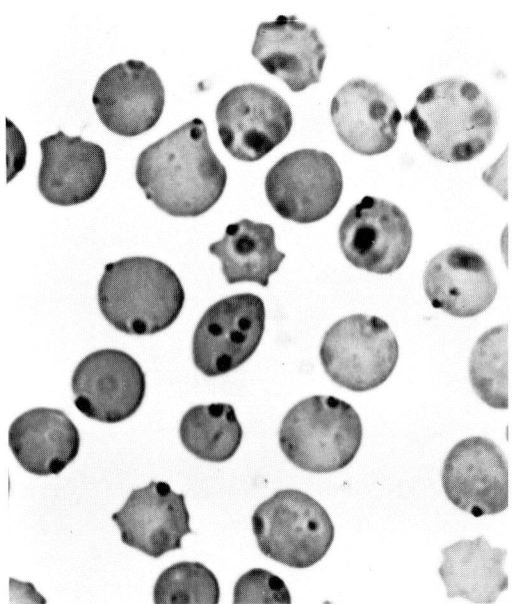

FIG. 9. Appearance of blood cells of a bovine infected with *Anaplasma marginale.*

ratory at Beltsville, Maryland, and eliminates the delay involved in sending blood samples to laboratories for analysis. The test may be done at the farm or ranch and the results are available within ten minutes. One drop of colored antigen is mixed with one drop of serum separated out of a blood sample; macroscopic colored clumps indicate a positive reaction.

Because much of the symptomatology is similar to that of other bovine diseases, caution must be maintained during diagnosis. Anemia and jaundice are indicative of gastrointestinal poisoning, acute parasitism, hepatic malfunction, and eperythrozoonosis. High temperature and rapid or labored breathing are symptoms of pneumonia, hemorrhagic septicemia (shipping fever), blackleg, and leptospirosis. Rapid death is a prime indication of anthrax in cattle.

Prophylaxis

Prophylaxis is accomplished chiefly by three means: (1) sanitation during routine surgical procedures to prevent mechanical transmission, (2) arthropod vector control, and (3) vaccination to prevent anaplasmosis. It behooves every stockman to recognize his responsibility for preventing infection and to design his management program accordingly.

Management procedures include slaughter of recovered and carrier cattle as soon as economically feasible, separation of the herd into age and functional groups, and testing of purchased breeding stock to disclose latent carriers. Valuable cattle that are reactors should be kept at least 300 feet apart from uninfected animals and given lengthy tetracycline therapy to destroy the pathogenic organism.

The production of a vaccine to protect cattle appears to be the long-awaited breakthrough in the battle to control anaplasmosis. A commercial vaccine now available is an attenuated (killed) preparation of *A. marginale* organisms. The manufacturer recommends that young animals (3 months of age or older) be given two injections of the vaccine at six-week intervals, followed by annual revaccination.

8
Anthrax

ANTHRAX, or splenic fever, is a subacute or acute communicable disease occurring in one form or another in all warm-blooded animals, including man. The disease is caused by a bacterium called *Bacillus anthracis* and is characterized by sudden death, bloody discharges from the body openings, and gross enlargement of the spleen. Cattle, sheep, goats and wild herbivores are most often infected while on pasture; swine and smaller domestic animals usually acquire the disease from contaminated feed.

Historically, anthrax has been known to livestock producers since Biblical times. It was the first disease described which involved a demonstrable bacterium and also the first reproduced by inoculation of bacilli grown artificially. Because of the great interest in this disease by early scientists, it was the first for which a protective inoculation was produced, successfully protecting livestock exposed to the virulent stage of the bacterium.

Geographically, anthrax occurs around the world and in many climatic zones. The disease is not uncommon in Old World pastoral communities, where close grazing brings livestock into frequent contact with soil areas where the disease is endemic. In the United States, areas in California, South Dakota, Nebraska, Louisiana, Arkansas, and Texas are considered anthrax districts, but the infection may appear spontaneously in any state, in any year. In anthrax districts, the disease constitutes a perennial problem, making its appearance during a more or less definite period of the year known as the "anthrax season." This season is usually late summer and early fall, and is associated with the prevalence of biting insects and with hot weather following a long wet period. However, isolated cases or sporadic outbreaks may occur at any time and in other sections of the country. The monetary losses to the livestock industry from this disease are considerable, and are incurred by vaccinations and other preventive measures as well as by mortality.

Etiology

Anthrax is caused by *Bacillus anthracis,* a spore-forming, nonmotile, rod-shaped organism. In the mammalian body, the bacterium reproduces rapidly and forms encapsulated rods with elliptical spores located centrally within the cells. When the organism is exposed to the oxygen of the air, the spore rapidly develops and the vegetative cell dies. The spore is resistant to heat, cold, drying, and many chemical disinfectants. Spores have been known to survive in laboratory preparations for over 50 years, and in conditions normally found in the soil, as well as in water and on cured animal hides, for many decades. Spores from these sources have been shown to grow and to produce the disease when introduced into a suitable environment. The vegetative stage of the bacillus is virulent and will multiply rapidly in the animal body. In this stage, however, the bacillus has little resistance to heat, drying, and disinfectants.

Transmission

Most outbreaks of anthrax occur when animals are on pasture. It has been observed that outbreaks frequently follow hot, dry summers with scant growth of herbage, necessitating close grazing. During dry seasons, swamps, ponds, marshes, and bottom lands dry out and become available for pasture. In close grazing, roots, in many instances with infective soil clinging to them, are consumed by the animals along with vegetation. Periods of rainy weather followed by extremely hot days also appear to favor the occurrence of the disease. Heavy losses from anthrax often follow floods and periodic inundations of low-lying lands, during which the organisms may be spread widely to uninfected areas from a normally locally-infected enzootic district. Streams carrying contaminated water from canneries, slaughterhouses and other sites where livestock products are processed may be foci for the spread of anthrax during times of flood and overflow. Anthrax may also be spread from one area to another, or from one country to another, through the interchange of infected objects closely associated with animal life, such as hair, hides, wool, bone meal, fertilizer, forage and other material. The last outbreak of anthrax in the midwest, where it is usually not enzootic, was traced to contaminated bone meal coming into this country from Belgium.

Governmental inspectors endeavor to prevent the introduction of anthrax into the United States through regulations governing the sanitary handling and control of animal products, animal by-products, and hay and straw of foreign origin.

Anthrax may be transmitted from one animal to another by biting flies, other biting insects, and contaminated instruments. In spite of this, however, the most common method of transmission is through contaminated feed and water. Due to the ease with which modern transportation moves products from one part of the country, or one part of the world, to another, contaminated material may cause anthrax in a new area if viable spores are introduced and come in contact with a suitable host. The U.S. Department of Agriculture maintains a constant surveillance against anthrax, and has prepared maps showing those areas in the United States where the disease is enzootic, as well as areas where it has occurred sporadically. Yearly statistics are maintained by the Department of Agriculture and published periodically.

Factors Influencing Susceptibility

The young animals of all species are susceptible to anthrax, and there is no difference in infection rate due to sex. However, physical condition may have an influence on susceptibility. Animals in poor condition, especially if fatigued or suffering from an intercurrent infection, will be more susceptible than vigorous animals in good condition.

The Animal Health Division of the U.S. Department of Agriculture, through its studies of anthrax distribution in this country, has reported that other infectious diseases may reach epidemic proportions during outbreaks of anthrax. These diseases in the past were probably counted with anthrax mortality. Prior to the period of scientific bacteriology, anthrax organisms were thought to propagate in the soil of endemic areas. However, as the millions of microorganisms in the soil made isolation difficult, specialists adopted the "persistent-spore" theory. They overlooked the lack of viability of spores in the soils, and based their beliefs on the dried spore preparations that remained viable in laboratories for years.

The endemic areas of anthrax, where the disease occurs year after year, indicate a soil survival phase. Thus, applied research has incriminated a specific environmental situation involving soil, wet, then dry, weather, and a propagation phase of *Bacillus anthracis* in water-damaged vegetation or dried silt on limestone rocks and soil. This concept is opposed to the persistent-spore theory, as it infers that a viable organism in a vegetative stage reaches infective levels when sporulation conditions are optimum during warm, dry weather. Nonendemic areas provide few opportunities for the aerobic vegetative stage to produce large spore crops. Thus, well-drained good agricultural soils do not serve as endemic areas for anthrax. The organisms must exist in a dynamic state, forming new vegetative organisms when conditions are favorable and sporulating when the situation becomes adverse. Dilution and time are less important than an adverse environment, as serious outbreaks may be halted by one cold rain.

Symptoms

Anthrax may occur in four forms: peracute, acute, subacute, and chronic. The symptoms of anthrax vary according to species of animal affected and acuteness of attack. Therefore, it is necessary to describe the signs more or less specifically for each species and each form of the disease. The *peracute* form, sometimes called the fulminating type, is characterized by sudden death with few clinical signs and a rapidly fatal course. It generally occurs at the beginning of an outbreak in cattle, sheep and goats. Some animals in the herd are found dead without having previously shown any evidence of the disease. These probably are the most susceptible individuals; as the outbreak progresses and the organisms gain virulence, the remainder of the herd is exposed and natural resistance present at the beginning of the outbreak is soon overcome. If symptoms are noted, the animal will be seen to stagger, collapse, convulse for a few moments and die. Due to the fulminating character of the peracute stage of the disease, an animal is usually found dead, with bloodstained discharges from the mouth, nose and anus. If the animal has been dead for some time it will appear bloated. The bloodstained discharges will be rich in the anthrax organism and should be treated with great respect to prevent the further spread of the organism. The sudden death of cattle, sheep and goats in known anthrax districts should always be regarded with suspicion. An important indication of this disease is the lack of rigor mortis, even in cold weather.

In the *acute* form, the first sign of the disease is a rise in temperature to 104 to 108 F. In both the acute and subacute forms there is excitement and, many times, mental derangement. The excitement stage is followed by a period of marked depression. The sick animal will often stand apart from the rest of the herd, and pregnant cows and ewes may abort. Depression is followed by respiratory distress, trembling, staggering, convulsions, and death. The acute form usually terminates fatally in one to two days. Prior to death, lactating animals will dry up and, if the disease persists long enough, there will be a period of constipation followed by diarrhea which may be excessively hemorrhagic. In cattle, a period of marked excitement is followed by a period of bellowing, with anorexia, suspended rumination, and, if the disease persists long enough, edematous swellings of the neck, the thorax, the flank and the

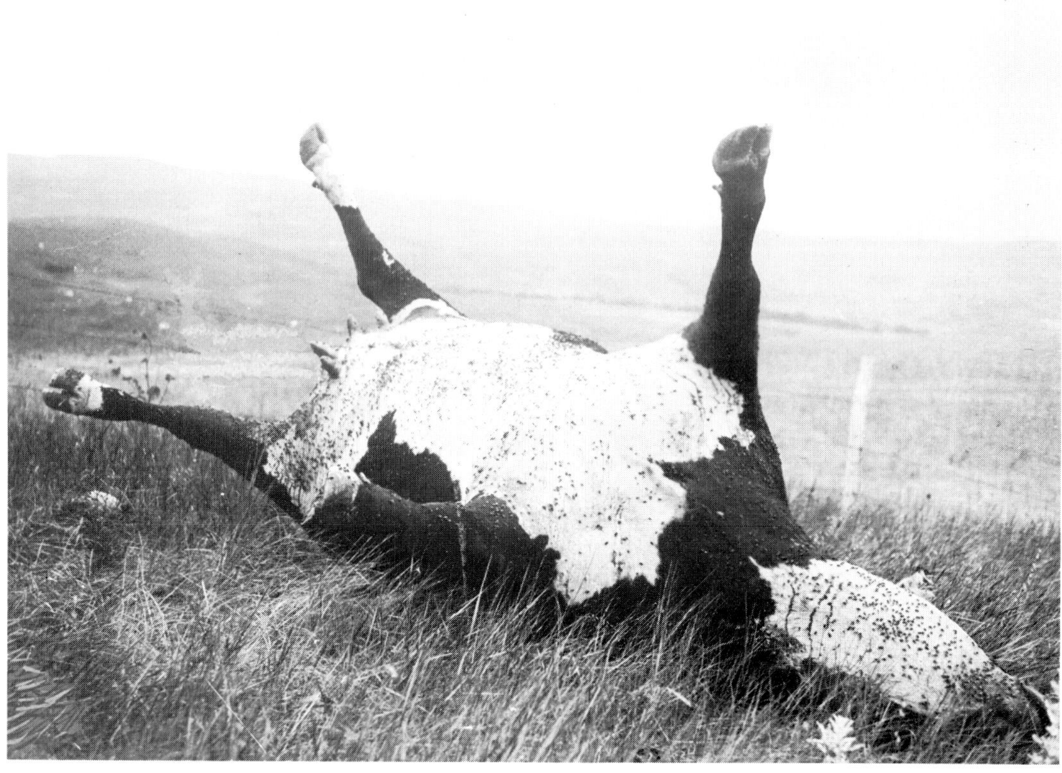

FIG. 10. Characteristic appearance of an animal that has died from anthrax.

lumbar region. In cattle, the disease may last longer than three days, but rarely. In sheep and goats, the disease is usually more fulminating and does not last as long as in cattle. In swine, the symptoms are not so fulminating as in other species and the symptoms appear less markedly. The temperature will be elevated to 107 to 108 F. The mucous membranes of swine will be cyanotic and pharyngitis, with hemorrhagic swelling in the larynx, difficult respiration and choking will be evident. Swine are more resistant to anthrax than any of the other domesticated farm animals. When the infection does occur in hogs, it usually follows feeding on an anthrax-infested carcass. Most swine show symptoms of the illness with rapidly progressive swellings about the throat, which in some cases may cause death by suffocation. A relatively large percentage of swine may become visibly sick for a few days, with or without moderate swellings about the throat, and then recover. When hogs develop anthrax from sources other than feeding on anthrax-infested carcasses, the same effects are observed, except that sudden death without visible symptoms is rare.

The *subacute* form of the disease differs little from the acute form except in duration of symptoms. In the subacute form, the animal may die in 3 to 5 days, or longer, but in some instances may recover. All of the signs prevalent for the acute form of the disease are seen in the subacute form.

The *chronic* form of anthrax may last for a considerable time before the animal finally succumbs. However, a significant number of animals may recover. It is not unusual in chronic cases for extensive areas of tissue to slough away, leaving large, denuded areas that must heal as open wounds. The best procedure in such cases is to destroy the animals; they will never be profitable and may serve as sources for spreading the disease to other animals. The chronic form of anthrax can occur in all species; however, it is most common in swine.

During warm months, when biting flies are most active, animals often show a subcutaneous form of anthrax characterized by local swellings in various parts of the body. Flies inoculate susceptible animals with the bacillus after feeding on infected animals. The cutaneous form may also be seen following vaccination, if vaccines containing attenuated spores, capable of producing localized anthrax, are used. Many outbreaks in recent years have been attributed to the use of such vaccines.

Pathology

The anthrax organism normally enters the body in the spore state. The organism germinates in the digestive tract, develops a capsule to prevent early phagocytosis, and begins to develop in the tissues of the body. When viable organisms are introduced into the body of the host through insect transmission, they are usually in the vegetative state and develop very rapidly in the vascular system. As organisms spread rapidly through the body, multiplying rapidly in the blood vessels, they produce a fibrinolysin. The bacilli rapidly clog capillaries, producing edema and hemorrhage. The fibrinolysin, a tissue-damaging substance, augments the rapid spread of the disease.

The postmortem lesions of anthrax are characteristic. The disease is characterized by edema, absence of rigor mortis, and rapid death. If anthrax is not suspected and a postmortem is actually conducted, the most important sign in all species except swine is enlargement of the spleen. The blood is usually of a tarry consistency and does not coagulate. Rapid putrefaction of the carcass is characteristic of anthrax. Gas forms in the intestine and the carcass may bloat excessively. The mucosa is cyanotic and blood exudes from the body openings. Usually, there are extensive hemorrhages under the skin; some are minute, while others may be extensive. The connective tissue is infiltrated with serous fluid, and all body cavities contain a considerable quantity of bloody fluid. A characteristic postmortem finding is the presence in the subcutaneous and intermuscular tissue of brightly colored, golden-yellow gelatinous exudate.

The lungs are red, hyperemic, and slightly swollen. The bronchi are filled with a bloody, frothy substance that exudes through the nostrils. In nearly all cases other than the exceptional peracute cases in cattle and sheep, there is distinct edematous swelling of the neck, chest, flank, lumbar regions and external genitalia. If an animal showing these signs is found dead, anthrax should be suspected.

Diagnosis

Any animal found dead in an enzootic area, having exhibited few symptoms, should be suspected of having anthrax. Any bloated animal with frothy, bloody exudates from the anus and nasal cavities should also be suspected of having anthrax. If a postmortem is done, the symptoms just listed will be important in the diagnosing of such a condition. In the field diagnosis, a stained blood smear examined under a microscope will quickly show the disease-producing organism and is positive proof of anthrax. When anthrax is diagnosed, great care should be exercised in the handling and disposal of the carcass, as the disease can be transmitted to man, often with disastrous results. Burning is recommended whenever possible, as feral animals may uncover buried carcasses and spread spores to other properties. Care should be used when moving carcasses, because body exudates are rich in infective spores and may contaminate soil over which the carcasses are hauled. If at all possible, carcasses should be burned where found.

Prevention

In areas of enzootic anthrax, the proper method of prevention is annual immunization of all susceptible animals kept on pasture. Vaccination should be done well in advance of the anthrax season, either with a spore vaccine or with bacterin. In enzootic areas the use of living spore vaccine is the most successful method of immunization; however, in areas where anthrax has not occurred previously, it is best not to vaccinate with live-spore vaccines because, once the premises are contaminated, it becomes necessary to vaccinate each year when a new crop of animals is turned onto the infected premises. In the past, stockmen have used bacterin and spore vaccine only to find later that, instead of reducing the incidence of the disease, they may have inadvertently established new foci of infection. In South Africa, a new type of spore vaccine made from avirulent, nonencapsulated, dissociated anthrax organisms was highly successful in producing immunity in sheep and cattle. Immunization is of definite value as antibodies produced by the introduction of the vaccine bring about precipitation of the capsular substances of the anthrax organism, making phagocytosis possible. This vaccine is manufactured commercially in the United States and has been used successfully in the control of anthrax for the past few years. It does not produce the reactions which follow vaccination with unattenuated spore vaccine.

By the use of vaccines and antibiotics, anthrax can be controlled. Only in an exceptional outbreak is it necessary to resort to unusual measures. In the infected herd, the apparently healthy animals should be isolated from the sick ones, immunized, and observed closely for signs of disease until immunity becomes established. Susceptible herds of exposed animals also should be immunized. Visibly sick animals should be treated promptly with injections of suitable antibiotics. Strict sanitary measures should be employed to prevent the spread of anthrax.

Vaccines are expensive and, in areas where anthrax is not a problem, most veterinarians recommend vaccination only when outbreaks occur. In endemic areas, however, anthrax can be effectively controlled by annual vaccination of all livestock plus control of movement of wild animals and strict application of sanitary measures. In an outbreak, vaccines help to control the disease, as protection develops in about eight days following vaccination. In the United States, a noncapsulated vaccine is widely used against anthrax.

In anthrax areas, cattle, horses, sheep and goats are vaccinated each year, and sometimes swine are included. Vaccination with the accepted type of immunizing agent will usually provide protection for a season, but not for more than one year; therefore, vaccination should be repeated annually.

Vaccines should be administered 4 to 6 weeks before the beginning of the anthrax season, and, if the season is exceptionally long, booster vaccinations should be given after six months. A veterinarian should be consulted about the time and type of vaccine to use in any given area.

State and Federal Regulations

Most states list anthrax as a reportable disease. Whenever anthrax has been diagnosed on a farm or ranch, state livestock sanitary officials will immediately post a quarantine on the premises. The states tend to regulate the use of immunizing agents and materials against the disease to prevent the seeding of an otherwise unknown anthrax district with live, viable spores. Any truck, car, or boxcar that has transported an animal that has died of anthrax must be thoroughly disinfected under governmental supervision. The federal government supervises a nationwide reporting system to locate those areas in which anthrax outbreaks do occur and to make this information known to other state and federal agencies. The federal government may also quarantine an infected anthrax district to prevent the movement of livestock during the dangerous seasons or during an extensive outbreak in a previously uninfected area.

9 Contagious Ecthyma

CONTAGIOUS ecthyma (scabby mouth) is a contagious disease specific for sheep and goats. It is caused by a filterable virus and is characterized by the formation of papules, vesicles, pustules, and scabs on the lips, nose, muzzle, udder and legs of sheep and goats. This disease is encountered in all parts of the world where sheep and goats are raised. The clinical symptoms are seen in late summer and fall in animals still on pasture, but later in the year in feedlots. The disease occurs most commonly in very young lambs in the spring, but rarely in mature sheep unless they have not been exposed to the virus in a previous season.

Historically, the disease was first described in Germany in the early 1920s. It was reported in Texas in 1929, and subsequently in all states where sheep and goats are raised. A successful vaccination was first reported in 1931.

Etiology

Contagious ecthyma is caused by a single strain of a virus universal in distribution. The causative virus is present in the scabs removed from lesions on the skin of sheep and goats. It is resistant to desiccation and may be found in dried scabs in a protected area many years after the scabs have fallen from an infected lesion. One attack of the virus develops immunity in sheep. Lesions caused by the virus are susceptible to secondary invaders, such as bacteria or screwworm flies, in the southwestern part of the United States, once the scabs have fallen off.

Transmission

The virus is transmitted by direct contact between lambs and kids, and by contact with contaminated feed and water. Young animals may become infected by nursing on dams with infected udders. Ewes and does themselves, nursing infected young, may develop lesions on the udder. In very young lambs, the initial lesion may develop on the gum line below the incisor teeth. The native infection is by direct transfer of the virus into the tissues by means of slight wounds. Grass seed, spear grass, or other prickly plants which cause small puncture wounds or abrasions are the means by which the virus is spread from animal to animal. The virus cannot enter the tissues unless an abrasion or other type of injury provides a portal into the mucous membranes or skin.

Factors Influencing Susceptibility

Sheep and goats are susceptible but no other ruminants have been shown to be affected by the virus causing contagious ecthyma.

Young lambs and kids are most susceptible to the virus of contagious ecthyma, but older sheep not previously infected may have the disease in a mild form. Sheep of any age are susceptible unless they have been previously infected; however, once a sheep or goat has experienced the disease, a lasting immunity is developed. In areas of mild winter weather, the disease usually strikes in the early spring months and continues until cold weather. In the higher parts of the country, however, lambs are not usually infected until they are brought in from summer range. In some areas, husbandry methods at times of castrating and docking may lead to the production of the pox-like lesions through contaminating the mouth and gums of young lambs by careless handling.

Symptoms

The first symptom is a slight swelling of the lips, followed by the appearance of small pustules which may break and exude pus. When these pustules dry, they form scabs which are yellowish-brown in color and may continue to thicken for a number of days. In approximately three weeks the scabs will detach themselves and fall to the ground. The virus in the scabs remains viable for a considerable length of time, especially if protected from direct sunlight and chemical disinfectants. The laceration occurring underneath the scab and on the membranes on the inside of the mouth may serve as a focus for secondary invaders. In some animals, the legs may be affected; where the inflammation spreads to the tissues between the claws of the hoof, severe lameness will occur. Lesions may also occur on the anus, vulva, and udder of infected ewes.

The incubation period of the disease is from 2 to 8 days, and many lambs exhibit extremely sore and swollen dental pads and lips. No other symptoms are noted in uncomplicated cases, except extreme thinness caused by lack of food. Because of the soreness of the lips and tongue, newborn animals fail to nurse and thus predispose themselves to any other stress factor which may be present.

Secondary infections on the legs and feet may cause serious suppurative wounds, often spreading up the leg. Sometimes lesions are seen on other wool-free parts of the body; reddish, raised, spongy areas occur in the mouth, the gums, the dental pads, and palate. Removal of the scabs leaves a raw, inflamed, bleeding surface. Young animals may find suckling very difficult, as the lips are immobile in badly affected cases and the animals may be in profound misery. Other complications may follow, producing separate sets of symptoms.

Pathology

Upon postmortem examination, lesions are primarily found confined to the mouth parts or areas of the skin not covered by wool, but in cases of a secondary infection one may observe ulcerative stomatitis, reticulitis, enteritis, necrotic pleural lesions with pleuritis, or necrotic foci in the liver. In some instances, the necrotic stomatitis may be extensive enough to cause a serious change in the shape or appearance of the lips of infected lambs. The disease produces typical lesions, but it may be confused with skin sensitization caused by other entities, such as mycotic dermatitis, photosensitivity, and poisoning or necrosis due to heavy metal poisons.

Treatment

None of the current treatments is of any significance in preventing contagious ecthyma, and, as the disease runs a benign course, it is advisable to attempt no treatment unless exceptional complications occur. In such cases a veterinarian should be contacted to provide the latest information about treatments.

Control

The control of contagious ecthyma takes two directions: the immediate isolation of infected animals and the cleaning of contaminated areas, and immunization.

Vaccination is quite effective. A vaccine made from the dried scabs of infected animals, diluted to a known strength, is used to vaccinate susceptible animals. It is wise, however, not to use a vaccine on premises where infection has never existed. Once the disease has appeared on a property it becomes necessary to vaccinate all susceptible animals every year, as the virus has been known to live in scabs removed from infected animals for as long as twelve years. Vaccination can be carried out at any time, but it is usually done when lambs are gathered for docking. The vaccine is usually applied to skin in a wool-free area. A successful immunization is indicated by a reddened area a few days after scarification, followed by a pustule and a scab. Since the infection is spread predominantly at lambing time, all ordinary preventive precautions should be used at this time, and susceptible animals should be vaccinated to prevent the spread of the disease.

Public Health Relationships

Although the disease known as contagious ecthyma is extremely rare in humans, it does occur through careless handling of lambs and sheep. Gloves should be worn when vaccinating lambs, as vaccinating accidents do occur. In human infection a papule develops, followed by a scab formation which heals in about three weeks unless complications occur. In some cases, especially where a human is bitten by a lamb suffering from this condition, lesions may develop on the hands and arms and regional lymph nodes may be involved. When this condition occurs, the healing process is protracted.

10
Bluetongue

BLUETONGUE is an infectious, febrile, catarrhal disease primarily of sheep and cattle and caused by a filterable virus related to that of African horse sickness. It is characterized by inflammation of the lips, gums, tongue and nasal mucosa, with a tendency to erosion and ulceration, congestion and capillary hemmorrhage of the coronary tissue of the hoof, and marked loss of weight.

The disease was first described from South Africa and was for many years believed to be confined to Africa south of the Sahara. In 1943, it was recognized in Cyprus and at the same time occurred in Israel. The disease appeared in the United States in 1948, but was not identified until 1952; for some time it was known as sore-muzzle, mainly because of the relatively mild nature of the symptoms.

Etiology

Bluetongue is caused by a filterable virus approximately 50 mμ in diameter. The virus is hardy and will remain viable in decomposing blood and tissues for a considerable length of time.

There are at least eleven strains of the virus, and each is antigenically distinct from the others. Thus immunity to one strain will not produce immunity to the other strains. The various strains differ in virulence. The low-virulence strains produce mild symptoms and tend to become weakened or attenuated by passage from animal to animal. The strains of high virulence retain their potency when passed in this manner.

All strains of the bluetongue virus will grow on chicken embryo and sheep organ tissue culture, and in this way can be attenuated to such an extent that they may be used to protect animals against their fully virulent counterparts.

Transmission

The disease cannot normally be transmitted directly from one animal to another, and, in the absence of insect vectors, healthy and sick animals can be housed in close contact without spread. Body discharges are not infective, and saliva and nasal discharges from sick animals can be rubbed into the mouths of healthy sheep without causing any further spread of infection. Infection can, however, be transmitted from sheep to sheep, or from cattle to sheep, by blood inoculation. Natural transmission is by bloodsucking insects. While it may sometimes be spread by mosquitoes, South African workers have incriminated night-flying flies (*Culicoides* sp.) as the chief vectors. In the United States, the virus is transmitted by the gnat, *Culicoides varripennis.* (Photomicrographs of infected gnats reveal that the bluetongue virus is carried in the salivary gland in quantities great enough to infect an animal in one bite. It is postulated that the virus multiplies in the body of the gnat.)

The transmission of bluetongue to cattle and sheep by the gnat is cause for great concern. Cattle exposed to virus-laden gnats have developed high levels of virus and corresponding antibodies in the blood. Although the symptoms were mild, the cattle maintained high levels of virus in the blood up to one year after infection. Sheep held in close contact with these cattle developed full-blown symptoms of the disease when exposed to gnats at the next fly season. Thus, it would seem that cattle, rather than gnats, are the reservoirs of bluetongue virus.

Factors Influencing Susceptibility

Bluetongue usually appears shortly after the beginning of the spring rains when the insect vectors become abundant, and it occurs most commonly in comparatively low-lying areas. Sheep and cattle of all ages are susceptible, except calves and lambs of immune dams which receive colostral immunity. The highest mortality in enzootic areas occurs in 1-year-olds, most of the older sheep and cattle being immune due to past exposure. The disease abates in the fall of the year, following the first frost.

All breeds of cattle and sheep are susceptible to bluetongue, but some breeds exhibit a degree of resistance. Within each breed individuals also show a variation in susceptibility. The strain of the virus is the most important variable in susceptibility and course of the disease.

Young animals whose dams have recovered from the disease have a passive immunity giving a measure of protection for two months or more after birth. Exposure during this time will produce very mild symptoms and protection up to about one year of age.

Symptoms

In Sheep

The incubation period is 6 to 9 days. The first symptom to be observed is a rise in temperature, which in most cases reaches between 105 and 106 F. This may be accompanied by unwillingness to feed, and rolling movements of the tongue or licking of the lips. This is followed after about 24 hours by a nasal discharge, salivation, and swelling of the lips. The nasal discharge is at first thin and watery, but soon becomes mucoid. As the disease progresses, the discharge dries up to form incrustations around the nostrils. The salivation varies in extent, but is frequently frothy and profuse. The nasal mucosa becomes congested and may ulcerate, in which case there is blood in the nasal discharge. The lips become swollen and tender, and bleed readily when handled, especially where the skin and mucosa meet. There is a tendency for the tissues to slough, and superficial ulcers form readily inside the lips and on the tip of the tongue. Deep ulcers filled with white necrotic material appear at any site where there is irritation, especially at the sides of the tongue opposite sharp cheek teeth, under the tongue, and on the dental pad. As the mouth lesions develop, the affected animals become unwilling to feed; if water is available they will stand with mouth immersed, though they may not actually be drinking. An edema of the face, ears, and submaxillary region has frequently been noted. The tongue may be greatly swollen, bluish in color, and protrude from the mouth so that breathing becomes difficult.

Shortly after the mouth lesions have fully developed, a lameness or stiffness of the limbs is observed. In mild outbreaks this may be the only symptom noticed in most animals. The lameness is due to a coronitis. The coronary band frequently shows intense congestion and hemorrhages into the horny tissues are common; a red or purplish band travels down the hoof with the growth of the horn. The skin in the interdigital cleft may be reddened or show a purplish discoloration.

Sick animals frequently adopt an attitude of torticollis, lying down with the head tucked around into the flank, comparable to the attitude of milk fever.

Secondary infections of the respiratory and digestive systems commonly occur, affected sheep showing symptoms of pneumonia soon after the development of the mouth lesions. Diarrhea, which may produce bloodstained discharges, is also seen in a number of cases.

The mortality rate is variable. In mild outbreaks it may be between 2 and 20 percent, but with virulent strains of the virus 90 percent of a flock may be lost. In most fatal cases, death occurs within six days of the first appearance of symptoms. Prognosis is difficult, as many severely sick animals recover completely while others which seem to be recovering may collapse and die at any time during convalescence. Recovered animals are usually considerably emaciated, taking a long time to regain full health. When the nasal or buccal discharges are fetid, or when diarrhea sets in, especially with bloodstained discharge, death is to be expected.

In Cattle

The symptoms often appear so mild that the herdsman will overlook the disease. In fact, experimental infection of cattle produces very mild symptoms, only lack of appetite and a slight fever. The natural disease, however, produces swollen lips, gums, and tongues, profuse salivation, stiffness and reluctance to move—in fact, all of the signs seen in sheep. Mortality in cattle is seldom reported but deaths have occurred following abortion and secondary infections.

Pathology

The bluetongue virus is transmitted by the bite of the *Culicoides* gnat from its mouth parts to the lips, nostrils, and ears of sheep and cattle. The virus rapidly multiplies. Viremia develops in the adjacent mucous membranes, causing swelling and disruption of capillaries, inflammation and ulceration of the mucous membranes of the nasal cavity, and localized inflammation of the skin.

Upon postmortem, the most striking changes noted are hyperemia, or reddening, and a gelatinous edema of the skin and mucous membranes of the respiratory and digestive tracts; cyanosis, or blue color, of the tongue; necrosis of areas on the tongue and lips; small hemorrhages in the muscles; hemorrhage around the coronary band; pneumonia; and often severe emaciation.

Diagnosis

Diagnosis is based on symptoms, lesions, and epizootiology. The outstanding features are fever, the swollen and hyperemic condition of the lips, nasal discharges, cyanosis of the tongue, ulceration in the mouth, foot lesions and stiffness, seasonal occurrence, and usually sporadic and noncontagious nature of the disease. To confirm the diagnosis, susceptible and immune sheep should be inoculated with either fresh or preserved blood collected from animals in the most acute stage of the disease. In the laboratory, the virus may be cultivated on chicken embryos and then inoculated into healthy sheep to produce the disease; this will confirm the diagnosis.

There is no specific treatment for bluetongue other than good nursing. Mouth lesions may be treated symptomatically. Infected animals should be kept in the shade as sunlight appears to aggravate the condition, and should be given soft easily masticated food. Recovery is followed by an immunity which lasts for over a year.

Prevention

In the past, South African workers were able to bring about an attenuation of some field strains of the bluetongue virus by serial passage through sheep; after 10 passages the only result was a mild febrile reaction followed by immunity. This was possible with the strains of low virulence; however, strains of high virulence retain their full power to cause disease when passed from animal to animal. Recent research, however, has revealed that, when highly virulent strains are passaged through chicken embryos, they quickly become attenuated and lose their ability to cause the clinical disease. Vaccines are made from the attenuated strains to protect animals against the disease.

It is of great importance in immunizing sheep and cattle that all known strains of the virus be used. There are eleven distinct strains, and immunity to one strain will not protect against subsequent exposure to any or all of the others. Strain and virulence are unrelated, but injection with an attenuated strain of the virus does protect against the virulent strain of the same virus.

In enzootic areas, control consists of annual vaccination of all sheep with a polyvalent vaccine at least a month before the vectors appear. Ewes should be vaccinated three weeks before breeding, as the vaccine may interfere with the brain development of the fetus and cause "dummy" lambs. Adverse effects do not occur with vaccination during the fourth or fifth month of pregnancy. Lambs may be vaccinated at 3 or 4 months of age when free of protection from colostrum. At the present time a vaccine for use in cattle is not commercially available.

It is possible to avoid infection by moving stock during the spring to relatively high well-drained ground where there are no *Culicoides* flies or other bloodsucking insects, or by providing adequate insect-proof housing at night. Burning smoke fires at night to drive away flies and dipping sheep in insecticides may also help. Segregation of sick animals is of little use in controlling the spread of the disease, but carcasses should be buried. Eradication of the disease in enzootic areas would appear to be almost impossible as cattle, the reservoir hosts, maintain the virus for long periods of time and over the winter. Control of gnats is not feasible due to their numbers and prevalence. Bluetongue may be controlled in enzootic areas by a program of strategic vaccination, and eradicated in sporadic outbreaks by tactical measures.

Bluetongue must be differentiated from contagious ecthyma, founder, photosensitization, and stiff lamb disease in sheep and from virus diarrhea, rinderpest, foot-and-mouth disease, and vesicular stomatitis in cattle. Otherwise, tactical measures will be of little value.

11
Infectious Papillomatosis

INFECTIOUS papillomatosis, or common warts, is a disease occurring in cattle, goats, dogs, rabbits and sometimes man in various parts of the world. The disease is characterized by the formation of warts, which are in effect benign tumors, consisting of fibrous cores covered to a variable depth with stratified squamous epithelium, the outer layers of which become hyperkeratinized. The papillomas, or warts, occur as single flower-like vegetations ranging in size from a pinhead to a large cauliflower 6 to 7 inches across. The vegetations may occur singly, in groups, or diffusely.

Historically, infectious papillomatosis has been known for centuries, but it was not until the turn of this century that research was undertaken on this disease. Shortly thereafter, it was reported that warts from cattle could be transmitted to humans; this has not been substantiated, however. In 1929, it was discovered that papillomatosis could be transmitted from one animal to another but only within the same species.

Etiology

Infectious papillomatosis is believed to be caused by one or more viruses possessing a high degree of host specificity. However, interspecies transmission does not occur under usual conditions, although experimental transmission between species has been reported. The filterable viruses can be isolated from the vegetative growth on the skin of infected animals. The microorganisms can be cultivated on chick embryo tissue culture, and a vaccine has been made from agents grown by this method.

The exact mode of transmission of infectious papillomatosis is not known; however, it is surmised that it is transmitted by direct contact from an infected animal to a non-infected animal through small abrasions on the skin. There is further evidence that indirect transmission of the virus may occur through improperly cleaned bleeding needles and instruments used by careless herdsmen. It is believed that the virus gains entrance through small injuries in the skin and by direct contact of the injured areas with infected animals, and that it is transmitted indirectly from animal to animal by means of halters, nose leads, leashes, and other articles contaminated by contact with diseased animals. Indirect transmission may also result through contaminated hands of attendants and contaminated instruments of restraint. Biting insects may also play a role.

Factors Influencing Susceptibility

Infectious papillomatosis is most often seen in calves and young cattle under two years of age, although adult bovine animals may become infected. In goats, the disease is most prevalent in animals over one year of age. The disease appears more frequently among stabled animals than among those allowed access to pasture or range. As transmission is favored by direct contact, the condition is often seen in several animals in the same pen, while other animals of the same age in different pens close by may not be affected. The incidence within a single pen, however, is variable, with extensive numbers of warts being found on some animals and none on others. There is no relationship of the disease with sex, condition of the animal, or feeding practices.

Symptoms

Infectious papillomatoses may occur singly or in clusters. The lesions may be hard or soft elevated masses. Many warts are small and rounded while others are broad, thin, long or club-shaped. Some warts become cauliflower-like growths, 7 or 8 inches across. These large growths are usually soft and give off a distinctive, offensive odor.

The warts are most frequently seen on the sides of the head, under the chin, and around the eyes, neck, dewlap, and shoulder of young cattle, but seldom on the legs. When a calf is infected with a large number of warts, or a few warts become excessively enlarged, the animal usually becomes unthrifty. Large warts are soft in nature, and thus are easily injured. As most warts receive a plentiful blood supply from the skin, they bleed easily when injured and the open wounds may become infested with parasites or contaminated by infective bacteria.

Warts may slough off spontaneously, and sometimes a new wart forms at the site where an earlier wart has disappeared; however, most animals are resistant to further infection once an infection has regressed. If warts become too large, they may break off at the base and become necrotic. The necrosis serves as an irritant which aids in the sloughing-off process.

Pathology

Infectious papillomas are benign tumors consisting of a fibrous core covered with stratified squamous epithelium. Upon postmortem examination, animals affected with an extensive infestation of warts show whitish cauliflower-like masses on the skin. In some adult dairy cattle, warts may be found in the teat canal, and in bulls the disease may produce a fibrous papilloma on the penis or prepuce. Growths are often seen on the vulva and in the vagina of heifers, but it is doubtful whether this particular condition is related to infectious papillomatosis. Warts are occasionally seen on the teats of cattle, and are relatively distinct, invariably hard and cornified, and grayish or black in color. Warts may be sufficiently numerous on the udder to cause difficult milking. Warts on the udder are usually somewhat larger and more flattened than those on other parts of the skin. As they are usually hard and dry in consistency, they are fairly easily removed by treatment. Frequently, warts have been seen to spread from the original site to cover large areas of the body, either in the form of numerous nodules

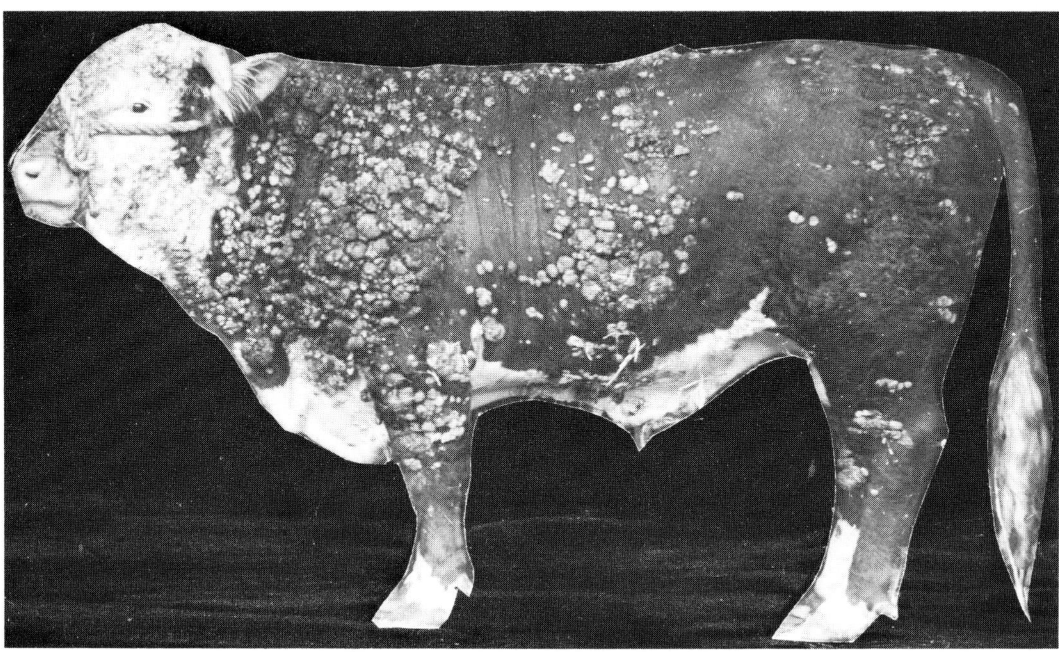

FIG. 11. Generalized infectious papillomatosis. (From Jensen, R., and Mackey, D. R.: *Diseases of Feedlot Cattle.* Ed. 2, Philadelphia, Lea & Febiger, 1971.)

or as large confluent masses which may be either hard or soft in consistency. The latter type bleeds easily, has a tendency to slough and gives off an offensive odor. Upon autopsy warts have also been found in the nasal openings of animals in the same herd, the agent apparently transmitted by the fingers of a person who held the animal or by an infected bull lead used as a means of restraint. The losses from warts are considerable. In young animals heavily infected with large warts, growth may be retarded. Greatest losses are the result of damages to the hides of slaughtered animals, brought about by the destruction of the hide where growth has occurred.

Diagnosis

Diagnosis of infectious papillomatosis, or warts, is not difficult, as the presence of dry, horny masses on the skin is significant. The warts affecting animals may clear up spontaneously with time. However, this time may be prolonged, and often there is need for curative treatment. There are indications that recovered animals are resistant thereafter. Surgical removal of several large warts is often followed by dry necrosis of the stump and a spontaneous sloughing of the remaining warts.

Treatment

With a small number of warts on a single animal, or where a few animals in a group are affected, it may be advantageous for the herdsmen to tie off the warts with a sterile thread or string. When this is done properly, the wart will be constricted at its base, dry necrosis will occur, and the wart will slough off; sloughing of all other warts on the body usually follows. Warts in cattle and goats sometimes respond to oil, acetic acid, or iodine applied locally before they become excessively enlarged.

If the condition is seen on a number of

animals, or if an excessively large number of warts occurs on one animal, it may be advantageous to seek the advice of a veterinarian concerning a program of vaccination to insure that other susceptible animals on the premises will not become infected. Wart vaccines are available from commercial sources. They are made either from wart tissue treated with formalin and suspended in physiological saline or from viruses isolated from such tissue and grown on chick embryo tissue culture. Wart tissue of bovine origin probably offers the most reliable vaccine source. These vaccines are given subcutaneously for prevention and treatment. The administration may be repeated at 5- or 10-day intervals, if necessary, but should be given only upon the advice of a veterinarian.

As the number of viruses actually involved in this particular condition is unknown, some commercial vaccines have proved ineffective. In such cases, good results have been obtained by subsequent treatment with autogenous vaccine made from tissues taken from the specific herd. This suggests that there may be immunologically different strains of a particular species.

Wart vaccine is administered subcutaneously or intracutaneously. It is claimed that a single injection will lead to rapid regression of warts in most cases. Papillomas on the udder and teats do not respond as well to vaccine therapy as do those on other parts of the body.

The viruses causing infectious papillomatosis appear to have a high degree of host specificity, and some of them even have specificities for particular kinds of epithelium within a single host. Although the viruses are host specific, all varieties are more prevalent within the young of the species affected.

For treating valuable herds that do not respond to other treatment, the veterinarian may recommend autogenous vaccine which is made from warty tissue taken from affected animals. Because it is prepared for individuals or a herd, autogenous vaccine should be used only in the herd from which it was collected.

Prevention

Tactical measures are as important as strategic methods in eliminating a source of infection once infectious papillomatosis has been diagnosed. These involve isolating severely infected animals so that they will not come into contact with susceptible animals.

Thoroughly clean barns, pens, chutes, and rubbing posts that infected cattle may have touched. Remove manure, burn contaminated bedding and rubbish, sweep and clean all free surfaces, being particularly careful to remove cobwebs, dust, and other debris before washing the area with hot water and lye.

Once the area has been cleaned of all extraneous material and allowed to stand fallow for a period of time, disinfect it by spraying a second time with a lye-and-water solution. Milk cows with warts on their teats and udders should be milked after all others in the herd have been milked. Clean and disinfect the milking machine teat cups and inflations before reusing. Where cows have been milked by hand during the treatment period, milkers should take stringent precautions to clean their hands with strong soap before milking other cows. In this way, there will be less mechanical transmission from cow to cow.

12
Epididymitis of Rams

THIS IS A specific bacterial disease of sheep characterized in the ram by epididymitis, orchitis, and impaired fertility; in the ewe by placentitis and abortion; and in lambs by perinatal mortality. Though earlier investigations suggested that epididymitis was a bacterial infection, the cause remained obscure until 1952 when it was found to be due to an organism with the characteristics of the genus *Brucella* but differing somewhat from the other members of that group. The name *Brucella ovis* was suggested for the organism in 1956, but this name has not received complete acceptance due to the differences between the amino-acid metabolism patterns for this bacterium and that of other *Brucella* organisms. It is informally called "ram epididymitis organism," or REO.

Epididymitis has been recognized historically in most countries where sheep are raised; however, REO was first described in New Zealand in 1952. In the United States, ram epididymitis organism has been recognized as a major sheep disease in California for the past decade. The incidence in rams in commercial flocks in that state varies, but has been high enough in most flocks to be significant.

Etiology

A point of major importance is the relationship between epididymitis and ovine brucellosis. Epididymitis may be of *Brucella* or non*Brucella* etiology, and therefore particular attention must be given to the diagnostic tests for this condition. Although most cases of epididymitis are caused by REO, other bacterial organisms have been isolated from frank cases of epididymitis, and neoplasms have also been demonstrated. REO has not been incriminated as the cause of natural infection in any other animal species.

Transmission

A survey of infected herds has revealed that up to 87 percent of aged rams carry the infection, whether epididymitis is present or not. Therefore, opportunities for ram-to-ram transmission are increased during the mating season as clean rams acquire infection by serving ewes previously served by infected rams. The disease can be transmitted from infected to noninfected rams by direct contact in the absence of ewes, however.

Ram lambs as young as eight weeks have been shown to be susceptible to experimental infection by a number of routes, per os, per rectum and by application of the agent to mucous surfaces such as the conjunctiva and prepuce. While experimental infection of ewes by oral and intravenous routes has confirmed this susceptibility, the clean-cut clinical picture of the disease has not been produced by artificial exposure. However, active infection has developed in ewes after being mated with naturally infected rams. Contaminated pastures or barns do not appear to play an important part in spreading of the disease.

Active infection is more persistent in rams than in ewes. A high percentage of infected rams are capable of shedding the causative agent in the semen for several years.

REO is more frequently seen in older rams than in young rams; however, it has been seen at all ages. The disease occurs with equal frequency in rams used for service and in those never mated.

Factors Influencing Susceptibility

Although ram epididymitis organism is considered a member of the *Brucella* family, it has never been shown to be infective in other animal species or in man.

Symptoms

The most obvious clinical symptoms of REO are lesions of the epididymis, tunica, and testes of the ram, and placentitis in the ewe with abortion and perinatal death of lambs. The usual history of a ram with epididymitis shows that it has become less fertile though without gross abnormality of the reproductive organs. Later, when enlargement of any part of an epididymis becomes apparent, the animal becomes infertile. If only one side is affected, the ram may become fertile again within 4 or 5 years after first becoming grossly infected. In the ewe, the principal symptoms are abortion late in pregnancy, necrosis of the chorion and infection of the placenta. Lambs are usually born dead, or are weak if carried to full term. In recently infected rams, the lesions may develop with marked rapidity, the first detectable abnormality being a marked deterioration of semen quality associated with the presence of inflammatory cells and organisms in the semen. There is pyrexia, lassitude, and an increased respiratory rate, with acute inflammation and swelling of the scrotum and its contents. Following regression of the acute reactions, lesions may be palpated in the epididymis and tunica of the scrotum. Enlargement of the epididymis may be unilateral or bilateral, and the tail is involved more frequently than the head or body. The most prominent lesions are spermatoceles, containing partially inspissated spermatic fluid. These are variable in size and lie within the interstitial tissue surrounded by extensive fibrosis. The tunics frequently become thickened and fibrous and adhesions develop between the visceral and parietal layers, in some cases obliterating the cavity of the tunica vaginalis.

In the field, the condition is most often encountered when palpating the testes of the ram upon examination for infertility. The normal feel of the testes of a fertile ram is firm, like that of a firm rubber ball. In the case of a ram with epididymitis in the early stages, the testes may feel soft and flabby. In the later stages, the fibrotic lesions have developed to such an extent that the testes will feel very hard to the touch, with knobby protrusions along the length of the epididymis.

Diagnosis

There are three principle methods of diagnosis of infection in rams suspected of having REO. The first and most often used is scrotal palpation. The ram is set up on its hindquarters and the testes palpated through the scrotum. If any abnormality is palpated, the ram is considered to have epididymitis and subject to culling from the herd. The second primary method of diagnosis is bacteriological examination of the semen. This reveals any *Brucella*-like organisms upon culturing in diagnostic medium. Thirdly, serological tests, in particular a complement-fixation test, will reveal antibodies in the blood as the result of an infection from REO. Although substantial numbers of infected rams exhibit lesions that can be detected by palpation of the scrotal contents, this method of diagnosis is not always adequate since not all infected rams show such abnormalities. Further, all cases of epididymitis are not due to this specific bacterium.

Prevention

Although the REO is susceptible to several of the broad-spectrum antibiotics, it is unprofitable to treat rams for this condition. Once the growth of lesions has occurred, and rams are showing a degree of infertility, they will not respond to antibiotic treatment even though the organism may be eliminated from the lesion. Therefore, the incidence and spread of the disease may be reduced by regular examinations of rams prior to the breeding season and the culling of those with obvious genital abnormalities. The spread of infection may also be retarded by special management practices, such as isolation of young clean rams from older, possibly infected rams on the same pasture, particularly during the mating season.

A recently developed vaccine is now available for the immunization of rams against REO. The manufacturer recommends that ram lambs be inoculated at four months of age and again two months prior to their first mating season. The vaccination is to be repeated two months before each successive mating season. Since infection in ewes apparently originates from infected rams, lamb losses through infection of ewes are believed to be controlled best by vaccinating all rams. In a recent experimental project, no marked adverse effects were observed due to vaccination by this schedule, and the incidence of the disease has been significantly reduced.

13
Enterotoxemia

ENTEROTOXEMIA (overeating disease, pulpy kidney disease) is an acute, highly fatal poisoning of sheep, principally lambs, caused by absorption of a toxin produced by the bacterium *Clostridium perfringens,* type D. The toxin is produced in the intestinal tract; the condition is therefore an auto-intoxication. It is characterized by cerebral symptoms, convulsions, sudden prostration and death. Adult animals are less susceptible to enterotoxemia and the condition is most often seen in young, fat, fast-growing, greedy lambs in feedlots or on pastures. It has been very costly to the sheep industry around the world. However, effective control has evolved from good management practices and the use of biological products for immunization against the toxin.

Geographically, enterotoxemia is found wherever sheep are raised. Historically, the organism which causes enterotoxemia was first isolated and described at Johns Hopkins University from a decomposing human cadaver before the turn of the century. Since that time, *Bacillus perfringens,* as it was first called, has been isolated from a variety of conditions and has been given several names. For many years, the bacterium was known as *Clostridium welchii;* however, by universal agreement it is now called *Clostridium perfringens* and further designated by toxogenic type, as each type of toxin causes a different set of symptoms in different species of animals.

Etiology

Clostridium perfringens is a large, anaerobically cultured, nonmotile, encapsulated, hemolytic, gas-producing rod-shaped organism capable of producing at least six types of powerful toxins that are designated by letters of the alphabet. These endotoxins contain fifteen antigenic toxic fractions. Each is immunogenically distinct from the others and has been designated by a small Greek letter. There are several conditions in livestock that are produced by *Clostridium perfringens.* Usually, one fraction is present in quantity along with minor amounts of the other toxins in each specific disease entity.

Type A. This was first isolated from man and, although it has been reported in lambs and calves, it is relatively unimportant from the veterinary point of view. Type A is found in the intestinal tract of most warm-blooded species.

Type B. The toxins produced by type B *Clostridium perfringens* cause a condition known as lamb dysentery. This has been reported in colts and in calves but is primarily seen in very young lambs.

Type C. This type affects sheep, goats, cattle and pigs. It was reported in England as a condition called "struck" in sheep, and it causes hemorrhagic enterotoxemia of lambs, calves, and baby pigs in this country.

Type D. This type is the cause of a common and destructive disease of sheep, calves, and goats, and has been described in all sheep-raising parts of the world. It is known variously as enterotoxemia, pulpy kidney disease, and overeating disease. It has been isolated from lambs, sheep, calves and cattle.

Type E. Type E *Clostridium perfringens* causes dysentery and enterotoxemia in lambs and calves but is of little importance from the veterinary point of view.

Type F. This type causes a chronic enteritis in man. It is believed that the ability to produce toxic symptoms in livestock is related to the ability of the organism to produce high hyaluronidase, which is linked with the pathogenicity of the toxins.

Transmission

The predisposing cause of intoxication with *Clostridium perfringens* type D is overeating or gorging on highly nutritive feed ingredients; this causes a disturbance in the digestive tract and creates an ideal environment for the multiplication of the organism. This organism is commonly present in the stomach and intestinal tract in normal warm-blooded animals, and is found in the soil in all parts of the world. The immediate cause of the disease is the absorption into the blood circulation of a toxin liberated by the bacterium. The organism is worldwide in distribution and affects sheep of all ages, goats and calves. It occurs in all seasons of the year, under widely different types of husbandry.

The intoxication is perhaps most common in lambs 2 to 6 weeks of age and in weaned lambs in the feedlot or on lush, green pasture. Enterotoxemia frequently affects the most vigorous, fast-growing lambs in the flock. Outbreaks are commonly associated with an increase in feed availability, or with a change in type of feed.

Factors Affecting Susceptibility

While the prominent etiological role of type D toxin is generally recognized, the circumstances giving rise to rapid proliferation of the organism in the intestinal tract are not clearly understood. One common factor seems to be the ingestion of extensive amounts of feed high in carbohydrates, since undigested starch granules are frequently found in the intestinal contents of acutely affected lambs. Digestive disturbances associated with sudden changes in diet and with the transition to solid food by nursing lambs may be other factors. The intoxication is most often seen in the fattest, greediest lambs in the flock. In nursing lambs, the condition occurs when the ewes are on good pastures of grass, winter wheat or early spring alfalfa; among feeder lambs on rich clover pastures or in feedlots with a heavy grain ration, the most greedy eaters will suddenly die. This is directly related to management procedures, as many feeders are willing to sacrifice a number of animals to increase the growth rate of most of the animals in the feedlot.

When enterotoxemia is seen in mature sheep, it is usually associated with the management practice of turning sheep into corn fields or excessively lush pastures during extremely hot weather.

Symptoms

Lambs affected with *Clostridium perfringens* type D toxin usually do not exhibit visible symptoms. The disease may be acute, the animal being found dead in the morning after having been in good condition the previous night. In other words, the first indication of the disease is sudden death in the best-conditioned animals. Where symptoms are noticed, the first signs of illness appear a few hours before death. Lambs may suddenly jump, fall to the ground in a convulsive seizure and die. Others show symptoms of irritability, indicating an inflammation of the brain. Such signs as circling, pushing against fixed objects, or mental depression are often seen in the early stages of the disease. Lambs showing convulsions may have only a slight rise in temperature. In less acute cases, diarrhea may develop with recovery occurring in a few of the lambs. In these cases, loss of appetite, depression, vomiting, paralysis, followed by diarrhea which may persist for several days, bring about a rapid loss of weight with slow recovery.

Pathology

Clostridium perfringens type D bacteria are normally present in the intestinal tract of all mammals and abundantly found in the soil. Because of the acute nature of the toxemia, this condition must be differentiated from other infectious diseases causing sudden death in livestock. As *Clostridium perfringens* type D organisms are found in the intestinal tracts of most animals dying of acute symptoms, they are frequently found as postmortem invaders from the intestinal tract in the tissues of bloating animals. For this reason some caution is necessary in drawing conclusions based on the presence of the organism in tissues collected after death. It is found more often in the so-called gas gangrene infections than any other organism, although it is generally associated with other species of anaerobes in this process. When a young lamb overeats, atony of the intestinal tract provides the proper anaerobic environmental conditions for the rapid growth of *Clostridium perfringens* and the proliferation of the type D toxin. As the organism multiplies, it rapidly produces the toxin. Because of the atony of the small intestine, the toxin then is absorbed into the bloodstream and the symptoms and lesions listed above are rapidly produced. Since rapid death is one of the prominent signs of this condition, it is evident that postmortem lesions are of relatively little importance in those dying in the peracute stage. However, several postmortem signs are readily attributable to this intoxication. If a lamb is opened immediately upon death, there is usually little to be seen in the kidneys. However, the synonym "pulpy kidney disease" has often been attributed to this condition as 3 or 4 hours after death the kidneys appear swollen, dark red, soft and mushy with a consistency of strawberry jam. This is not a constant lesion, however, and is only seen in animals dead for several hours before autopsy is attempted. There is passive congestion of the lungs and the trachea. There is an increase in the fluid in the heart sac and it is often coagulated. There are diffuse hemorrhages, occasionally large blotches but most often very small dot-like hemorrhages, occurring on all of the intestinal organs, abdominal muscles, the diaphragm, and the thymus gland. The livers of animals dead for several hours appear friable, dark and congested; they are occasionally spotted with light-colored areas 2 to 4 mm in diameter. The urinary bladder is usually empty, and there is frequently an absence of solids or fluids in the intestinal tract but much food in the stomach.

Diagnosis

Diagnosis in the field is usually based upon sudden death in young, fat, vigorous, greedy lambs. However, because there are other diseases in which death occurs suddenly, an autopsy must be performed. Specimens taken by a veterinarian and sent to a laboratory should include urine and intestinal contents for confirmation of the type D toxin.

Prevention

It is difficult to treat enterotoxemia because death is rapid and usually the first symptom seen. However, the control of enterotoxemia may be effected by proper husbandry and by immunization. The method of control depends upon the type of husbandry exercised by the farmer or rancher. Grain rations should be reduced when the disease first appears and then gradually increased as the outbreak subsides. Sometimes losses can be minimized by carefully sorting lambs as to size and space at the feed trough to prevent the greedy ones from overeating. Grazing stock should be moved temporarily to other types of feed. Under range conditions the movement of lambs is not feasible; therefore, supplemental feeding of well-cured alfalfa is helpful in some cases. Sudden changes in type and amount of feed should always be avoided, as such changes tend to create overeating. When an outbreak does occur, type D antitoxin, which confers a temporary immunity, may be used to control the outbreak. However, losses in lambs up to about six weeks of age cannot be controlled in this fashion. The protection for such lambs is best accomplished by immunizing the ewes with two doses of *Clostridium perfringens* type D toxoid, the second dose being given about two weeks before lambing. The passive immunity conferred thus on the lamb lasts about six weeks, after which the lamb itself may be vaccinated; the first injection can be conveniently given at the time of docking. To provide effective protection, two doses separated by an interval of not less than four weeks are usually regarded as necessary. Immunity following the first injection takes about ten days to develop, while that following the second is not only stronger but develops more quickly. Six months after the second injection, a booster dose is sometimes necessary. Antitoxin gives an immediate immunity lasting 2 to 3 weeks. It is used to stop death losses in lambs following an outbreak of enterotoxemia and may also be used to immunize feedlot lambs on a short-term feeding basis for up to three weeks.

Bacterin is intended to stimulate the development in healthy animals of an immunity lasting 5 or 6 months; protective immunity requires ten days to develop. Bacterin, therefore, should be administered at least ten days before sheep are placed on full feed. There may be a reaction in the tissues at the site of injection. Because it may persist for at least thirty days, it is inadvisable to use bacterin if the animals are intended for slaughter within that time. Bacterin should not be injected into lambs under two months.

Antitoxin and bacterin should not be injected at the same time because the immediate immunity established by the antitoxin will prevent the body tissues from reacting to the bacterin. The antitoxin or bacterin is injected by aseptic means usually under the skin of the fleece-free area back of the place where the foreleg joins the body. Injections there help to prevent unnecessary lameness.

14
Hemorrhagic Enterotoxemia

HEMORRHAGIC enterotoxemia is an acute disease of young calves, sheep, goats, cattle, and pigs. It is characterized by sudden onset, a profuse hemorrhagic enteritis and sudden death. The disease is seasonal, with the greatest incidence in late winter and early spring.

Historically, this disease was first described in 1930 in England as a disease of adult sheep in an area limited to the Romney marsh area. It was called "struck" in that country because of the rapidity of the development of symptoms and subsequent death. More recently, it has been studied in sheep and cattle in the western part of the United States and has been isolated from an outbreak in pigs in Minnesota.

Etiology

Hemorrhagic enterotoxemia is caused by *Clostridium perfringens* type C toxin. The beta toxin of type C organisms is inactivated by trypsin, and this fact probably explains why the enterotoxemia is largely restricted to young, suckling animals. Type C is one of six antigenic types of *Clostridium perfringens,* and beta toxin produced by type C is the most potent of all these toxins. Toxin is produced in the intestine due to the favorable conditions for the growth of the organisms produced by enteritis; this is associated with overfeeding resulting in intestinal stasis, which rapidly favors the absorption of the toxin.

Transmission

Transmission of the *Clostridium perfringens* organism is universal, as this is a common soil contaminant and a normal part of the flora of the intestinal tract of most animals. The susceptible hosts are calves under two weeks of age, piglets under one week, adult sheep and goats and, occasionally, adult cattle. The factor influencing susceptibility is overeating, or enteritis from some other cause, causing stasis of the intestinal tract. Stasis allows for absorption of greater-than-normal amounts of toxin, with the rapid production of symptoms.

Symptoms

Type C intoxication of hemorrhagic enterotoxemia is usually fatal to vigorous suckling calves under two weeks of age and piglets under one week. It is characterized by sudden onset, hemorrhagic enteritis, bloody diarrhea and early death. Affected calves are commonly from dams that are heavy milk producers. It is believed that unfavorable, inclement weather at calving time has some influence on the incidence and severity of the disease. The disease also occurs in lambs and pigs under similar conditions. In pigs, the symptoms usually appear on the first or second day after birth, the heaviest mortality occurring on the second through the fifth day. The morbidity within litters varies and ranges from a single pig per litter to the entire litter. Most commonly, however, only some of the affected litters die. Diarrhea is consistently observed, except for peracute cases which suddenly collapse and die before the onset of diarrhea. In acute cases, most piglets die on the first or second postnatal day, and bright red, watery feces are evident. Cases with a subacute clinical course of two to three days have reddish brown liquid feces, whereas cases of a slightly longer duration have colorless, liquid feces in which particles of gray, necrotic debris may be seen.

Commonly, the syndrome is that of a fatal, nonhemorrhagic, diarrheal disease of several days' duration, recovery being rare. In calves, the most common symptoms are listlessness, weakness, and failure to nurse, accompanied by evidence of colicky pains such as kicking at the abdomen or uneasiness and rolling from side to side. A hemorrhagic diarrhea is evident after the other symptoms have begun. There is rapid progression of the symptoms through prostration, tetanic spasms, and early death. The normal course of the disease in calves varies from 2 to 24 hours and in many cases the animals die without overt signs being observed. The temperature remains normal to subnormal. Mild cases do occur; upon recovery, these animals fail to make normal gains but have a good antitoxin titer.

Pathology

Upon postmortem, the lesions are usually noted to be hemorrhagic in character. The prominent lesion is a necrotic, hemorrhagic, enterocolitis. The lumen of the intestine is filled with blood and tissue debris. Small hemorrhages occur on the thymus, the heart and the covering of the intestinal tract.

The lymph nodes show an appreciable degree of swelling and there are small pinpoint hemorrhages on the thymus gland and on the diaphragm. The heart sac contains an excess of fluid with some clotting, and the third stomach (in the case of calves) is distended with partially coagulated milk. The membranes of the stomach are inflamed and covered with a thick, tenacious, mucoid membrane. There may be areas of local necrosis throughout the intestinal tract.

Diagnosis

Diagnosis in the field is made on the history of sudden death in calves under two weeks of age and pigs under one week of age. Supportive diagnosis is made upon postmortem signs. However, positive diagnosis is confirmed only by demonstration of the type C toxin in the intestinal contents and by isolation of the *Clostridium perfringens* organisms from scrapings of the intestinal walls. The veterinarian can advise as to the method of preserving the intestinal content for transmission to a diagnostic laboratory.

Prevention

Hemorrhagic enterotoxemia can best be controlled by vaccination of the breeding herd of cattle with type C toxoid. It is recommended that two doses be administered, four weeks apart, the first year, and that booster doses be given annually. Vaccination of dams confers passive immunity to the offspring, via the colostrum, lasting 3 to 5 weeks. Calves from nonimmunized dams can be immunized with antitoxin soon after birth. Cows should be immunized with the toxoid 2 to 4 months prior to parturition, with a booster injection 3 to 5 weeks following the first injection.

In sows, a similar course should be followed. Because of the sudden onset and rapid course in piglets, it is usually not considered profitable to vaccinate baby pigs; they must obtain passive immunity from the sow through the colostrum.

15
Botulism

BOTULISM is a fatal disease caused by the toxin of *Clostridium botulinum* and characterized by rapidly progressive motor paralysis. It is not a bacterial infection, but rather an intoxication caused by the ingestion of a preformed toxin, usually in decomposed or "spoiled" animal or vegetable matter. As a disease of man, judging by ancient edicts warning against their consumption, it was first ascribed to the eating of blood sausages. The peculiar form of neuroparalysis liable to follow the eating of such sausages was first accurately described in Wurthemberg in 1735; the actual term *botulismus* or sausage poisoning appeared in the medical literature of southern Germany about 150 years ago.

It has been recognized as a disease of domestic animals since 1917, when it was first noted in horses. Veterinarians were quick to point out the striking similarity of botulism in man, limber neck in chickens, and forage poisoning in horses. Upon observation, it became evident that at least some of the outbreaks diagnosed as forage poisoning in horses were actually from *Clostridium botulinum.* Of course, other outbreaks undoubtedly were encephalitis of viral origin. Botulism in other species seems to be relatively infrequent. This is due, in part, to species resistance to the toxin and also perhaps to other factors such as eating habits. For example, outbreaks in cattle have been caused by feeding on carrion, as a result of perversion of appetite due to mineral deficiency. In any event, cattle, sheep, swine, dogs, and cats are commonly regarded as relatively resistant to botulism. Wild ducks are susceptible, and large numbers have died from the disease. The disease has been reported in captive mink and the common laboratory animals. Guinea pigs and mice are very susceptible, and are the animals of choice with which to demonstrate the disease experimentally. Current thinking regarding botulism as a naturally occurring disease in swine is that it is of no great importance, due to modern feeding practices. However, *Clostridium botulinum* is widely distributed in nature, being found in soils, especially those well fertilized with animal wastes, and in fruits, vegetables, decaying organic matter, aquatic and emerging vegetation and moldy hay.

Etiology and Transmission

The organism responsible for the production of the toxin causing botulism is generally referred to as *Clostridium botulinum.* On the basis of its proteolytic abilities, it is now commonly subdivided into two groups and designated as either *Clostridium botulinum* (nonproteolytic) or *C. para-botulinum* (proteolytic). However, for purposes of general reference, both groups will be referred to collectively here as *Clostridium botulinum.*

Clostridium botulinum is a motile, gram-positive, rod-shaped bacterium occurring singly or in short chains. Spores are generally terminal or subterminal. Growth requires strict anaerobic conditions, such as those found in necrotic or decaying organic matter. Growth occurs within a wide range of temperatures up to body temperatures, but is perhaps optimal at about 90 F. *Clostridium botulinum* is commonly found in the soil and in the intestinal tract of healthy animals. Here it causes no harm, but, once the animal dies, the bacteria multiply rapidly and produce the toxin which causes intoxication when consumed by another animal.

Since botulism is fundamentally an intoxication rather than an infection, it is not transmissable from animal to animal in the usual sense. This is in spite of the fact that massive doses of toxin-free spores may rarely result in sufficient germination, multiplication, and toxin liberation, in vivo, to produce the disease. Several types of botulism toxin have been described, as have some subtypes. Variation in cultural features does not appear to be closely related to type of toxin produced; that is, type B may be formed by proteolytic or nonproteolytic strains, while in either proteolytic or nonproteolytic strains more than one type of toxin may be formed.

Even though the toxin is said to resist a degree of acidity equivalent to that of the gastric juice and to be impervious to the action of pepsin or trypsin, some animals are particularly resistant to oral doses of the toxin. This may be due to the fact that there is slight absorption of the toxin through the small intestine of these animals. Further, it is possible that the bacterial flora within the intestine has a deleterious effect on the toxin.

Factors Affecting Susceptibility

Botulism is rarely seen in livestock in the United States; in fact, it is more often seen in man than in animals. However, the intoxication may be seen in cattle, sheep, horses and chickens. Swine are resistant to the condition.

In areas with a phosphorus deficiency, cattle and sheep may chew on the bones of dead animals in whose carcasses *Clostridium botulinum* has multiplied and produced toxin, thereby incurring botulism. Forage poisoning of cattle and horses is due to botulism toxin that has developed on decaying silage and hay. Thus, starvation, mineral deficiencies, or any other factor associated with the ingestion of toxin-contaminated material predispose to the condition.

Symptoms

Naturally and artificially affected animals appear to be affected alike. After the latent period of 8 to 72 hours, a progressive weakness of the voluntary muscles appears, usually beginning in the head and neck regions and spreading backward over the body. The weakness, leading to paralysis, is manifested in the disturbance of several functions. The most obvious, of course, is the disturbance of locomotion. Weakness in the forelegs often appears first, followed by involvement of the hindlegs and ultimately prostration due to complete paralysis of all limbs. The muscles of the throat are often affected, resulting in inability to swallow and in excess salivation. The ears may droop more than usual, adding to the appearance of depression. Vision may be impaired. Superficial reflexes appear to be affected only in that motor responses become progressively weaker. The activity of smooth muscle is not affected, and the chief effect upon the circulatory system is a fast and uneven pulse. Ultimate involvement of the respiratory muscles results in cyanosis, anoxia, coma, and finally death of asphyxia. Cases of botulism which survive may require weeks or even months for complete restoration to normal health.

Pathology

There are few postmortem lesions to be noted other than infrequent hemorrhages in the lungs and the general signs associated with high temperature. There may be froth in the trachea, but this is not a common sign.

Diagnosis

Diagnosis of botulism is generally based on history, symptoms, absence of gross lesions, and laboratory diagnosis of the offending toxin. Occasionally, the source of toxin can be demonstrated in the stomach of animals dead from the intoxication. For example, the eating of carrion can sometimes be determined at necropsy by noting the presence of maggots in the gut. When this is true, it may lead to the source of the intoxication.

Clostridium botulinum occasionally may be isolated from animals with botulism, but not with sufficient regularity to be of much value as a diagnostic procedure. Therefore, negative results do not preclude the possibility of botulism.

Treatment and Control

While the toxins of *Clostridium botulinum* are immunogenic, they may be used to produce not only antitoxin but also toxoids. To be of value in the prevention of botulism in animals, antitoxin must be used early in the course of the disease. The use of such products in swine is not practical, however, even in garbage-feeding enterprises, because of cost and the low incidence of the disease which, in turn, is apparently due to the natural resistance of swine to botulism. Cattle and sheep raised in phosphorus-deficient areas, however, can be immunized by the use of polyvalent toxoid. For best results cattle and sheep should be vaccinated each spring before being turned out on pasture or range.

Spoiled canned goods, spoiled garbage, and carrion appear to be the commonly incriminated media in which botulism toxin is formed. Thus, in spite of the fact that swine are known to be relatively resistant to the action of the toxin, they should not knowingly be fed such products. Any food considered unfit for human consumption should not be fed to animals; this should be considered the first step in preventing botulism. The toxins are thermolabile, so boiling of garbage for thirty minutes should destroy the toxins. The spores, on the other hand, have great thermal resistance which apparently varies with the strain, the pH, and other conditions of the medium. The botulism spores survive for considerable lengths of time under dry heat, and freezing has little effect on either spores or toxin.

In view of the ubiquity of *Clostridium botulinum* and its ability to survive under most natural conditions, there seems to be little hope of completely eradicating botulism. On the other hand, the disease should be found only under uncontrollable circumstances.

16
Blackleg

BLACKLEG is a sporadic, acute, infectious, noncommunicable disease of livestock. It is characterized by gas-filled swellings in the heavy muscles, especially of the hindleg, which crepitate or crackle when palpated. This disease is sporadic in nature and affects mainly young cattle and sheep, although occasionally goats and wild ruminants may be affected. Blackleg is caused by *Clostridium chauvoei,* one of the gas-producing organisms commonly contaminating pastures and feedlots.

Geographically, blackleg has been found in all parts of the world where cattle are raised and where cattle and sheep are pastured on low-lying, marshy pastures or, more frequently, on well-irrigated pastures.

Historically, blackleg is one of the older diseases known to cattle; however, it was not until 1875 that a positive diagnosis of the condition was made. Prior to that time it had been confused with anthrax, but in 1875 the disease was finally differentiated and the organisms causing the disease were cultured.

Etiology

Blackleg is one of the clostridial diseases. It is caused by *Clostridium chauvoei,* a gas-producing, spore-forming, gram-positive, rod-shaped bacterium. The microorganism occurs singly in cultures and the spore develops subterminally. In the natural state, the spore form is most often found on contaminated pastures. The vegetative form, however, may be found in the diseased muscles of animals that have died of this disease. The organism growing in the animal body produces a toxin which is not, however, as potent as the toxins produced by other clostridial microorganisms. There are several antigenic strains of the blackleg organism but there are no differences between the sheep and cattle strains. The spore stage of the microorganism is resistant and will remain viable on pastures, contaminated feed and bedding for a considerable length of time. *Clostridium chauvoei* exists in the soil and is ingested on the forage from the contaminated pastures. Multiplication of the vegetative stage takes place in the intestinal tract of farm animals, and the spores enter the bloodstream where they circulate until a focus is established. At that time the spore organisms change into the vegetative state and rapidly develop, causing the gross appearance of the disease. The spore-forming organisms are found in most parts of the United States but primarily in those areas where low-lying pastures, at times marshy or swampy, predominate.

Transmission

The primary source of infection is usually considered to be ingestion of contaminated spores which enter the digestive tract with contaminated feed and water. Wound infections, whether from tick bites, scratches, wire cuts, animal bites, or any other traumatic experience (such as castration or docking), provide a means of entry of the organism into the bloodstream. Soil infection is considered to be the primary source since spores of the microorganism are found both outside and inside the body of an infected animal. If the pasture has become infected, it remains so permanently.

In sheep, wounds of any kind, whether accidental (as from shearing cuts, injury from fences, and similar causes) or intentional (as from docking, castration, or vaccination procedures) are to be looked upon as potential avenues for the entrance of the disease-producing organisms. Microorganisms commonly enter the body when sheep are dipped for scab, lice or sheep ticks, immediately after shearing. Too often this is a careless operation, resulting in scratches and cuts of the animal's skin, and the dip serves as a focus for the collection of microorganisms which may then enter the body through the lesions described. When this occurs the results are often disastrous, as treatment is generally ineffective after the disease has once developed. The disease may occur in ewes from infection of wounds of the genital tract produced at lambing time. In rams, lesions have appeared about the head from infection of wounds received when butting and fighting. Grass cuts on legs of both sheep and cattle may serve as means of infection through the skin.

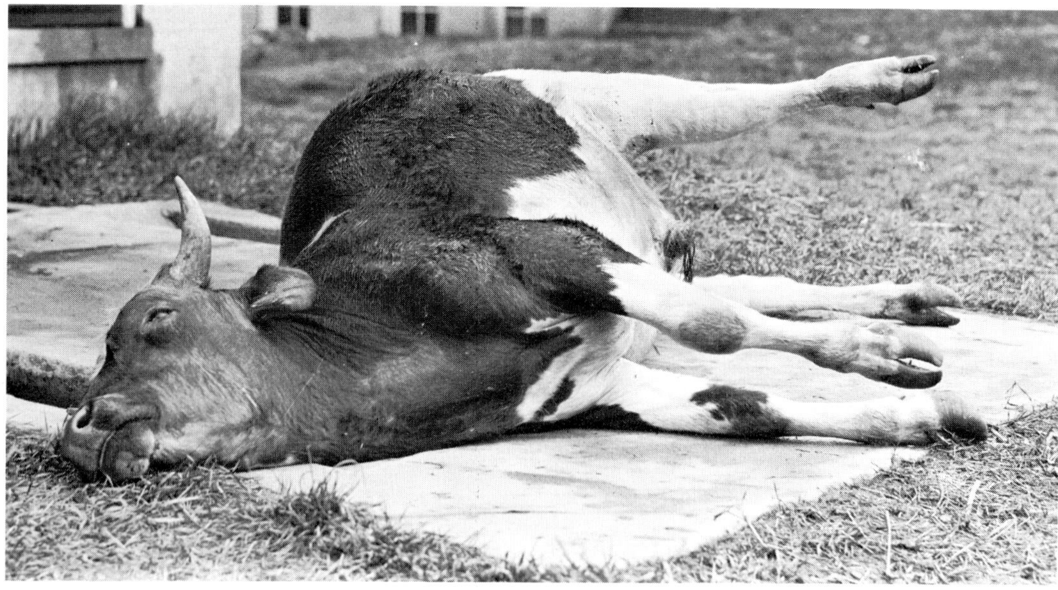

FIG. 12. A young steer that has died of blackleg.

Factors Influencing Susceptibility

Young cattle from 4 months to 2 years of age suffer from blackleg, as do sheep and goats of most ages. However, cattle which have not been vaccinated against the disease or which have not been in an area where the disease is prevalent may succumb at an older age. Wild ruminants (such as deer), swine, and laboratory animals are also infected upon occasion. Older cattle are usually resistant to the disease because they have either recovered from an inapparent bout of infection, or because they have not had access to an infected area and thus have not experienced the disease-producing organisms. In this way, a measure of resistance may be considered a part of disease prevention. There is no evidence of physiological immunity to this disease nor is there a relationship due to sex or breed. The disease is most often seen in well-nourished young cattle at about the time of weaning. Most cases appear in the fall, early winter and spring, but they can occur at any time regardless of weather or feeding conditions. Herd outbreaks commonly occur among unvaccinated beef calves soon after weaning in the fall. Livestock maintained on cultivated land, especially irrigated pastures, or on low, swampy regions are more susceptible to the disease than are cattle or sheep maintained on dry, upland pastures. Cattle presumably contact infection through ingestion of contaminated food, soil or water rather than from the introduction of the microorganism through wounds or injuries, while the latter is the case with sheep.

Symptoms

In cattle, symptoms appear in most cases sporadically or spontaneously, unassociated with wounds or other injuries. Affected animals are usually in good condition, and the disease appears when they are turned out to pasture. The incubation period is from one to five days, usually less than three days, and the course of the disease is rapid, from 24 to 60 hours. There is an acute rise in temperature to 106 F. If symptoms are seen, the animal will appear lame and will resent movement. The swellings appear commonly in the hindlegs or hip regions and are hot and painful. Later, the swellings are cold, and the animal does not evidence pain when they are palpated. The animal may be found lying on his side, with legs extended and the swellings filled with gas. There will usually be a dry, crackling sound as the result of this gas accumulation under the skin. The skin will appear dry and dark over the areas where gas is noted. The animal will appear dyspneic, that is, respiration will increase rapidly and there will be a rapid, thready pulse. Just prior to death, the temperature will fall and the animal will become comatose. In most cases, the symptoms appear so quickly that the first sign of disease is a dead animal.

The symptoms in sheep are different from those in cattle. In sheep, age is not a factor in incidence of disease. Sheep of all ages may be affected, from lambs a few days old up to ancient ewes and rams. A considerable time may elapse between ingestion of the spores and the manifestations of the symptoms in sheep. While spontaneously developed lesions may occur in sheep of all ages, serious outbreaks usually follow such traumatic farm operations as shearing, crutching, dipping, docking, and castration. Because of the slow development of the disease in sheep, they are not often found dead without premonitory signs. These signs include lameness, reluctance to move, crepitating swellings on various parts of the body, rise in temperature, and inability to stand, following which the animal will die quickly.

Pathology

Once organisms of blackleg have entered the body from the spore state, they tend to localize within the crypts of the intestines where they find an anaerobic atmosphere in which to develop. Once they enter the circulation, however, they circulate until they localize in injured or poorly drained muscle tissue. There, the development of necrotic tissue provides a favorable environment for the growth of the vegetative stage of the bacterium. Toxin liberated by the vegetative stage of the microorganism causes local necrosis of the muscles in the area surrounding the foci of infection. The gas produced breaks up the tissue and provides a gaseous, hemorrhagic inflammation which then is evidenced by crepitation. The toxins liberated cause high temperatures, rapid respiration, degenerative changes, and death.

There is little putrefaction as the result of a gross infection with *Clostridium chauvoei* organisms. However, large crepitant swellings or changes may occur, although on occasion such changes may not be extensive. Upon excising the skin, the muscle color is dark, with light streaks and gas pockets which produce a pungent, rancid odor. The fluid exuding from a cut portion of skin will be frothy as a result of gas bubbles within the fluid. It is best, if blackleg is suspected, not to open the skin. If the skin is removed, however, it will be hemorrhagic immediately under the surface. In sheep, since lesions of the spontaneously occurring type are often small and deeply situated, they may be easily overlooked upon autopsy and the condition may be confused with other clostridial diseases. Thus, an accurate diagnosis can be made only by laboratory examination of specimens taken from the sheep at time of autopsy. However, any time young cattle are found to have died suddenly and exhibit gas-filled lesions or swellings of the muscles, primarily of the hindlegs, without any other symptoms, blackleg must be suspected.

Treatment and Prevention

Young cattle with symptoms of blackleg are seldom observed in time to save them. However, as the disease is not so spontaneous in sheep, they may be treated successfully with a variety of broad-spectrum antibiotics; in those areas where expensive animals are kept for breeding purposes, the use of an antiblackleg serum which provides temporary protection may also be used. The veterinarian should be contacted immediately whenever blackleg is suspected.

Because blackleg is a disease both sporadic in nature and enzootic in various parts of the country, once it has been diagnosed immunization must be done yearly on infected premises. Blackleg bacterin is used extensively and is safe and reliable for both cattle and sheep. A single injection confers immunity lasting for several months. Where heavy infection of premises necessitates early vaccination of calves and lambs—before they are old enough to produce strong, active immunity—a second vaccination must be given at about six months of age or at the time of weaning. In sheep, vaccination is used not only as a routine measure in blackleg areas but also as a preventive at the beginning of an outbreak to check further losses. As further means of controlling this disease, whenever animals die of blackleg it is wise to bury the carcasses deeply, to cultivate all known blackleg-contaminated ground and to keep young animals out of such areas until they have been effectively immunized.

The bodies of animals that have died are the chief source of soil infection. They harbor the microorganism in large numbers and liberate them from artificial and natural body openings. For this reason, any dead animal should be promptly burned or buried, and with few exceptions the sick should be slaughtered and disposed of in the same manner. Disinfect all woodwork or utensils that have come in contact with the infection. The surface of the ground may be made safe by burning it over with a heavy layer of straw. Because of the vitality of the spores of blackleg, pastures may remain infected for years, even when kept free of cattle. In some regions, where contamination of the soil is limited, the disease may be avoided by a change of pasture. It seems possible that, in time, an infected pasture may become free of microorganisms if all animals feeding upon it are vaccinated.

17
Bacillary Hemoglobinuria

BACILLARY hemoglobinuria, or redwater, is an acute infectious disease of cattle and sheep, and rarely swine, caused by *Clostridium haemolyticum.* It is characterized by high temperature, depression, rapid hemolysis, hemoglobinuria or blood in the urine (from which it gets its name), intestinal hemorrhages and death in 24 to 36 hours.

Historically, the disease was first observed within the United States in 1916. Since that time it has been described in various parts of the western range areas in the United States, Mexico, Chile, and many other warmer parts of the world.

Etiology

Bacillary hemoglobinuria is caused by *Clostridium haemolyticum,* a large rod-shaped bacterium producing a potent toxin. This toxin is actively hemolytic and can cause rapid death in animals infected with this microorganism. The spores produced by the vegetative stages of this microorganism vary in their resistance from strain to strain; however, most are rapidly killed by oxidizing disinfectants. The causative organisms are ingested in feed or water and ultimately become lodged in the liver as latent spores, where under favorable conditions they multiply and cause a large infarct from which the hemolytic toxin is released in large amounts. In the terminal stages of the disease, bacteremia develops in addition to the toxemia. The incubation period of the disease varies from 7 days up to several months but, once clinical signs are observed, the course is rapidly fatal. The spores of *C. haemolyticum* may remain dormant in the liver until some injury provides a favorable medium for rapid reproduction and proliferation of toxin.

Redwater is often thought to be associated with liver flukes, as the disease is encountered in cattle and sheep reared in swampy, poorly drained pastures in the range states of the west. It has been diagnosed in many cattle-producing areas in the southeast and in the middle south, and in countries of South America and, indeed, various parts of the world. It occurs mainly in the summer months; however, sporadic cases may occur throughout the winter. In affected areas, susceptible additions to herds come down rapidly following entrance into a contaminated herd if they have not been previously vaccinated against the disease.

Transmission

Bacillary hemoglobinuria is primarily spread by the movement of cattle from infected to noninfected ranches, by the intermingling of cattle from infected ranches or farms with those on ranches formerly free of the disease, and possibly by contaminated cattle trucks and boxcars. The disease is primarily spread through the ingestion of latent spores in feed and water. The spores ultimately lodge in the liver where they undergo development when favorable conditions exist. Invariably in the liver of affected animals, an infarct, or a large lesion, is demonstrated, and within the lesion the vegetative stages of the bacterium develop and produce a toxin. The incubation period depends apparently on some as yet undetermined factor or factors in the liver favorable to the multiplication of causative organisms. It is generally thought that liver-fluke invasion may be a factor producing local necrosis, thus providing a favorable anaerobic focus within which the latent spores may begin their development and production of potent hemolytic toxin.

Bacillary hemoglobinuria is primarily a water-borne disease of cattle and sheep pastured on swampy or poorly drained pastures, although the disease has also been identified in hogs. Forage harvested from such areas also may occasionally be infectious. The prevalence of the disease depends largely on climatic conditions. In temperate areas it is a disease of summer and fall, although exceptions may occur. In subtropical and tropical areas, it may occur throughout the year.

In cattle, the symptoms may be seen from six months of age to advanced age; however, most cases occur after one year of age. This pattern is primarily due to the fact that the spores picked up from a contaminated pasture do not have a chance to develop within a liver lesion until the animals have picked up wandering flukes or other organisms to provide a focus for development within the liver. Thus, this is not a disease of very young animals.

Factors Influencing Susceptibility

Bacillary hemoglobinuria is most often seen in late spring and during the summer and fall, when waters in swampy areas reach their peak. It is most common in years of plentiful rainfall, when the organism in the spore stage becomes widespread in marshy areas. It is not a disease of young animals. Transmission of the organism is always by ingestion of contaminated water, grass or hay, and the nature of the pasture is often not material to the method of transmission. Mechanical transmission from contaminated to noncontaminated areas may occur through wandering dogs and other feral animals.

Symptoms

Cattle affected with redwater disease rapidly lose their appetites and rumination ceases. When this occurs, milk secretion is reduced and defecation is retarded with resulting constipation. Affected animals stand apart from the herd, with their backs arched and abdomens tucked up. The coat becomes dry and lusterless, the eyes become sunken, and the animal appears to be in distress. The muzzle is hot and dry and the mucous membranes are yellowish or icteric. Respiration is slightly advanced, with shallow breathing. There appears to be pain on respiration and the animal will grunt when forced to move.

The temperature rises to 106 F but may drop to a subnormal level sometime prior to death. The pulse is increased but weak, and as the disease progresses the animal becomes subnormal in all respects. In the latter stages of the disease in cattle, the feces become soft and diarrheic, urination is frequent and copious with a well-marked reddish, port-wine color, and rapid dehydration follows. The erythrocyte count is decreased appreciably. Within approximately 36 hours of the onset of symptoms, death usually occurs due to acute toxemia. The mortality exceeds 95 percent in animals not receiving antisera or antibiotic treatment.

In sheep, the symptoms are similar to those in cattle but much more difficult to detect. Death usually results from anoxia due to the rapid and extensive destruction of red blood cells by the toxin.

Pathology

Rapid rigor mortis and hemorrhage from the nostrils and anus follow death. The conjunctiva becomes yellowish and the entire body takes on a yellowish, icteric color. There are small hemorrhages throughout the subcutaneous tissues. The lymph nodes appear to be swollen and the liver is extremely enlarged, yellowish in color, soft and friable to the touch, with a large infarct usually located near one end.

Diagnosis

In the field, diagnosis is primarily based upon the history of the area, the season of the year, and postmortem appearance, primarily of the liver. In the liver the infarct is especially diagnostic, and organisms may be recovered from such an infarct by laboratory diagnosis.

Prevention

Treatment is difficult due to the speed with which this disease develops; therefore, immunization and sanitation are the primary preventive measures. Immunization may be accomplished with *Clostridium haemolyticum* bacterin prepared from whole cultures of high toxin content. These bacterins will confer a solid immunity for about six months. In areas where the disease is seasonal, one preseasonal dose is adequate; where the disease occurs throughout the year, semiannual immunization is required. When the disease is already prevalent in a herd or flock, it is sometimes expedient to treat all animals with antisera to alleviate the full brunt of the disease. Blood transfusion is indicated for extremely anemic animals, and supportive treatment with palliative handling and care is expected. Proper sanitation includes keeping animals away from swampy areas which have been incriminated as contaminated and refusing to feed hay from such infected areas.

18
Tetanus

TETANUS, or lockjaw, results from a wound infection of deep tissue with *Clostridium tetani.* It is characterized by intoxication accompanied by spasmodic and tonic contractions of voluntary muscles. All common types of livestock are susceptible to tetanus except poultry. A list of the more highly susceptible animals would include men, horses, mules, sheep and goats. Swine are more obviously susceptible when young since the highest percentage of cases occur at an early age; however, this may be at least partly due to the greater opportunity for infection at that time through the practice of clipping needle teeth. The distribution of the disease is essentially worldwide, but it occurs most commonly in old farming areas with large livestock populations and where manure is commonly returned to the land. Tetanus occurs more often in tropical and subtropical regions than in the colder parts of the world.

Clostridium tetani and the disease it produces are of historical interest. The disease has been known and greatly feared for centuries. As early as the fourth century B.C. physicians believed tetanus was caused by the wind. In 1884, scientists produced tetanus in a rabbit using materials from a person who had died of lockjaw. It was shown that toxins produced by *Clostridium tetani* when injected into rabbits would produce the disease. Later it was shown that immunization against the toxins could be obtained by the injection of small doses of blood serum from experimentally infected animals. Such a serum could neutralize the toxin both in vitro and in vivo. Thus it was in connection with tetanus that (1) anaerobic techniques were first used, (2) bacterial toxins were first demonstrated, and (3) the foundation for serum therapy was first laid.

Etiology

Tetanus is caused by the toxins of *Clostridium tetani.* The vegetative form of the organism is a slender, gram-positive, anaerobic rod. Spores are usually terminal in location and 2 to 3 times the diameter of the vegetative rods, giving the sporulated rod the appearance of a spoon or drumstick when seen microscopically.

Clostridium tetani is commonly found in the soil and in the feces of most animals. The spores are resistant, especially when protected from light and extremes of heat, and exist almost indefinitely in the soil.

As are other clostridial species, this microorganism is anaerobic and finds suitable conditions for growth in deep wounds, where two toxins are produced by the growing bacteria. One of the toxins is a hemolysin and of slight importance in producing the symptoms of the disease. The other, however, is a neurotoxin causing the characteristic symptoms of tetanus.

Transmission

Clostridium tetani gains entrance to the body via wounds. The disease commonly results from deep, penetrating, or puncture wounds, those in which there is considerable tissue damage and those grossly contaminated with soil or manure. Probably the most common port of entry in lambs, calves, and pigs is via castration wounds. Occasionally, the infection gains entrance into the body at the unhealed navel shortly after birth, via the dental alveoli during eruption of teeth, or possibly through wounds caused by unclipped needle teeth. There remains a small number of cases in which no likely portal of infection can be demonstrated; these are often referred to as idiopathic tetanus. Some such cases probably result from infection of small wounds which heal before tetanus appears.

Adult animals often acquire the infection through parturition wounds, dental caries, wire cuts, nail stab wounds, shearing cuts, dehorning wounds, castration, or any number of traumatic experiences.

Symptoms

The incubation period for tetanus is from 1 to 3 weeks following infection. The first symptom is a mild muscle stiffness which may be localized but is more often general. The progress of the disease is generally rapid enough, however, that the signs are distinctive within 24 to 36 hours. The characteristic manifestation, from which the disease is named, is that of tonic or tetanic muscle spasms. Although all muscles are affected, the stronger ones overcome the weaker or opposing muscles and produce the attitudes characteristic of the disease. The contraction of the muscles of the back, neck, and tail produce orthotonos and even opisthonos; contraction of the muscles of the limbs produces a sawhorse attitude, the extensor muscles being stronger than the flexors; and contraction of the muscles of mastication causes lockjaw. Difficulty in locomotion may be manifested first in turning or backing, but the animal soon finds it difficult to walk or even stand. Pigs often show unusual erectness of the ears and all animals exhibit some protrusion of the third eyelid. Spasms of the muscles of respiration permit only shallow and therefore rapid breathing. A fast heart rate may be quite noticeable. Animals often fall to the ground with head thrown back and all muscles rigid.

As the disease progresses, the animals become apprehensive and sensitive to sensory stimuli. Sudden movements, sharp noises, or slaps will intensify muscle spasms or protrusions of the nictitating membrane. Toward the end of a fatal attack, the temperature may increase to 108 to 110 F. The disease is almost always generalized and fatal. This is especially true of very young animals, although the mortality averages 80 percent among adults. There is a prolonged convalescent period for those that recover. Death is undoubtedly due to anoxia from interference with respiratory and cardiac functions.

Pathology

Under favorable conditions, the spores, having been carried into the wound, become vegetative, multiplying and forming toxins at

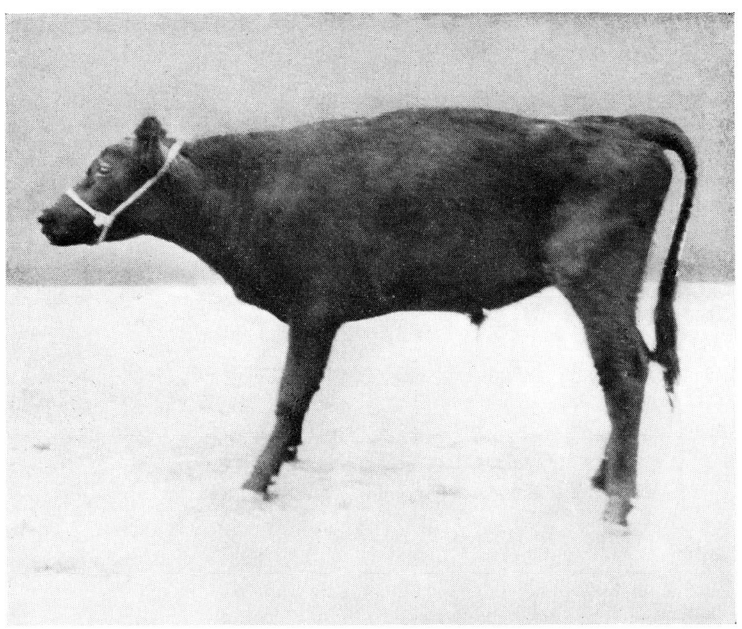

FIG. 13. Tetanus following castration. Sawhorse attitude, extended head and neck, and raised tail are all apparent. (From Gibbons, W. J.: *Clinical Diagnosis of Diseases of Large Animals.* Philadelphia, Lea & Febiger, 1966.)

the original site. The toxin includes tetanolysin, a hemolytic portion, and tetanospasmin, the more important lethal fraction. Tetanus toxin is one of the most poisonous substances known. The organisms show little tendency to spread to other parts of the body. However, the toxin apparently passes by diffusion into the surrounding medium, into the bloodstream, and then spreads to the central nervous system where it seems to produce its most dire results.

There is no unanimity of opinion regarding the route by which the toxin reaches the brain; however, it is thought that its route is via the arterial blood after absorption from the site of local infection by the lymph.

The incubation period for tetanus is usually 1 to 3 weeks but occasionally is shorter or much longer. The length of the incubation period is probably influenced not only by the number of infecting organisms but by the conditions set up in the contaminated wound, particularly by the amount of tissue damage incurred. It has been shown that washed spores of the tetanus organism when injected into healthy tissue do not germinate, presumably because the oxygen tension is too high in such tissue. However, if a culture which also contains toxin is injected, germination does occur and the disease results. Likewise, it has been noted that the disease results with regularity when washed spores are introduced with some irritant solution. Thus, it appears that tetanus spores germinate only in dead or injured tissues, or those altered in a way resulting in lowered oxygen tension. In addition, it has been observed that tetanus toxin adversely affects leukocytes and thus interferes with phagocytosis of the spores.

Rigor mortis appears early following death from tetanus. However, no significant gross lesions are characteristic for this disease. The blood is usually dark red and may be poorly clotted. Pulmonary congestion and edema may be noticeable and a few hemorrhages may be found in the serous membranes of the chest cavity. Necrosis at the site of injury may be so slight as to be unnoticed.

Diagnosis

Despite the fact that there are no characteristic gross lesions in tetanus, the diagnosis usually presents no particular difficulty. The symptoms are not likely to be confused with those of any other diseases except strychnine poisoning, eclampsia, lead poisoning or rabies. However, the last three have additional symptoms which should easily clear up any confusion. Symptoms of tetanus are often accompanied by a history of recent castration or the presence of a contaminated or infected wound. Therefore, clinical diagnosis is based upon history and symptoms. It is confirmed at autopsy by the absence of significant gross lesions and, in the event the infected wound can be demonstrated, by the presence of the characteristic bacteria. It is seldom necessary to go beyond the clinical examination to establish the diagnosis of tetanus.

Treatment

Tetanus is more common in some areas of the country than in others. However, even in the regions where the disease is rarely encountered, exposure should be expected when large numbers of animals are docked, castrated, or dehorned. In such instances instruments should be kept sterile, wounds disinfected, and any common holding yard moistened to hold down spore-laden dust. Following such procedures, all stock should be given antitoxin and turned out onto grass pasture, if possible.

All animals injured by nails, wire or other sharp objects should be considered infected and antitoxin should be administered. The wounds must be cleaned, drained and dressed to prevent further complications. The use of tetanus antitoxin in the range of 1500 to 3000 units is appropriate in all animals whenever the skin is broken for any reason. This treatment provides passive immunity for up to two weeks, usually long enough to protect the animal until the wound heals.

In the event exposure cannot be avoided, or symptoms are suspected, then antisera may be used to provide a concentration of antibodies for immediate protection. However, in most instances the period of protection to be desired is longer than that provided by antisera, so that either antitoxin or toxoid should be used in addition.

Tetanus toxoid will provide active immunity to the disease, but in older sheep and cattle annual booster injections are recommended. Although a single injection of toxoid will provide appreciable immunity, three injections about three weeks apart will provide excellent immunity in swine. Due to individual variability, however, annual boosters are recommended for breeder stock.

Prevention

There is no practical means of eliminating the spores of *Clostridium tetani* from the environment. Losses from tetanus, though generally sporadic, may be enzootic due to heavy concentrations of spores in the soil and inadequate precautions against the disease.

There are three points at which attempts can be made to break the cycle of the disease: (1) Since tetanus is a wound-infection disease, every effort should be made to prevent unnecessary wounds by removing from the environment any sharp objects such as bare nail points, wire, splinters, broken glass or projecting boards. It is important for swine producers to clip the sharp points from the needle teeth of newborn pigs. (2) A clean environment should be provided so far as possible; that is, maternity pens should be periodically sanitized and kept as free of manure as possible, umbilical cords should be tied off and treated with antiseptic soon after birth, and all livestock should be turned out onto clean pastures. Castration, dehorning, and docking operations should be performed with every reasonable precaution to prevent infection. (3) If all these precautions fail or cannot be properly carried out, the possibility of immunization remains.

19
Malignant Edema

MALIGNANT edema is an acute, usually fatal, infectious disease of cattle, sheep, goats, swine, and man. The disease is caused by *Clostridium septicum* and is characterized by swellings within the body, usually located around a wound, where pathogens have entered or localized in the tissues. The disease produces marked prostration, and is often fatal in 1 to 4 days.

Historically, this disease was one discovered early by Pasteur and co-workers. They cultured the causative bacteria from the blood of a cow in 1877. Koch later produced the disease in cattle and went on to describe the organism in great detail.

Geographically, the organism is worldwide in distribution and found wherever cattle and sheep are raised. However, the disease is not so prevalent on the American continent as it is in Europe and Asia.

Etiology

The cause of malignant edema is *Clostridium septicum*, a short, plump rod that grows actively in penetrating or lacerated wounds; it grows anaerobically and produces gas deep within the muscle tissues. The etiology is similar in both man and animals. Closely allied with the causative organism are any number of *Clostridium* organisms found in the soil.

Transmission

The organism gains entrance to the body through cuts, lacerations, and penetrating wounds caused by castration, docking and shearing, vaccination with unclean needle, abortions and deliveries in contaminated surroundings, broken bones, wire scratches, and the bites of animals. The most susceptible hosts are cattle, sheep and swine, although horses, mules, dogs, and men are also susceptible. There are no premonitory factors affecting susceptibility, and there is no relationship associated with either sex or age. The disease may occur in all species of animals at any time. Although this is an infectious disease, it is not considered a contagious disease.

Clostridium septicum, the microorganism causing this disease, exists in all fertile soils and in the intestinal tract of herbivorous animals. Whether it multiplies in the soil, or whether it merely exists there as spores after being formed by the vegetating organisms in the intestinal tract of animals, is not known. Infection ordinarily occurs through contamination of nonaerated wounds, but many cases of this disease cannot be accounted for in this manner.

Symptoms

The period of incubation of malignant edema is from 2 to 5 days after a wound has become contaminated. Sometimes the condition may occur more rapidly, depending upon the infecting dose and the extent of the wound. Usually within this time edema-like swelling, primarily involving the subcutaneous tissues and the skin, occurs. The organism spreads rapidly and the lesions may become emphysematous. Blood-tinged fluid may escape at the point of injury or can be withdrawn by hypodermic aspiration. Lameness, fever, increased pulse rate, congestion of the conjunctiva, and marked toxemia appear almost in the order given. Death may occur in 1 to 4 days after the appearance of the initial lesions. In those cases where the disease is prolonged, a profuse, foul-smelling diarrhea may be noted. Where a genital infection follows abortion or delivery of a dead fetus, swelling of the labia, necrosis of the vagina, and external edema, gravitating to the ventral abdomen, may occur. Following castration symptoms may develop within a few hours or not until several days following the operation. The symptoms will first appear as swelling with serosanguineous exudate from the incision. Later the swelling becomes more extensive with extension downward to the ventral area. The affected animal will become toxic, develop a high temperature, show signs of dyspnea and die.

Pathology

The malignant-edema organism, *Clostridium septicum*, gains entrance into the body with dirt through penetrating wounds. There it finds suitable foci for growth in the necrotic tissue resulting from the trauma. The toxin produced causes edema and gas production which further disrupts the muscle tissue. Upon postmortem, a massive edema due to straw-colored or brownish fluid in the area of the wound is noted. The muscle tissue appears reddish-black and gas bubbles are evident throughout the area. The gas bubbles tend to be subcutaneous rather than intermuscular, as in the case of blackleg. There is usually edematous fluid in the body cavities and in the pericardial sac. Other signs are generalized hyperemia and cyanosis of the tissue. In the field the condition is diagnosed primarily through a history of traumatic wounds, plus the typical lesions and symptoms listed. However, positive diagnosis can only be made by laboratory isolation of the causative organisms.

Treatment and Prevention

Because of the rapid appearance of symptoms and the acute nature of malignant edema, treatment is not recommended. Therefore, prophylaxis depends on sanitation and immunization against this disease.

Immunization is accomplished by using bacterins composed of a combination of organisms. It has become a common practice to include the organisms of both malignant edema and blackleg in a single bacterin for protection against both diseases. Lambs and calves should be vaccinated at the time of castration, and again at about six months of age, for best results.

Because malignant-edema organisms continue to multiply for some time after sporulating in the carcasses of dead animals, it is a wise procedure immediately to destroy all carcasses suspected of this disease either by deep burying or burning. A wise precaution against the disease is strict asepsis during such operations as castration, docking, surgery, inoculation or injection.

20
Shipping Fever

HEMORRHAGIC septicemia, or shipping fever, is an acute or subacute infectious disease of cattle, sheep, swine and rabbits, characterized by several different syndromes including acute septicemia and pneumonia, and following shipment or stress. The cause is believed to be a poorly understood complex of viral and bacterial agents. However, *Pasteurella multocida* and *Pasteurella hemolytica* have been isolated most often from animals in the febrile stage of the disease.

Historically, shipping fever was first described in Germany. In 1880, it was described in the United States and *Pasteurella multocida* was incriminated as the causative organism. In 1912, a bacterin was produced that was partially successful against the disease. In 1917, scientists at the United States Department of Agriculture first used the term "shipping fever" and divided the disease into three types. Today, there is still confusion about the exact etiology of the syndrome.

Geographically, the disease is encountered throughout the world, frequently causing great economic losses. In the southern United States the acute septicemic form of the disease is most prevalent, while in northern states the respiratory form is most often encountered. The disease occurs frequently in feeder cattle and sheep, especially when subjected to the stress of shipment. Therefore, shipping fever is most common in those areas of heaviest animal production.

Etiology

The etiology of shipping fever is fundamentally difficult to elucidate as the disease has multiple causes. The pattern of the disease suggests that the causative agents are divided into three main categories—stress, virus infection, and bacterial infection. Within each of these categories the various elements appear to be nonspecific, so that the typical shipping-fever syndrome might be the result of any combination of the factors listed. The signs of the disease are not usually acute when only stress and a viral agent are present; however, when a bacterial agent is also present, the signs include pronounced involvement of the respiratory tract.

The bacterium *Pasteurella multocida,* a nonspore-forming, gram-negative rod, is often considered to be the precipitating cause of the disease, but the symptoms are seen only in cattle and sheep subjected to stress. The disease results when bacteria invade the respiratory tract of animals with lowered resistance due to stress and predisposing viral infection.

The virus, parainfluenza 3, has been isolated frequently from nasal secretions and lung tissues of young animals affected with shipping fever. It is antigenically related to a strain of parainfluenza 3 isolated from children with influenza.

The stress factors associated with shipping fever cover a wide range of environmental agents. Cold, stormy weather often triggers the syndrome, but the disease has also been seen during hot weather, especially if associated with such contributing causes as prolonged transit, castration, dehorning, weaning, vaccination, or sudden change of diet. Purely physical forms of stress may lead to an outbreak of the disease on a farm or ranch where the livestock have not been shipped or driven long distances.

Transmission

Recent research into the causes of shipping fever has revealed that the microorganisms associated with the disease can be found in the respiratory tract of normal animals. Therefore, transmission is most likely to be by contact and by consumption of contaminated feed and water. When animals are coughing, droplet transmission of the infection is significant. Very young calves have a measure of resistance to shipping fever, but tend to lose that resistance at about four months of age. Calves may become infected from the teats of cows at an early age but not show symptoms until much later.

Although shipping fever may be seen in several species, whether or not the disease can be transmitted from one species to another is not known.

Shipping fever may occur in all seasons of the year, but most cases are seen in the fall, the time of greatest movement of feeder cattle and lambs. The crowded feeder cattle routes become heavily contaminated, and this, plus the stress of shipping, provides increasing exposure of all animals to infection. Stockyards, sale barns, trucks, railroad cars, and feed yards become so heavily contaminated that healthy or recovered animals may become carriers and disseminate the disease widely.

Factors Influencing Susceptibility

In recent years the increase in the incidence of shipping fever has been attributed to the younger age at which feeder animals are shipped. Calves and lambs weaned just before being shipped are more susceptible because they are excitable, experience a drastic change in feed, and have less resistance than older animals to infection in general.

Predisposing factors are of a major importance in susceptibility to shipping fever. In recent years much work has been done in tracing the progress of the disease from time of diagnosis backward two or three weeks to discover the environmental or physiological conditions that had been present. Throughout these studies certain factors reappeared a number of times and have been termed the *predisposing factors* of shipping fever. The following are the most prevalent:

1. Physiological and emotional changes to which cattle and other animals are subjected during shipping.
2. Excitement, exhaustion and change in feed and water.
3. Irritation of mucous membranes by dust.
4. Overcrowding and long periods of feed and water deficiency.

5. Adverse changes in weather conditions, such as those occurring in autumn or spring.
6. Confinement in drafty or humid and poorly ventilated barns.
7. Malnutrition (mainly vitamin A deficiency, since vitamin A is helpful in maintaining healthy mucous membranes).
8. Shipment of recently weaned calves and lambs.
9. Stress—a specific syndrome occurring in the body as a result of hormonal influence in response to nonspecific factors.

When one animal becomes infected, the virulence of the organism is increased when transmitted to another animal. There is always the danger that an animal added to a clean herd may be a carrier and readily transmit the disease. No relationship has been found for parasites as a predisposing factor in this disease. Age and sex have little effect on susceptibility.

Recently, more evidence has been pointing to the fact that shipping fever is a complex disease caused jointly by a virus, bacteria and environmental stress. From the current work being done, it seems possible that a virus is the major cause with bacteria playing a secondary role, as it is difficult or impossible to cause the disease by inoculation with an isolated culture of the *Pasteurella* organism alone. However, *Pasteurella* organisms can be found on mucous membranes of healthy animals, indicating that another factor must be present to cause the appearance of frank symptoms of the disease.

Symptoms

Shipping fever is primarily a respiratory disease, varying from a mild form to rapidly fatal pneumonia. In the peracute type there is an incubation period of 2 to 5 days, during which the animal is depressed, stands apart from the others and eats or drinks little. The muzzle appears dry and the hair coat begins to look rough. The temperature rises to 104 to 108 F, and the pulse becomes rapid. As the disease progresses, the affected animal develops a discharge from the eyes and nose, and has difficulty breathing. The ears droop. Lactation stops, the animal becomes prostrate, and death may occur in 12 to 24 hours following appearance of symptoms.

In the acute type there is more pronounced pulmonary involvement, with thick, copious nasal exudate, rapid breathing, hemorrhage from the nose, soft cough and respiratory rales. The fever will be high; the animal will not eat, and rapidly loses weight. At times hemorrhagic diarrhea will develop and the animal will dehydrate rapidly. There may also be nervous involvement, evidenced by erratic movements.

In the chronic type the animal will have recovered from shipping fever, sometimes without treatment, but will have lost weight and will retain some of the respiratory symptoms. The mortality rate of chronic cases is variable but most animals do not live more than a few months following an acute course of the disease.

The symptoms of shipping fever may vary from feedlot to feedlot just as the appearance and course of symptoms may vary among individual animals. In some feedlots the symptoms of the disease may be evident upon arrival of a shipment, while in others the respiratory signs may not appear for several days. Usually, symptoms appear within the first two weeks, but the rate at which signs appear in the animals will be variable, as will the morbidity and mortality rates. The morbidity usually does not exceed 20 percent at any one time and, with prompt and adequate treatment, the mortality seldom exceeds 5 percent of affected animals.

Pathology

The pathogenic agents of shipping fever affect the entire respiratory system. With the first rise in temperature, a mucous nasal discharge develops and fills all of the paranasal sinuses. A few hemorrhages and some edema may be found in the mucosa of the larynx and upper part of the trachea. Death results from extensive bronchial involvement, pneumonia, and septicemia.

The pathogenic agents localize in the upper respiratory tract and, because of the lowered resistance caused by stress, are able to invade the mucosa; this leads to generalized septicemia. At necropsy, the most prominent observation is that of pneumonia. However, there is inflammation throughout the nose, sinuses, larynx and trachea. The lungs are distended with fluid or fibrin, and the chest cavity contains an excess of straw-colored fluid. There may also be evidence of blood in the stomach and intestines.

Diagnosis

The diagnosis in the field is mainly based upon a history of predisposing factors, clinical signs, and, if necessary, postmortem signs. Laboratory diagnosis may not be positive, but the demonstration of *Pasteurella* organisms in the blood or spleen is presumptive of shipping fever.

Typical signs of pneumonia, fever, loss of weight, nasal discharge, and loss of appetite in cattle about 10 days following a stressing experience are the basis for a diagnosis of shipping fever.

Shipping fever in cattle closely resembles contagious bovine pleuropneumonia both clinically and at postmortem examination, although the pleuropneumonia spreads through a susceptible population with great rapidity. Shipping fever is generally most often observed in cattle following shipment over long distances or in newly weaned calves. The clinical signs and severity of the disease may vary from death in 3 to 5 days to recovery without treatment. The diagnosis is complicated because of the number of diseases which can be confused with shipping fever.

Acute dyspnea is characteristic of fog fever and anaphylaxis but the onset is usually more sudden, the dyspnea more severe, and the lungs more diffusely affected in shipping fever. Chronic shipping fever may resemble chronic emphysema and lungworm infestation but, in shipping fever, dry crepitant rales are characteristic and are usually localized in the ventral parts of the lung. Infectious bovine rhinotracheitis affects only the upper respiratory tract except in cases where it spreads to the lungs as a secondary infection.

The diagnosis of shipping fever in swine and sheep is similar to that in cattle. In swine, shipping fever is confused with and similar to acute enteric salmonellosis, but the latter—although accompanied by pulmonary involvement—is usually distinguished by signs of septicemia and enteritis. In sheep, viral pneumonia is of minor importance because *Pasteurella* occurs mainly as the secondary bacterial infection.

Prevention

Bacterins, aggressins, and vaccines used for prevention of shipping fever are still considered by many to be the first line of defense. Individuals using these methods attribute any reported lack of efficiency to improper administration, namely, that the bacterin is not given the proper length of time before shipment. It is recommended that immune sera be injected before shipment and again upon arrival at destination. This procedure will provide an immediate immunity lasting for up to three weeks.

Bacterins have been effective in controlling *Pasteurella* organisms from becoming viable in the body. Good immunity probably occurs between the sixth and ninth day; therefore, the bacterins should be administered 10 days prior to the shipment. Sometimes three injections should be given to provide adequate protection, especially in valuable stock. As previously mentioned, no means of complete immunity can be devised until the relationship between *Pasteurella* organisms and viruses have been demonstrated.

Sanitation is probably the most important means of prevention known. If the predisposing factors could be eliminated (and most can), the occurrence of the disease would be lowered. Proper management of premises and herds can prevent serious outbreaks of the disease. Among the most important management factors are:

1. Vaccination with immune serum.
2. Adequate, warm, dry and clean quarters for the animals.
3. Adequate nutrition.
4. Vaccination with bacterins.
5. Proper care during and after shipment of animals.
6. Treatment of sick animals. They should be isolated from the rest of the herd or flock, given a light nutritious diet, and protected from stress.

Young recently weaned calves may be given tranquilizers to ease the trauma of separation, but this practice is of questionable value. In many feedlots, the managers (with the approval of their veterinarians) routinely treat all newly arrived animals with either sulfa drugs or antibiotics in drinking water as a means of preventing the disease.

Immune sera, bacterins, and vaccines have been used, either alone or in combination, to combat shipping fever. These products are still being used and have many advocates, but controlled experiments indicate that they have little, if any, lasting value and that there is considerable evidence of their inefficiency. Because of the serious nature of this disease and its similarity to several other diseases of economic importance, the diagnosis, treatment and control should be promptly delegated to a veterinarian.

21
Parainfluenza

PARAINFLUENZA is an acute upper-respiratory infection of cattle caused by a virus. The disease is characterized by fever, serous nasal discharge, coughing, and lacrimation. The virus causing parainfluenza has been incriminated as one of the complex causing shipping fever, although additional stress factors and secondary bacteria are required for the serious disease picture to result.

Parainfluenza is of recent origin; the virus causing the condition was first isolated in 1958. However, the disease is widespread. A recent survey of market cattle held at various slaughterhouses indicated that at least 70 percent of the slaughtered cattle in all parts of the country were carrying antibodies to this disease.

Etiology

Parainfluenza is caused by a virus called myxoparainfluenza 3. This virus is sometimes the only isolate from cattle exhibiting a coughing, shipping fever-like syndrome, although its full importance as a clinical entity is not well known.

The parainfluenza virus is transmitted by droplet infection from infected to susceptible cattle. Field evaluation and serological sampling of market cattle and recently transported feeders suggest that the infection may appear as a mild or inapparent form, a specific acute respiratory infection, or a frequent concurrent invader with other bacterial and viral agents.

Factors Influencing Susceptibility

Infection with parainfluenza virus is widespread and apparently occurs during infancy, calves possibly receiving the infection from the dam. The severity of the course of the disease is affected by stressing conditions superimposed upon the virus. In colostrum-deprived calves, clinical signs, temperature response, and lesions of pneumonia have been demonstrated. In such instances the virus has been obtained from lungs with lesions of pneumonia with no complicating bacteria present.

The disease is usually benign when found as a single entity; however, with complicating bacterial agents the severity increases appreciably. Any other type of stress adds to the severity of the condition.

Symptoms

Clinical signs after exposure run a course of 5 to 8 days. Lacrimation, conjunctivitis, increased mucoid nasal discharge, inappetence, and general malaise are observed. Uncomplicated parainfluenza infection is characterized as an upper-respiratory infection of sudden onset, with a fever ranging from 104 to 108 F. Early in the infection, many animals will show an initial high fever with no other evidence of clinical illness. In some animals the elevated temperature persists for 25 to 48 hours, and may be followed by prompt recovery. Most animals remaining febrile for more than two days show anorexia and mild depression, and develop a dry, hacking cough with a clear, serous discharge.

There is concurrent hyperemia of the upper nasal and conjunctival mucous membranes with a slight flow of tears from the medial canthus of the eyes. Animals not infected with secondary bacterial invaders or with other virus infections and not subjected to undue stress promptly recover. Experimentally, this initial syndrome can be duplicated with intranasal installation of nasal culture; however, all animals so inoculated will not contract the disease. It is felt that some stress factor must be present to produce parainfluenza routinely, as observed in the field.

An increase in respiration is a common clinical observation, and labored breathing is present in some cases. There appears to be no hypersalivation in uncomplicated cases and diarrhea is not noted. Morbidity may reach 100 percent, although fatalities in uncomplicated cases are virtually nonexistent.

The temperature is monophasic and the early leukopenia is followed, in protracted cases, by a leukocytosis caused by secondary invaders. Since the infection is usually associated with stress and is of short duration, its importance rests with the fact that it lowers body resistance, thus complicating other diseases, or allows secondary bacterial invaders to produce serious disease and death losses. The virus is assumed to be of importance in the all-inclusive syndrome called shipping fever. It is thought that control of parainfluenza virus will help to abort many of the so-called epizootics of shipping fever.

Diagnosis

Diagnosis can be confirmed by virus isolation and tissue culture inhibition study. Presumptive diagnosis can be made from history, clinical symptoms, and failure to isolate any causal bacterial pathogens. An acute or mild upper-respiratory infection of short duration with concurrent leukopenia and absence of other findings is suggestive of parainfluenza.

As with other viral diseases, there are no specific therapeutic agents. Antibiotics are of value only in preventing complications due to secondary invaders. Good sanitation and management practices should be followed, and any sudden changes and stress procedures should be avoided.

Cattle exposed to an aerosol spray of parainfluenza virus produce clinical respiratory signs, including pneumonic lesions, febrile response and leukopenia.

Prevention

A successful vaccine has been produced to protect young cattle against mycoparainfluenza 3. That the vaccine has been effective is evidenced by the increase in hemagglutination-inhibition titers of vaccinated animals. Several inactivated virus vaccines are commercially available and can be used on very young calves. Two injections, intramuscularly, 21 days apart prior to shipment or stress provide solid protection.

Vaccines are recommended for the protection of healthy animals against the respiratory disease. Because of the possibility that maternal antibodies persist in calves until 4 or 5 months of age, vaccination is particularly recommended at 2 or 3 weeks prior to weaning of beef calves. When this procedure is not practical, calves should be vaccinated at weaning and held in isolation in order to develop resistance. Such resistance should be allowed to develop before the calves are stressed by shipment and/or exposure to virulent microorganisms.

Vaccination of calves showing signs of fever and respiratory distress should be delayed until after treatment has cleared up the symptoms and animals are in satisfactory condition.

22
Swine Erysipelas

SWINE erysipelas is an infectious disease of young swine, mainly, but is manifested in various ways in cattle, horses, fish, birds, laboratory animals, and humans. The causative organism, *Erysipelothrix insidiosa,* has been incriminated as the cause of nonsuppurative arthritis in lambs and calves, post-dipping lameness in sheep, acute septicemia in turkeys, and erysipeloid in man, as well as in diamond-skin disease, arthritis, and heart disease in swine.

Swine erysipelas does not often result in severe herd losses from death, but the great economic loss comes from the general unthriftiness of animals that have recovered from a mild attack or are suffering from the chronic form of the disease.

Geographically, erysipelas is worldwide in distribution and is considered a serious economic disease wherever swine are raised. In the United States, swine erysipelas has been reported from every part of the country and from most states.

Historically, the microorganism now known to cause swine erysipelas was first isolated from a mouse in Europe in 1878. The disease was first described in swine in 1885 and in humans in 1887.

In the United States, the specific organism of swine erysipelas, formerly named *Erysipelothrix rhusiopathiae,* was first isolated in 1921 by scientists at the Bureau of Animal Industry from a tissue injury in a Texas hog. The organism was obtained from a specimen of skin showing a "diamond-skin" lesion. Such lesions, typical of those described in European countries as the result of infection with swine erysipelas, had been observed in the United States for many years, but the disease was called diamond-skin disease. Swine erysipelas was not considered to be present in this country before the isolation of the organism. After this discovery, other workers isolated the organism from lesions in the joints and other tissues of the bodies of swine. It was then recognized definitely that swine erysipelas existed, apparently in a chronic form, in certain parts of the United States. While the infection appeared to be confined principally to the corn belt, it perhaps existed in many other states in a chronic, low-grade form.

Etiology

Swine erysipelas can be readily isolated from all tissues of pigs showing symptoms of the disease and from the tonsils of normal swine.

The causative microorganism, *Erysipelothrix insidiosa,* is small and rod-shaped, either straight or curved. It is gram-positive and may have a beaded appearance when viewed under a microscope. It is nonsporeforming, nonmotile, and may form long filaments that do not branch. It survives for long periods in decaying flesh and in water, and is resistant to such preservative processes as salting, smoking and pickling. The bacterium is susceptible to caustic soda and the hypochlorites, but is resistant to formaldehyde, phenol, hydrogen peroxide and alcohol.

The microorganism causing swine erysipelas is considered by many to be a saprophyte and to live and multiply in the soil when conditions are favorable. The bacterium will multiply well in warm alkaline soil containing considerable amounts of humus, but will die rapidly in acid soil.

Transmission

Swine erysipelas is an insidious disease, and the manner in which it spreads is not entirely understood. It is likely, however, that the disease requires considerable time to make any appreciable headway when introduced into an uncontaminated area. In certain parts of the United States it has probably existed in a chronic form for many years, gradually increasing in virulence until favorable conditions prevail, at which time it is manifested by the acute type of the disease.

Since the bacteria can survive for long periods in certain soils, the recurrence of swine erysipelas can readily be brought about by conditions favorable to the microorganisms. On some farms where infection exists, the disease may recur irregularly over a period of several years, although it may not appear on other farms where the soil is similarly infected. No satisfactory explanation has been made for these differences. Once an infection has appeared on a farm, however, a potential danger exists that it will reappear in subsequent years.

It is not definitely known whether infection proceeds directly from animal to animal or whether the bacteria excreted by an infected animal must pass some part of their life outside the animal body, or otherwise undergo some change, before they are capable of reproducing the disease in susceptible animals. It is generally agreed that cultures of the bacteria will reproduce the disease only occasionally when injected into swine. It is also generally held that some unknown factor in addition to the microorganism itself is necessary to bring about infection. The erysipelas microorganism enters the body primarily through ingestion with contaminated feed and water. The infective agent may also gain entry through abrasions on the skin and mucous membranes; it has been theorized that it may enter the mucosa through lesions caused by parasites. Insect vectors have also been incriminated in the dissemination of this disease to experimental animals, but the significance of this to the farmer is unknown.

During an attack of the disease, the causative agent can be found in the blood, urine, and feces. Thus the surroundings of the animals soon become heavily contaminated. Animals affected with the chronic form of the disease may also pass it on to others.

The swine erysipelas microorganism may be harbored in some parts of the bodies of apparently healthy animals, i.e. the tonsils and parts of the intestinal tract. Possibly this is a result of a previous mild infection and recovery, or the organisms may have been picked up from contaminated soil without resulting infection. Such healthy animals may possibly be dangerous to others or may subsequently develop the disease themselves if their resistance is lowered by stress.

The disease occurs most often during the spring, summer and fall, every year, because in this country sows farrow every month of the year and thus there is a continuous supply of new pigs susceptible to infection.

In the case of arthritis in lambs and calves, the causative agent, *Erysipelothrix insidiosa,* gains entry into the body through slight wounds and scratches and through the untreated navel at birth. Microorganisms may also gain entry at the time of castration, docking, or dehorning unless care is taken to disinfect all wounds and to control the dust in sheep pens and holding yards.

Erysipelothrix insidiosa is a common contaminant of dipping vats to rid range sheep and cattle of external parasites. Such vats provide a focus from which the microorganisms gain entry into the animal body through small cuts and abrasions, leading to post-dipping lameness. The bacteria localize in the joints and in the laminae of the hoof to produce the lesions causing the lameness.

Factors Influencing Susceptibility

Swine of all ages are susceptible to the disease, from suckling pigs to adult animals. The causative microorganism has also been found to affect a variety of fish, birds and animals, including man. In some parts of this country, the disease is of economic importance in both sheep and turkeys. That the bacterium is infective to man is evidenced by the number of cases reported in veterinarians, butchers, and livestock handlers, for whom it is considered an occupational hazard. The so-called fish handlers' disease is caused by infection with the swine-erysipelas microorganism found on the skin of many salt-water fish.

Although it does not bear spores, the erysipelas microorganism contains a waxy substance which is resistant to adverse conditions. In a cool, dark place it will remain active for a month or longer. In smears on glass exposed to direct sunlight, it will survive only a few days, but will remain alive for many days in water. The microorganism is very sensitive to heat, however. At 111 F it is destroyed in 4 days, at 125 F in 15 minutes, and at 130 to 137 F (far below ordinary cooking temperatures) in several minutes.

Living erysipelas microorganisms have been found in putrid material after four months. In the flesh of swine, the bacteria are resistant to destruction and have been found living in a carcass buried for 280 days. The microorganisms are only slowly destroyed by salting and pickling, and they have been found alive after 26 days in strong brine.

Since the disease often manifests itself in a low-grade infection, and since it has been shown that animals affected with the chronic form may, in certain circumstances, pass it on to normal hogs, it is apparent that animals with mild infection should be removed from the herd when discovered.

Stress is a factor in erysipelas. Swine experiments have indicated that both vitamin deficiency and ascariasis favor development of erysipelas and may account for some sporadic cases in winter. It has been proved that the incidence of the disease is lowest during the winter months and highest in the hot summer. Whether high temperature and humidity increase the pathogenesis of the microorganism or decrease the animals' resistance, or whether both are factors, has not been determined.

Although swine of all ages are susceptible to erysipelas, suckling piglets of immune dams are not affected for the first few weeks after birth. It has also been postulated that when the dam is affected with chronic arthritis the period of passive immunity will last until the piglets are three to four months of age. However, young pigs are most susceptible to the disease, and swine over three years of age are rarely affected. Older animals acquire immunity following either subclinical or inapparent infection.

Factors with a direct bearing on susceptibility are often one or more of the following: (1) virulence of the bacteria, (2) natural resistance of the pigs to the infection due to maternal antibodies or to subclinical exposure, (3) genetic influences, or (4) stress. Stress as a factor of susceptibility may be related to nutrition, atmospheric conditions, overall sanitation on the property, and the virulence of the bacteria in the natural environment. Because the disease-causing bacteria are present on the tonsils and excreted from the intestinal tract of normal pigs, it is possible for swine to be reinfected following weather conditions favorable for reproduction of the microorganisms in the soil, as it has been demonstrated that the saprophytic development takes place in the top four inches of the soil. Thus, rooting pigs are exposed to great numbers of the infecting microorganisms.

Factors altering the physiological state of the pig can often be associated with an outbreak of swine erysipelas. Such predisposing causes are fatigue, sudden changes in diet, excessive fattening, exposure to cold, high humidity or warm temperatures, and overfeeding with succulent, high-energy feed.

In handling diseases of swine, owners should always contact state and local veterinarians; this is particularly important in combating actual or suspected outbreaks of swine erysipelas.

Symptoms

The clinical symptoms of swine erysipelas appear in acute, subacute and chronic forms although subclinical, inapparent, or unobserved signs may occur.

Acute Swine Erysipelas

This condition is characterized by sudden onset, and many swine in the herd may be affected at the same time. Only a few may be visibly sick, while others may run high temperatures (105 to 110 F). At the higher temperatures some pigs will shiver as though chilled. Affected hogs lie in their bedding, and, although their eyes are clear and they appear alert, they are reluctant to move. If forcibly disturbed, they start off with considerable activity but protest loudly. Since the tissues of the joints are involved in the disease process, many infected swine are undoubtedly in pain when they walk. They make an effort to keep their feet under them, which makes the backbone appear long and strongly arched. After moving about a bit, they drop down on their bedding again. Where considerable swelling at a joint is noted, there may be exostoses (bony growths) which do not disappear when the disease subsides. Animals thus affected are the so-called knotty-legged hogs, or chronics, which harbor the disease organisms in their joints and may act as spreaders of the infection.

Most animals are reluctant to eat in the early stages of the disease, and will cease eating altogether as the condition progresses. Often infected pigs will stop eating and regurgitate. The feces will become hard and scanty but later diarrhea may develop. Diarrhea is more common in young animals than in older animals.

Several hogs may die quite suddenly. They may appear well at feeding time one evening and be found dead the next morning. There have been cases where entire herds have died; this is rare at present in this country, although it is not uncommon in unvaccinated herds in erysipelas districts of other countries. As a rule only a few hogs die, some make a complete recovery, and the rest remain unthrifty chronics. The mortality is rarely over 10 percent, but in any given outbreak the morbidity may approach 100 percent.

In hogs acutely ill with swine erysipelas, shortness of breath caused by pulmonary edema (a waterlogged condition of the lungs) may be noted. At times swellings about the snout make breathing difficult. Nausea and vomiting are not uncommon. Some 24 to 48 hours after the onset of the disease irregular red patches, neither tender to the touch nor swollen, may be noted on the lighter parts of the skin. Such areas may remain localized or may enlarge and run together until the greater part of the body surface is involved. Death is sudden, usually preceded by respiratory distress brought about by the pulmonary edema and heart weakness. The temperature drops, and the mucous membranes become cyanotic.

The so-called diamond-skin disease, characterized by regular rhomboidal lesions, sometimes appears in acute cases, in which event the affected swine die within three days after the onset of the disease. Such lesions on the skin are often associated, however, with a less severe type of swine erysipelas where the symptoms are milder and rapidly subside after the appearance of the characteristic skin eruption. Unless complications set in, hogs affected with the mild type of erysipelas usually recover within two weeks. Where the diamond-skin lesions extend over considerable areas, however, there may be a dry gangrenous sloughing of large portions of skin. The ears and tail are often lost in this way. Loss of the tail, which is the more frequent, may be the only apparent evidence of infection past or present. Skin lesions are difficult to see except on light-colored breeds of hogs or on the light parts of dark breeds.

The swine that do not die of the disease are often left in a condition unprofitable to the owner. Many have swollen joints, and these animals are discounted by packer-buyers. Hogs that do not develop enlarged joints may become dehydrated and gaunt. These are often called race-horse pigs by owners, because they eat a great deal but do not fatten as profitably as normal hogs. (Swollen joints may appear as an independent manifestation of the disease. All joints may be enlarged, but those of the knee, hock, and toes are most frequently affected.)

At times the only indication of infection is a dry, scaly dermatitis, nonparasitic in character, which fails to clear up in response to changes of feed or the application of parasiticides. Such lesions disappear as a rule upon the administration of specific antiserum, alone or in combination with living culture, or with antibiotic treatment.

Mortality is generally highest in the 1- to 3-month-old age group; but, again, all ages are susceptible. In the peracute cases death may occur without noticeable symptoms. Most often death occurs 3 to 7 days following the first signs of sickness. If the animal lives beyond that period, it either recovers or becomes a chronically infected carrier. Mortality is low among chronic carriers except in those affected with valvular endocarditis.

Subacute Erysipelas

This condition exhibits clinical symptoms less severe in effect than the acute. The swine do not appear ill; temperatures may not be elevated as high or as long; appetite may be unaffected; skin lesions may appear but will be less evident and easily missed; and, if visibly sick, the pigs will not remain so for the same length of time as the acutely affected.

Chronic Erysipelas

This follows acute infection and is characterized by necrotic changes involving loss of portions of the skin, ears, tail, and feet. Valvular changes in the heart occur and, of most importance, arthritis appears.

The areas of necrotic skin are dark, dry, and firm; they eventually become separated from the healing underlying tissue and fall off, leaving an ugly scar. Secondary infection usually occurs and slows the healing process, which extends over many weeks.

Localization of the infection on the heart valves can give rise to symptoms of cardiac insufficiency and will be most noticeable following exertion.

Chronic arthritis results in joints with various degrees of stiffness and enlargement. Interference with locomotion ranges from slight to complete, depending upon extent of damage and number of joints involved. It has been observed that apparently healthy pigs in affected herds may develop arthritis in spite of treatment, at a later date. All chronic cases of swine erysipelas are the result of some degree of acute infection.

Acute nonsuppurative arthritis in lambs and calves is manifested by painful, slightly swollen hock, stifle, elbow, knee, and hoof joints. Although most cases recover in a few weeks, growth rate in young animals is adversely affected by their unwillingness to move about and graze. In a few lambs, the infection persists and causes permanent enlargement of the joints. Such animals are usually unthrifty and many are condemned when sent to slaughter.

Most outbreaks follow such traumatic events as castration, dehorning, and shearing. The erysipelas microorganism gains entrance through skin wounds and localizes in the joints. The incubation period is constant and lameness is noted 9 to 10 days following exposure.

Post-dipping lameness is prevalent in older sheep and is an extension of infection which gains entry into the body through small cuts or abrasions on the feet and legs. These small wounds result from grass and wire cuts, or from contact with the rough surface of the dipping vats. The erysipelas microorganism is a common contaminant and will reproduce in most dipping solutions unless adequate copper sulfate is added. Once the bacteria gain entrance, the resulting infection spreads to the laminae of the hoof, causing acute pain and lameness.

Erysipeloid is a wound infection in humans due to *Erysipelothrix insidiosa.* The incubation period is 2 to 5 days, and is usually manifested by a localized, swollen, hot and painful lesion. In some cases the infection may extend to nearby joints, but in most cases there is no suppuration and inflammation subsides in a few days. In rare instances there may be a generalized septicemia accompanied by skin eruptions.

Pathology

In most instances, the microorganism causing swine erysipelas enters the body by way of the digestive tract. However, in a significant number of cases the bacteria gain entry through the skin. Regardless of route of entry, the microorganisms multiply rapidly and bacteremia results in less than 24 hours. The severity of the infection is determined by the degree of virulence of the bacteria and the resistance or susceptibility of the host.

Few pathological lesions distinguish acute swine erysipelas from other septicemias, with the exception of individual skin lesions. Lymph nodes may be enlarged, the liver and spleen may be congested, and the mucosa of the stomach and small intestine may be slightly inflamed. If the joints are involved, there will be an increase in the amount of fluid and the tissue within the joint capsule may appear inflamed.

Swine afflicted with the chronic type of erysipelas have enlargement of one or more joints, with an increase in synovial fluid and thickening of the joint tissues. In severe cases the joints may be calcified and ankylosed. A gangrenous process may involve the skin, the ears, the tail, and the feet. Many internal organs show evidence of chronic inflammation, and there will often be vegetations on the heart valves; the localization of the microorganisms, and the irritation they cause, produce granulation tissue and fibrin which adhere to the valves. Such vegetations often interfere with normal heart function and lead to the death of the host.

In cases of nonsuppurative polyarthritis in lambs and calves, post-dipping lameness in sheep and erysipeloid in man, the causative agent enters the body via a skin wound, rapidly multiplies, and causes a generalized bacteremia. As with swine, severity of infection varies with the virulence of the bacteria and the resistance of the host; however, in most instances there is extension of the infection with localization in the joints. The pathological appearance of the affected joints is similar to that seen in swine.

Diagnosis

Diagnosis in the field is usually based upon a history of sudden illness and other symptoms, prevalence of the disease in the area or on the farm, and postmortem findings.

The diagnosis of swine erysipelas presents difficulties, but in areas where it has become prevalent veterinarians, through clinical observations supported by laboratory findings, have been able to recognize it with a fair degree of accuracy. The disease is at times confusing, however, because it may manifest itself in many ways. The problem is one for the consideration of a veterinarian.

Symptoms and manifestations aiding in diagnosis are sudden onset, typical skin discoloration, dehydration, evidence of pain on moving, reluctance to move unless forcibly aroused, enlarged joints, eczema, sloughing of patches of skin, high temperatures. The eyes may be clear and the squeal vigorous.

Specimens from suspected outbreaks of swine erysipelas may be forwarded to a diagnostic laboratory for bacteriological examination. Generally, laboratory tests are considered to be more applicable to herd problems than to the diagnosis of the disease in individual animals. When erysipelas is suspected in a herd, a number of animals should be bled and the diagnosis delayed until the representative serological picture of the herd has been obtained. It must be remembered that the chronic form of swine erysipelas may be present in a herd also affected with some other acute disease, and that a positive identification of the swine erysipelas bacterium does not rule out the possibility of another infection.

Treatment

The biological control of swine erysipelas may be attempted by several methods: (1) hyperimmune serum, (2) serum plus virulent culture of *E. insidiosa,* (3) avirulent or attenuated bacterins. The use of serum plus culture is not currently approved in all states; the serum-culture product is available only in certain states where swine erysipelas is common and disease control authorities have authorized its use. Commercial manufacturers of this product are allowed to sell the product only in those states where its use is authorized, and, in some instances, only when the order is accompanied by a certificate of permission from the chief veterinary official of the state. Most of these states are in the midwestern part of the country. The restrictions on the sale of the culture have been imposed in the belief that it is unwise to distribute virulent organisms in areas where swine erysipelas is not prevalent.

Where the simultaneous serum-plus-culture method is approved, swine may be injected at any time and at any age when an outbreak appears. The product will not cause abortion in sows when used during the later stages of pregnancy. Although baby pigs suckling immune dams are temporarily immune, they may be inoculated at 2 to 3 weeks of age. The duration of immunity on the average lasts for six months, and in most instances this will be long enough for the pigs to reach market weight. Gilts have been found to be immune for up to eight months. Thus, breeding stock may be inoculated at later dates for more persistent immunity.

Hyperimmune serum may be used at any time in swine because there is no danger of spreading the disease by this means. Normal pigs injected with serum receive immediate passive immunity of about two weeks' duration.

Bacterins are safe because they do not infect other species of animals but do confer an immunity of relatively short duration. In most instances, this is a useful procedure as the pigs will be protected until they are marketed. Doses of 10 to 30 cc of serum are used as early in the course of the disease as possible when an outbreak occurs.

Live-culture strains of swine erysipelas bacteria of low virulence but high immunizing potential are currently being used extensively in the United States in avirulent vaccines. An oral type of vaccine of low virulence is also available commercially. These vaccines usually provide immunity for up to one year. Serum alone is effective only when given early in the acute stage of the disease; after the disease once establishes itself and becomes chronic, the value of serum is limited.

Prevention

Swine erysipelas is difficult to eradicate due to the insidious and widespread distribution of the microorganism, its association with a wide variety of animals, and its ability to adapt to either a parasitic or saprophytic existence. The control of carrier animals is of utmost importance to the farmer, and no replacements should be brought onto a farm without a thorough knowledge of the herd of origin and without isolating the new animals for at least 30 days.

Animals should be maintained in uncontaminated areas under modern conditions of practical husbandry where special attention is paid to housing, nutrition, sanitation, and immunization procedures. When an outbreak does occur, treatment should be initiated as quickly as possible, dead animals safely buried, exposed animals isolated, and the exposed area decontaminated before restocking with susceptible animals.

23
Hog Cholera

THE ANNUAL expense of hog cholera to the swine industry in the United States exceeds 50 million dollars. This disease occurs in every state and in every country where hogs are raised, except in those that have undertaken vigorous and continuing eradication measures. In the United States, hog cholera is the target of an all-out federal-state cooperative eradication program.

Hog cholera, also known as swine fever, is a highly infectious, contagious, generally fatal disease caused by a filterable virus. It is characterized by generalized hemorrhages, loss of appetite, fever, reluctance to move, high morbidity, and high mortality. The infection usually runs an acute course but may become chronic. Lesions may be mild or absent in chronic cases but severe to extreme in acute and subacute infections.

Swine are the natural hosts for the virus of hog cholera and are the only animals in which the disease is known to occur naturally. Although individual animals may be immune, all breeds of swine are susceptible to the virus even though there may be a degree of susceptibility due to the virulence of the virus.

Historically, hog cholera has been reported to be a serious problem in this country since 1830. Some reports indicate that the disease was prevalent before that time in Ohio, but there is some confusion about the dates. In any event, hog cholera has devastated the hog population of the United States by cyclic epidemics several times during the past 150 years. Because of conflicting reports and theories, it was not recognized as a specific disease until 1860, while the virus nature of the disease was not recognized until 1903. Five years later U.S. Department of Agriculture scientists developed a virus-serum immunization program which was widely used in the midwest. In 1940 a tissue vaccine was introduced, and in 1942 the crystal-violet vaccine was introduced and widely used. With the beginning of the cooperative hog cholera eradication program in 1962, the interstate shipment of modified virus vaccine was halted.

Etiology

The etiological agent causing hog cholera is a filterable virus which may be found in the blood, urine, feces, and nasal and oral secretions of hogs infected with hog cholera. The virus has a particle size of 22 to 30 $m\mu$, is classified among the smaller of the filterable agents, and appears to be spherical in shape. It will grow well in living swine tissue and has been adapted for growth in rabbit tissue, but will not grow on embryonated chick eggs.

The virus is destroyed by a 2 percent creosol solution in 60 minutes, and a 3 percent solution of sodium hydroxide in combination with 2 percent milk of lime kills the virus in 15 minutes. Heat will rapidly kill the virus, but it will withstand freezing and will persist for months in dry or refrigerated tissue.

The virus lives best in an acid solution. It will survive in meat products for months and will live at least six months in pickled, salted and smoked meats. Putrefactive processes destroy the virus in about five days, except in the bone marrow where it survives at least 15 days. When it enters the pig's body, the virus passes to the bloodstream and develops there to produce a viremia or blood infection. The blood of the pig becomes infectious within 24 hours after the virus enters its body. The virus may be demonstrated in the urine and feces usually within 48 hours. The secretions of the eyes and nose become infectious by the third day.

Transmission

Hog cholera does not occur in a herd unless the specific virus is introduced. The most certain way to do that is to bring infected hogs into a herd. Any hog added to a herd must be considered a potential source of danger until it has been isolated long enough for the disease to develop if the hog had been exposed to the virus. Swine vaccinated with either virulent virus or with modified live-virus vaccines may spread hog cholera to susceptible hogs.

Because infected swine discharge the virus from their bodies in urine, feces, and secretions of the nose and eyes, manure, bedding and dirt are contaminated.

Infected hogs shipped to market to get rid of them, or hogs recently vaccinated with virulent vaccine, may contaminate public stockyards, unloading chutes, railroad cars, and thus provide means by which susceptible hogs are exposed to hog cholera.

Hog cholera may be carried to a farm in contaminated feed, litter, manure, or other material from public stockyards, from infected farms, or in improperly cleaned trucks. Infected material may adhere to other animals, wagon wheels, tires, and shoes.

Apparently healthy carriers may spread cholera by both direct and indirect contact. Bloodsucking parasites may also play a role in transmission of this virus disease when it occurs in herds in isolated areas for the first time.

Garbage containing scraps of uncooked pork and bone also can serve as a means of transmission if fed to a susceptible herd.

Factors Influencing Susceptibility

Early studies indicated that sex, age, type of housing, feed, weather, and chemicals were not factors in the susceptibility of swine to hog cholera. Swine of all ages are subject to infection by the virus, although there may be some individual and variable resistance to the disease. Young suckling pigs nursing immune dams are protected for a short period of time, but the antibodies found in colostrum may persist long enough to interfere with the stimulation of active immunity by vaccination. Care must be exercised in the selection of a vaccine to prevent this from happening.

Stress from any cause has a bearing on susceptibility, as the lowering of general body

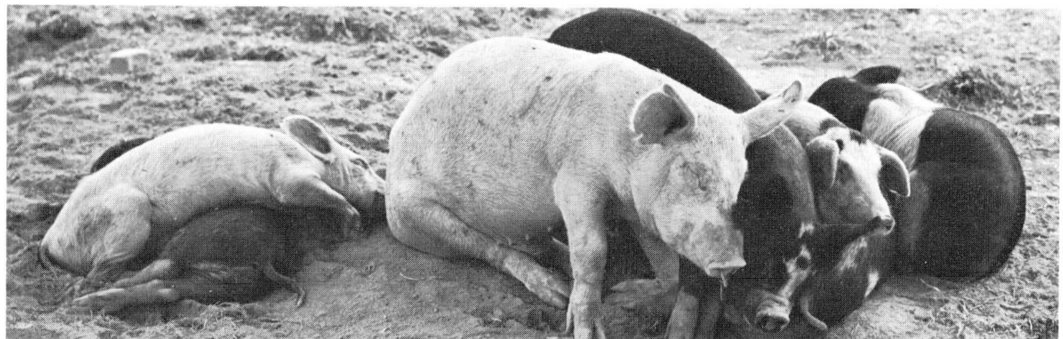

FIG. 14. A distressing picture of young hogs suffering from hog cholera huddled in a characteristic manner in the barnyard.

resistance may predispose to the disease. Hog cholera appears to be cyclic in appearance, being most prevalent in the hot summer months.

The severity of symptoms will vary depending on the virulence of the virus. Investigators have recognized that a group of strains is characterized by high virulence and another by low virulence. Hog cholera of low virulence is becoming increasingly prevalent; in some states in the midwest, over one-third of the outbreaks are apparently caused by viruses of low virulence.

Symptoms

Hog cholera has been recognized in four types or syndromes: peracute, acute, subacute, and chronic.

The peracute type is incriminated when hogs are found dead or die within a few days after the first symptoms are noticed.

With the acute type, animals die in 5 to 19 days. The subacute type lasts from 20 to 30 days with symptoms similar to the acute type, and, in chronic disease, the course is protracted and the symptoms milder. However, survivors of the latter two types are usually stunted in growth, fail to gain efficiently, and are a source of economic loss to the producer.

The incubation period for hog cholera virus is 5 to 8 days, but may vary from 2 to 12 days. Often the virus is found in body secretions within two days following entry of the virus into the body.

The first symptoms usually noted by a producer are a reluctance to move about and a tendency to huddle as if seeking warmth. Sick pigs usually eat very little and have a fever ranging from 105 to 108 F. In the early stages there may be constipation but diarrhea is associated with this disease. In the later stages there will be weakness of the hindquarters, discoloration of the skin of the abdomen due to hyperemia, and dehydration.

Pathology

The virus of hog cholera is invasive as well as virulent. It apparently enters the body through either the upper digestive tract or the respiratory system. Under natural conditions, it is quite probable that most infections develop from exposure of the oral mucous membranes to virulent viruses contained in infected food or water. The virus is capable of penetrating the unbroken membranes of the respiratory and tonsillar areas and entering the bloodstream.

Once the virus has penetrated into the tissues, it is picked up by either the lymphatics or the capillaries and becomes attached to white blood cells. The infected cells carry the virus to regional lymph nodes, where it causes destruction of some cells, hemorrhage, and swelling of the nodes. About three days after exposure, the leukocyte level of the blood is appreciably reduced and a temperature develops. The virus rapidly spreads to other organs and glands, causing small localized hemorrhages accompanied by swelling and ulceration in the mucous membranes of the large intestines. The hemorrhages are due to degeneration of endothelial cells of capillary walls. Lesions produced in the capillaries of the lungs and intestines predispose the animals to secondary bacterial invaders. The virus will be found in the blood, urine, feces, and ocular, nasal, and pulmonary exudates.

Postmortem lesions will be insignificant in the peracute type of the disease. In the acute disease, hemorrhage of the circulatory system and swollen lymph nodes are the most significant gross lesions. Large purplish areas are often seen on the lungs and small pinpoint hemorrhages are characteristically found on the surface of the kidney.

Chronic cases usually do not exhibit the lesions of classical hog cholera except for the button ulcers in the large intestines.

Diagnosis

The field diagnosis of hog cholera is based upon the recent history of the herd with particular reference to exposure, observance of high morbidity and mortality, the vaccination status of the herd, and significant symptoms and lesions.

Laboratory confirmation is based upon evidence of leukopenia, microscopic examination of the brain for perivascular cuffing and the fluorescent antibody test to demonstrate the virus.

Positive diagnosis in controversial cases depends upon inoculating suspected material into both susceptible and immunized swine. Inoculations of animals other than swine are of no value in the diagnosis of hog cholera.

Treatment

The first measures used to control hog cholera in the United States included the use of a virulent virus plus anti-hog-cholera serum. This method was useful in the control of large outbreaks, but at the same time was the means by which the virus was seeded in fields, pens, barns, and other animal enclosures. The virulent virus vaccine has now been banned in all states and is no longer available. At the present time three types of prophylactic agents are available for use in this country: anti-hog-cholera serum, modified live-virus vaccine, and killed-virus vaccine. Each has its uses, but for most effective results hog-cholera vaccine should be used only in healthy animals. Because of individual differences, degree of immunity may vary from animal to animal.

Anti-Hog-Cholera Serum

Anti-hog-cholera serum (or antibody concentrate), made from the blood of hogs highly immunized against the disease, provides immediate immunity to nonexposed hogs. This immunity lasts two to three weeks or more, depending on the pig and the amount of serum used. Since the effect is temporary, it is normally used only to provide emergency protection to susceptible pregnant sows or to pigs afflicted with some other disease and therefore too weak to tolerate full vaccination. Use of too much serum may block action of other vaccines, thus preventing development of immunity.

Modified Live-Virus Vaccine

Modified live-virus vaccines are prepared by repeated passage of virulent virus through different hosts until the disease-producing ability of the virus is greatly reduced.

To produce immediate and lasting protection, it is recommended that anti-hog-cholera serum be used with all modified live-virus vaccines.

Pregnant or nursing sows should not be vaccinated with these vaccines. Pigs freshly vaccinated should be isolated from unvaccinated animals and from pregnant or nursing sows for a period of 21 days.

Killed-Virus Vaccine

Killed-virus vaccines are made from live virus inactivated by chemical treatment; there is no danger of spread. Anti-hog-cholera serum should not be used with these vaccines.

Killed-virus vaccines produce immunity lasting several months. However, since immunity does not become established for about three weeks after vaccination, these vaccines should not be used on pigs that have been exposed to hog cholera.

To obtain maximum immunity, pigs must be fully susceptible. Suckling pigs acquire some resistance from immune sows, and therefore should not be vaccinated until at least two weeks after weaning. Breeding stock should be revaccinated every six months.

Killed-virus vaccines can be safely used on pregnant sows and unthrifty pigs, if vaccination is necessary.

The use of anti-hog-cholera serum and the various hog-cholera vaccines is subject to certain other limitations. For example, pigs with anemia may develop shock following the use of anti-hog-cholera serum. In rare cases, some normal pigs in a herd may be particularly susceptible to hog cholera. Vaccination except with killed-virus vaccine may cause these animals to develop the disease, even though the same vaccine immunizes other pigs. Infectious diseases (swine influenza, bacterial pneumonia, swine dysentery, malignant edema, swine pox, erysipelas, enteritis, rhinitis, and other diseases) may reduce a pig's ability to develop immunity.

Pigs treated with anti-hog-cholera serum alone, and vaccinated later with modified live-virus vaccine—with or without serum—may not be immunized, because the protective antibodies of the first serum treatment may not have disappeared by the time the pigs are vaccinated. These antibodies block the action of the vaccine and prevent immunization.

Prevention

Due to the great economic losses to the swine industry caused by hog cholera year after year, a national hog-cholera eradication program has been initiated through state-federal cooperative efforts. The program consists of four phases with the objective of completely eradicating hog cholera from this country. The state-federal cooperative program was begun in 1962, and has a target date for all "hog cholera free" states by 1972.

Ending vaccination has long been recognized as a necessary, but crucial, step in the eradication campaign. Vaccines help control hog cholera but, because they can also cause the disease, vaccines must be eliminated when the risks outweigh the benefits.

Federal regulations now establish the cutoff dates for interstate shipment of hog cholera vaccines as of July 1, 1969, and for vaccinated hogs as of January 1, 1970. Elimination of vaccination will eliminate the major cost of hog cholera and, hopefully, management will prevent the disease.

The state-federal eradication program is based upon nine points: vaccination, shipping regulations, reporting, quarantine, disposal, disinfection, cooking of garbage, prohibition of virulent virus, and information. Details of this program can be obtained from agricultural extension agents or local veterinarians.

24
Brucellosis

BRUCELLOSIS is a contagious bacterial disease of cattle, swine, goats, sheep, man, and secondarily of other animals. It is characterized by abortion, sterility, genital infection, and the formation of localized lesions in various body tissues. It is of public-health importance due to the debilitating disease (undulent fever) in man. All breeds of cattle, including beef cattle, are susceptible to the disease. The frequent occurrence of brucellosis in dairy cattle is associated with close housing and intensive management methods, rather than with susceptibility factors. Likewise, the frequency in swine is due to foraging and eating habits rather than to particular susceptibility.

Brucellosis in goats is no longer a significant problem in this country because of the successful eradication of the disease by the test-and-slaughter method. Sheep brucellosis has not been a problem in the United States, although it is a problem in some places in Europe.

Historically, brucellosis was recognized as a contagious disease for many years before the causative bacteria were isolated. The *Brucella* microorganisms were first isolated in 1887 from humans in the Mediterranean area, suffering from a malady known as Malta fever. Later, the organisms were isolated from goat's milk and cheese in Malta, in 1905, and named *Brucella melitensis.* In 1897, *Brucella abortus* was isolated from aborted fetal membranes and fetal stomach contents in Denmark. Brucellosis of swine, formerly called contagious abortion of swine, was recognized as a specific disease when *Brucella suis* was isolated in 1914 in the United States. In 1930, a strain of *Brucella abortus* of low virulence but good immunizing properties was isolated and ultimately used to make Strain 19 bacterin, used worldwide to immunize young calves against the disease.

Geographically, brucellosis occurs in most swine-raising areas of the United States and in most countries of the world where swine exist in the domesticated or wild state. The disease is encountered in cattle throughout the world and is of major economic importance to cattle producers.

Etiology

Although each class of livestock is primarily infected with a particular species of Brucella, each of the three *Brucella* species is capable of infecting any class of livestock and humans. Thus, brucellosis must be considered as one disease-control problem for all livestock, not three different control problems. All three species are related serologically, morphologically and culturally.

Brucella suis is the primary cause of brucellosis in swine as it is the species most often isolated from infected herds. However, *Brucella melitensis* and *Brucella abortus* are capable of causing infection in swine under natural conditions of exposure.

Brucella abortus is the principal cause of brucellosis in cattle, although the other species have been isolated upon numerous occasions.

All species of Brucella affecting livestock are coccoid in shape, gram-negative, and have characteristic growth requirements. *Brucella abortus* requires increased carbon dioxide tension for isolation, while the others grow well under ordinary laboratory conditions. Although all species are similar, they exhibit individual differences to certain dyes.

All species are susceptible to pasteurization temperatures, and will quickly die if exposed to drying and direct sunlight. However, the bacteria are resistant outside the animal body when maintained in cool, moist surroundings. They have been found to remain viable in aborted fetuses at freezing or near-freezing temperatures for up to 824 days, although such conditions are seldom present under normal circumstances. The microorganisms are also susceptible to most common disinfectants if properly used.

Transmission

The bacteria causing brucellosis are shed in the milk, especially the colostrum, and in uterine discharges several days before abortion and up to several months following parturition. Some adult females may spread bacteria during the entire gestation period without exhibiting any other sign of the disease.

Brucellosis in cattle is commonly transmitted by close association with contaminated animals and environment. Fetuses and placental material resulting from abortion caused by brucellosis are heavily infected with the disease-causing bacteria, and are readily available to any other susceptible animal. The contaminated material may remain infective for a long time, thus increasing chances of spread. Since *Brucella* commonly enters the body through the alimentary canal, the disease may be spread by animals licking the genital organs or the placenta or vaginal discharge of an infected animal. The conjunctiva and mucous membranes of the nose, as well as the vagina, provide for convenient entry. Infection may also result from the ingestion of contaminated grass, water, and dry roughage.

Transmission from bull to cow during natural service has been demonstrated, although this route of infection is rare unless the bull is shedding viable bacteria in the semen. Semen from a contaminated bull used for intrauterine artificial insemination is a common source of infection.

Swine brucellosis is transmitted chiefly by direct contact. Therefore, an infected animal from a new herd can spread the disease into the herd where it is introduced. An animal may become a carrier if, at a show or fair, it comes in contact with carriers.

The disease is transmitted from boar to female during natural service. Ingestion of the products of abortion, food and water contaminated with vaginal exudates of infected and aborting females, milk from infected sows or gilts, or other infected material is an easy means of entry into the alimentary canal.

Young animals born to dams that are carriers will be covered with viable bacteria and may spread the disease through a crowded barnyard. Calves and piglets nursing from infected dams may spread the bacteria throughout an area with their feces, particularly if unconfined.

It is often difficult to discover how brucellosis has gained entry into a herd. However, it must be realized that the infected female, usually a healthy carrier, is the most common vector for spread, both within the herd and from herd to herd. Precautions must be exercised to insure that new animals introduced into a herd are free of brucellosis, and to quarantine and test the new animals to be sure that they were not incubating the disease at the time of purchase.

Dogs, birds, and feral animals may occasionally be incriminated as spreaders of brucellosis by dragging infected, aborted fetuses from one property to another. Improperly cleaned vehicles used to transport animals may be sources of infection for susceptible animals, as may unsanitary sales barns, show rings, and holding yards.

Factors Influencing Susceptibility

Season of the year, climate, and weather apparently are of little significance as factors of susceptibility to brucellosis. Age and sex, however, are important. Although all males are susceptible to infection, bulls appear to be quite resistant while boars are very susceptible to brucellosis. Females are much more susceptible than males, but all females are not equally susceptible. Some are naturally immune and resist infection even if exposed to a massive dose of bacteria. Some have moderate immunity, and others have none.

Young calves and piglets appear to have a natural resistance to brucellosis and seldom become infected, although they may harbor the bacteria temporarily and spread viable microorganisms in their feces until weaned. In some instances, young animals have been infected at birth and have carried the microorganisms until maturity, at which time the usual symptoms appeared. In most instances the fetus infected in utero, however, loses the infection before reaching six months of age. Brucellosis may, therefore, be considered a disease of mature animals.

The progress of the disease is dependent upon the individual. Most animals are readily able to resist the disease before reaching sexual maturity, but as they approach maturity their susceptibility increases. Sexually mature bulls seem more resistant than sexually mature heifers or cows. Pregnant cattle are more apt to get the disease than nonpregnant ones, and their disease is more severe.

Symptoms

Of the primary symptoms of brucellosis, in cows, the act of abortion is the most characteristic, although all infected pregnant animals will not necessarily abort. In addition to abortion, the birth of weak calves, retained placenta, and vaginal discharge are prevalent symptoms. Any of these may be followed by temporary or permanent sterility or temporary infertility. In animals infected while open, symptoms are generally absent. Udder infection frequently appears in animals infected by artificial insemination. Clinical symptoms may or may not be apparent in infected bulls. The prominant signs are, generally, enlargement of one or both testicles, loss of sexual desire, and infertility. These are usually accompanied by infection of one or more of the accessory sex organs, which can be determined only by rectal examination.

If an animal has some resistance to the disease, or if the infection is of low virulence, the disease has a tendency to localize, without clinical symptoms, in the udder or supermammary glands; in these cases the bacteria may persist for life, reappearing in the uterus during pregnancies.

Usually the first suspicion of brucellosis in a herd is unexplained abortion or return to service by a previously bred female. The disease is insidious in its manifestations and the signs of impending abortion are no

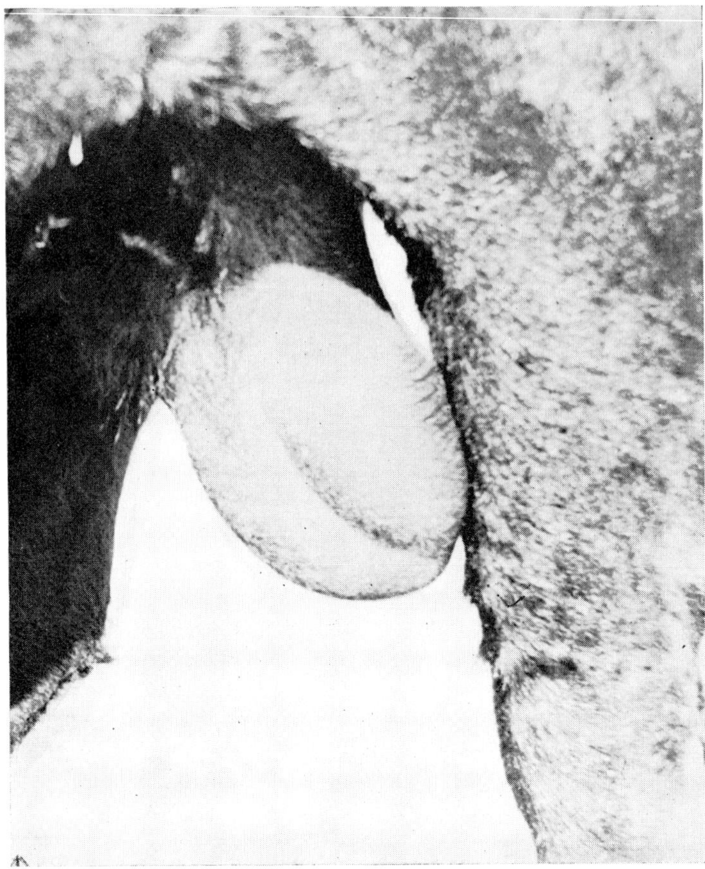

FIG. 15. Orchitis in bull due to brucellosis. (From Gibbons, W. J.: *Clinical Diagnosis of Diseases of Large Animals.* Philadelphia, Lea & Febiger, 1966.)

different from those of normal parturition, except that they may occur at any time during the gestation period depending upon the time of infection. Some females may abort early without any warning signs, although usually the abortion occurs during the latter stages of pregnancy.

The incubation period is variable and depends upon the age of the female and the stage of pregnancy at which infection occurred. The younger the fetus at the time of infection, the longer the incubation period. Experimentally, when the exact time of infection is known, abortions have occurred at varying lengths of time after two weeks of incubation.

The establishment of a carrier state in cows is usually associated with a reduction in milk production, dead calves at term, retained placenta, and metritis. Also, in this chronic stage of the disease, there may be lameness due to accumulations of bacteria in joint capsules, causing swelling and pain. In the male, there may be enlargement, hardening, and even abscess formation in the testes, with resultant pain and lowered sexual drive.

The classical clinical manifestations of *B. suis* infection are abortion, birth of stillborn or weak pigs, infertility, unilateral or bilateral orchitis, posterior paralysis, and lameness. Decreased sexual drive is occasionally observed in affected boars.

Abortions have been observed as early as 22 days following natural service to boars disseminating *B. suis* in the semen. Early abortions are usually overlooked under field conditions, and the first indication of infection is a large percentage of sows or gilts showing signs of estrus 30 to 45 days after service terminating in conception. Little or no vaginal discharge is observed with early abortions. Abortions during the middle or late stages of gestation usually occur in females that acquire infection after pregnancy has advanced past 35 or 40 days. The persistence of genital infection in females varies considerably. *Brucella suis* usually persists a minimum of one month in the nongravid uterus. In a group of sows bred to boars disseminating *B. suis* in the semen, several shed the microorganism in vaginal discharge for at least 30 months. An apparently abnormal vaginal discharge is seldom observed in sows with uterine infection. The percentage of females eventually recovering from genital infection is relatively high.

Infection of cattle with *Brucella suis* is rare; it is usually localized in the udder or nearby lymph nodes with no clinical symptoms. There is little information on *Brucella melitensis* in cattle, but limited studies show that it causes udder and uterine infection with occasional abortion.

Pathology

After they invade the body, the microorganisms enter the bloodstream and are carried to various organs and tissues where they multiply freely. The udder, uterus, testicles, seminal vesicles, lymph glands, and spleen are most often affected. Abscess formation is common in affected organs and tissues.

During pregnancy, the microorganisms localize in the supermammary lymph nodes and udder, and then infect the placenta and fetal fluids. They localize in the epithelial cells of the chorion where they cause necrosis and eventual death of the fetus, and subsequent abortion. The appearance of the placenta is leather-like, thickened, and brownish in color, with marked necrosis of the cotyledons. After or just prior to abortion, bacteria appear in the mammary glands and their lymph nodes.

In bulls and boars, bacteremia results from localized infection of the seminal vesicles, testes, and epididymis. In many males the infection becomes chronic, leading to permanent destructive changes in the testes and to infertility.

Diagnosis

The diagnosis of brucellosis is based upon isolation of infective bacteria from the vaginal exudates of aborting females, from the tissues of aborted fetuses, from semen of infected males, and from the milk of lactating females. The field diagnosis may be made by one or more diagnostic screening laboratory tests, followed by serological examination for antibodies. A rising titer is significant in adult animals, but of little value in positive diagnosis in immature animals who may have received antibodies transferred from the dam in milk.

Treatment

Viable bacterins have been shown to be of value in the control of brucellosis in cattle, but have been of little use in combating the disease in swine. When coupled with a program of test and slaughter, calfhood vaccination has been of inestimable value in eradication programs in this country.

In 1930, scientists in the U.S. Department of Agriculture isolated a strain of *Brucella* characterized by low virulence and high antigenic properties, called Strain 19, now used on a worldwide basis.

Calfhood vaccination with *Brucella abortus* Strain 19 vaccine (bacterin) is effective in increasing resistance to the disease. However, resistance is not complete in all cases, because of individual differences, and will break to some extent in the presence of massive exposure. In most calves, the immunity does not decline with the passage of time. Caution must be exercised, however, in the use of the vaccine, as some calves carry a persistent titer into adult life. This causes consternation in regulatory agencies, as it is difficult to tell the difference between a vaccination titer and a frank infection titer. Thus, older calves and adult cattle must never be vaccinated with Strain 19. Most young calves lose the vaccination titer by the time of sexual maturity, although the immunity persists for life.

Young female calves should be vaccinated between the ages of 2 to 4 months, but regulatory officials do not recommend the vaccination of bull calves. The veterinarian must vaccinate and identify all calfhood vaccinates.

Prevention

Calfhood vaccination, associated with the intensive application of milk-ring and serological tests in a manner prescribed by governmental regulatory agencies, has proved to be practical and successful in combating brucellosis on a nationwide basis. To be efficiently maintained, these procedures must be coupled with modern sanitary measures aimed at preventing contact of susceptible animals with infected animals and material.

A national cooperative swine brucellosis eradication program is currently being conducted in this country. The program is based upon a voluntary herd validation program. Details may be obtained from veterinarians.

The state-federal cooperative plan for the eradication of brucellosis in cattle is one of the most important regulatory programs now in operation in this country. The dairy industry is responsible for persistent calfhood vaccination, annual testing of adult cattle, and accurate maintenance of records in order to sell milk on the open market and to obtain the coveted "Certified Brucellosis-Free" status.

There are several options by which "Certified Brucellosis-Free" status may be obtained, but to be retained all herds must be tested according to USDA rules and regulations as set forth in *Recommended Uniform Methods and Rules—Brucellosis Eradication.* This publication may be obtained from state or federal veterinarians, or from local accredited veterinarians.

25
Leptospirosis

LEPTOSPIROSIS is an infectious bacterial disease of cattle, swine, sheep, dogs, cats, rodents, wild animals and man. The spirochetes causing the disease are enzootic in wild animals, which serve as natural reservoirs for the microorganisms. The disease may be transmitted from animal to animal and from animal to man, but progression usually stops with man.

Historically, the microorganisms causing leptospirosis were first seen in man in 1905, but the infective nature of the bacteria was not recognized until many years later. They were isolated from humans that died following rat bites, and were found in the kidneys of rats. Leptospires were isolated from cattle in 1944, and from swine about 1950, although symptoms attributed to leptospires had been recognized for many years.

Geographically, the disease now known as leptospirosis has been diagnosed worldwide in domesticated livestock, in wild animals, and even in snakes. In the United States, leptospirosis is particularly widespread in dairy cattle and swine, although persistent testing reveals that beef cattle are not immune to the disease.

Etiology

Leptospirosis is caused by one or more serotypes of bacteria called *Leptospira,* the smallest of the spiral-shaped, slender rods called spirochetes. These cells are difficult to see and are visible only with the dark-field microscope or when special stains are used.

Serotype is the term used to designate the subdivisions of the genus *Leptospira,* rather than the usual species or strains. This variance from the usual classification is based upon antigenic structure revealed by serological investigations. There are currently 70 serotypes, and more will doubtless be discovered as investigation proceeds. Only about ten of the known serotypes have been isolated in this country.

The primary cause of leptospirosis in farm

animals is *Leptospira pomona,* although other serotypes have been found in isolated outbreaks. The leptospires commonly found in the dog, *Leptospira canicola* and *Leptospira icterohaemorrhagiae,* have on occasion been isolated from cattle, swine, and man.

Leptospires are susceptible to drying, extremes of pH, and extremes of heat and cold; they will not withstand exposure to strong sunlight. They have low resistance to physical and chemical agents and are susceptible to iodine, calcium hypochlorite, and the cationic detergents.

Transmission

Carrier animals which have become urinary shedders after acute, mild, or, more often, inapparent infection serve as dangerous foci of infection. Direct infection results from contact with the urine of these shedders, while indirect transmission occurs when the bacteria are excreted into water or moist soil where susceptible animals subsequently come into contact with the contaminated environment.

Regardless of the serotype of *Leptospira,* or the species of animal involved, the symptoms produced are much the same except for variations due to individual resistance. The microorganisms gain entrance to the body through skin abrasions, through mucous membranes and conjunctiva via aerosols of infected urine splashed from hard surfaces or puddles, and through the intact skin.

Leptospirosis is spread to calves and piglets through the milk of infected dams. In adult animals the primary spread is through contaminated feed and water. Animals are infected by drinking from ponds or sluggish, slow-moving streams contaminated by urine from barnyards or feedlots. Infection may sometimes be spread from cow to cow via contaminated milking equipment.

Arthropods have been incriminated as spreaders of leptospirosis, but they are not considered to be important vectors of the disease. The spirochetes are motile, and may penetrate the unbroken skin of animals exposed to contaminated water long enough for the skin to become softened.

Leptospires may survive for several weeks in the external environment with such optimal factors as mild weather, stagnant ponds and streams, and moist neutral soil of suitable chemical composition.

Factors Influencing Susceptibility

In young animals, leptospirosis is often fulminating and fatal. In older animals, however, the disease is usually mild or inapparent. The disease occurs in all breeds and in both sexes, with age the usual determinant of the severity of the symptoms. Young calves are usually infected by their dams. Piglets, on the other hand, are infected by rooting in heavily infected soil in barnyards or feedlots. Adult cattle are often infected by contact with the urine of swine on the same property. Lambs are commonly infected when they first begin to graze on contaminated pastures where either cattle or swine have been kept.

The disease may be spread from infected herd sires to susceptible females during the breeding season. A carrier animal provides a ready source of infection for young animals produced on the property and for susceptible replacements. Swine carriers may continue to shed viable *Leptospira* in the urine for six months or more, while cattle may shed the bacteria for up to three months.

The season of the year, the climate, and the weather are not important as far as susceptibility is concerned. However, crowding animals into small areas and mixing animals of different ages do have an influence upon the spread of the disease.

Symptoms

The clinical signs and symptoms of leptospirosis vary considerably among species as well as among individuals within a species. The symptoms may resemble those of several other serious livestock diseases, thus requiring careful differential diagnosis.

Leptospirosis in cattle is characterized by fever, prostration, jaundice, blood in the urine, abnormal milk, lowered milk production, and lack of appetite.

In swine, the symptoms of leptospirosis are mild and often inapparent. Abortions and the birth of weak pigs are the most obvious and often the only evidence of the disease.

Leptospirosis is usually divided into three forms—acute, mild, and chronic—depending upon the severity and duration of the clinical signs.

The incubation period is relatively short, from 7 to 9 days. The acute form of the disease usually is seen in calves, is sudden in onset and is fatal in 2 to 10 days; animals surviving this period usually recover, but their growth rate is retarded and they are slow to gain weight. The temperature rises to 105 to 107 F and persists for up to 56 hours. There is jaundice on the second or third day, and blood in the urine is followed by anemia. Because of the fever there is lack of appetite, and rapid loss of weight. Increased respiratory rate and difficult breathing are common signs. Most of these symptoms are associated with the rapid destruction of red blood cells; when the blood count falls below two million, death is inevitable.

The acute form is usually not as severe in adult cattle as in calves, although most of the clinical signs appear. In addition, however, lactating cows develop bloody milk, with a dramatic drop in production, although the udder remains soft and pliable. Pregnant animals may abort at any stage of pregnancy, but most commonly during the last three months of gestation. Infected cows that recover usually produce dead or weak calves at term. Because the symptoms in older cattle are mild and vary greatly, the first suspicion of the disease may be associated with abortions in the herd or flock.

The mild form of leptospirosis, usually seen in older cattle, has similar but less severe symptoms. The temperature is not as high and the observable signs may persist for only a few days. The only observable signs may be a slight drop in milk production and transitory blood in the urine.

In the chronic form of the disease, microscopic changes occur in the kidneys. Although abortion may occur during the last month of pregnancy, the usual sign is a mummified fetus or a weak calf at term. Retention of the fetal membranes following abortion is a common observance. Chronic loss of weight and persistent anemia are sequelae of this form.

The acute form of leptospirosis in swine is characterized by the small number of animals developing any clinical signs of disease. The infection spreads through a herd, as evidenced by serological examination, but only a few will be acutely ill at any one time. These animals demonstrate various levels of lack of appetite, fever, and diarrhea for a period of a few days.

In the chronic form in swine, the principal signs are abortion during the latter stages of gestation and birth of weak pigs at term. Metritis and lowered fertility have been associated with the disease, as have jaundice, anemia, hyperirritability and transitory incoordination. Pigs farrowed at term but so devitalized that they die within a few hours are characteristic of this form of leptospirosis.

Pathology

Leptospires which enter the animal's body invade the circulatory system and rapidly multiply. Within 2 to 5 days, the microorganisms may be found in all organs and in the blood and urine.

Within 7 to 10 days bacteria may be demonstrated in the peripheral blood with difficulty, but antibodies may be detected in the serum. After the appearance of antibodies, the spirochetes localize in the kidney tubules and continue to multiply; they are shed from the body in urine. During the time when the

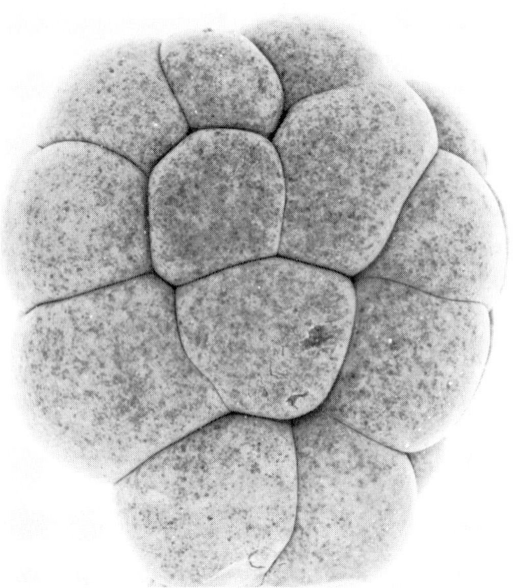

FIG. 16. Kidney of heifer affected with acute leptospirosis. (From Jensen, R., and Mackey, D. R.: *Diseases of Feedlot Cattle.* Ed. 2, Philadelphia, Lea & Febiger, 1971.)

bacteria are rapidly multiplying in the bloodstream, destruction of red blood cells causes hemoglobinuria, or red urine. At necropsy there is generalized jaundice, anemia, and mottling of the liver. The kidneys appear swollen and congested, with small pinpoint hemorrhages covering the surface. The bladder often contains dark brown urine.

Diagnosis

Diagnosis is usually based upon clinical signs and herd history, but, because of the similarity of symptoms to those of other serious diseases, a differential diagnosis may be desirable. The most rapid method of diagnosis in the field is the slide agglutination test; this is performed by a veterinarian, using serum from an animal and prepared diagnostic antigens. When more definitive diagnosis is required, a blood sample must be sent to a laboratory. The most rapid laboratory diagnosis is based upon demonstrating antibodies in the serum. Demonstrable antibodies first appear in the serum on about the sixth day of infection and titers continue to increase during the active phase of the infection. As soon as the microorganisms are no longer shed via the urine, the serum antibody level declines to a more or less stable level and persists at that level for life. Because bacterins and live attentuated cultures also result in persistent titers in the serum, a single positive serological titer will indicate only an exposure to the organisms or to the antibodies in colostrum or bacterins; it should therefore not be considered of diagnostic significance. Laboratory confirmation of a field diagnosis requires the observation of a rising antibody titer over a period of time from consecutive serum samples. Serum samples should be examined as early as possible and at weekly intervals until a definite trend has been noted. Antibodies are usually demonstrable in the urine about three weeks following infection.

Treatment

Calves nursing cows that either have recovered from the clinical stages of this disease or have been vaccinated with a bacterin receive a degree of passive immunity lasting up to two months. The leptospiral antibodies are concentrated in the colostrum, and the calves usually demonstrate a higher antibody titer than their dams.

Leptospirosis may be prevented, or at least controlled, by the judicious use of bacterins which, under favorable conditions, provide immunity for six months or more. It has been observed, however, that some animals are afforded only partial immunity and become occult carriers of the disease unless they receive a second booster injection after an interval of one to two weeks, but no longer. It is good policy to vaccinate all replacement animals added to a herd or flock, and routinely to vaccinate all animals on a yearly basis.

Due to the peculiarity of the development of the disease in swine, sows should be vaccinated during the breeding season or after farrowing, but not during gestation; they should be revaccinated at each breeding season.

Prevention

Prevention of leptospirosis is based upon breaking the cycle of transmission of bacteria and eliminating reservoirs of infection. The first step is to prevent contact of susceptible animals with infected urine. This may be achieved by proper sanitation, modern methods of manure and urine disposal, drainage of low swampy areas, fencing of stagnant ponds and sluggish streams. Other husbandry methods include segregation of livestock by species and age groups, isolation of sick or aborting animals, and disinfection of all buildings or pens where sick or aborting animals have been housed.

All animals should be fed and watered under sanitary conditions to prevent contamination of racks, waterers, feed containers, feed, and water with urine from carriers. Especially, avoid feeding livestock on the ground.

It is particularly important to isolate all replacement or new animals until they have passed two successive negative blood tests at least 30 days apart.

Some animals that have recovered from leptospirosis may be inapparent shedders of bacteria for varying periods of time. Thus, they should be isolated from healthy animals until laboratory tests reveal that they are no longer carriers of infection. The veterinarian may recommend treatments in the light of recent advances, but, in the past, antibiotic therapy alone has not been sufficient to eliminate the disease.

26
Salmonellosis

SALMONELLOSIS is an acute or chronic contagious disease caused by one or more species of bacteria of the genus *Salmonella.* Salmonellosis is characterized by moderate fever, profuse hemorrhagic diarrhea, gastroenteritis, respiratory difficulties, intense septicemia, and in some cases a prolonged state of unthriftiness. Salmonellae have been isolated from outbreaks of infection in all of the common domestic animals and man. Several hundred species of *Salmonella* are capable of producing infection in mammals, birds, fish, reptiles, and particularly rodents. Among the various strains certain species tend to be host adaptive, while others show no host adaptation at all.

Geographically, salmonellosis is worldwide in distribution and is found particularly where swine and cattle are maintained in crowded conditions. Within the United States, salmonellosis is more common in the corn belt of the middle west than in other parts of the country. However, the disease is metropolitan in distribution and is found wherever animals are found.

Historically, salmonellosis is one of the oldest reported diseases of swine. The true nature of the condition was not discovered until 1885, when it was described as being identified with hog cholera. However, with the isolation of the virus cause of hog cholera in the early 1900s, the true nature of the disease associated with *Salmonella* organisms was discovered. Salmonellosis in cattle was first observed in the United States in 1902, and has since been found in all parts of the country and in other countries where cattle are maintained.

Etiology

Salmonellosis in livestock can be caused by one or more species of *Salmonella.* The most prevalent cause in cattle is *Salmonella typhimurium,* closely followed by *Salmonella dublin* and *Salmonella newport.* The most prevalent cause of the disease in swine is *Salmonella choleraesuis.* Although the pig is considered the reservoir for *Salmonella choleraesuis,* this species has also been recovered from man, cattle, dogs, poultry, and wild animals. The disease is more common in young animals than in adult animals. The mortality is much higher in the young than in the old, although both young and adult animals may frequently be debilitated. Carrier animals exist among adults, and the infection may persist in an inapparent form in these animals for many years. Such animals, however, may develop active clinical signs if subjected to stressful conditions such as inclement weather, poor nutrition, and other infectious diseases causing debilitation.

Transmission

The primary route of infection for salmonellosis is through the alimentary tract. The infective bacteria are introduced into the alimentary tract through contaminated feed and water. Animals actively excreting the microorganisms during the acute stage of the disease, or carrier animals excreting the microorganisms, are primary sources of infection. Secondarily, feed contaminated by urine and fecal material of rodents is a frequent source of spread of salmonellosis. This disease may be considered to be associated with mismanagement, as related to the transmission of microorganisms to young animals. Young calves and pigs maintained in less-than-optimum sanitary conditions, associated with older animals, crowded into filthy barnyards or holding yards, are particularly susceptible to the disease through the bacteria deposited in the soil in fecal material of older, carrier animals. There is little evidence that prenatal infection occurs with this disease. However, if the dam is suffering from clinical salmonellosis during parturition (indicated by acute diarrhea, high temperature, low milk yield, and almost complete loss of appetite), she is likely to be excreting salmonellae in the colostrum. The number of animals affected in this manner is low; observations on clinically normal dams soon after parturition show salmonellae in the feces, on the udder and on the teat surfaces, but not in the milk. In most instances, young animals obtain the infective microorganisms from the surface of the teats while nursing. Salmonellae may often be demonstrated in the feces within 24 to 36 hours after birth.

In addition to direct dam-to-offspring transmission, *Salmonella* microorganisms in the environment of young animals can result in infant infection at an early age. It is usual to bring recently born calves and piglets into a shed, barnyard, or holding area for preliminary inspection. Calves are often placed in small enclosures for varying periods of time. After a day or two, the cow may return to the herd. The calf is allowed to suckle for a short period only, prior to being sent to slaughter or mixed with older calves. Young pigs, however, are usually confined in a farrowing area in a barn or shed which has been used for many previous farrowings and may not be as sanitary as it should be. These maternity and/or feeding areas usually get perennially heavy traffic, and, if there are adults in the herd excreting *Salmonella,* the enclosures can quickly become grossly contaminated. Furthermore, these areas usually favor persistence of the microorganisms. Observations on premises where outbreaks have occurred show that in most cases the feeding equipment is grossly contaminated, as are the water troughs and containers.

Without equivocation, however, the most persistent means by which salmonellosis is transmitted is the carrier animal. Carriers seed the soil and equipment within an area with the microorganisms, for direct and indirect transmission to susceptible animals. The bacteria causing salmonellosis in livestock may also cause food poisoning in humans, by the heavy contamination of foodstuffs with fecal material inadvertently handled with them.

Factors Influencing Susceptibility

Observations for the presence of *Salmonella* microorganisms have been made on both calves and pigs sent to slaughterhouses. In most instances, the mixing and mingling of hogs held in the pens at sale barns and in holding pens at packing plants provide the means for extensive exposure and spread of salmonellae from animal to animal; salmonellae were isolated from the drinking water of the pens and from the feed containers. At slaughter, animals were found to be contaminated by *Salmonella* species highly pathogenic to man. Overcrowding of young calves, particularly during inclement weather in poor housing, has also been found to be conducive to the spread of infection. Some calf enclosures are unsatisfactory because regular or even inefficient cleaning is virtually impossible. If housing cannot be readily cleaned, particularly between groups of calves, it would be advisable to resort to some sort of temporary shelter. Excessive crowding during transportation is another means by which salmonellosis is readily transmitted. There is no evidence that debilitated animals are more likely to harbor salmonellae than apparently healthy animals; therefore, it is likely that animals maintained in overcrowded, unsanitary conditions are exposed to excessively high numbers of *Salmonella* microorganisms and transmit them with regularity.

Recent evidence shows that young calves are able to excrete more organisms than older calves. The importance of initially isolating young or recently bought calves from older animals then is evident. The isolated calves are likely to obtain better supervision, particularly when being taught to drink or if requiring treatment. It is advisable to feed young calves with separate utensils and also to clean and disinfect isolation pens or sheds between groups of animals. Purchase of calves in small groups direct from another property minimizes the risk of acquiring infective animals.

Salmonellosis may develop in feedlot cattle any time in the fattening period, but it occurs also in adult dairy cows and, still more frequently, in calves. While the disease may occur during any month of the year, the incidence is high from June through October. Age is a definite factor influencing susceptibility to salmonellosis; however, breed and sex are of no significance. Salmonellosis is more prevalent in dairy animals than in beef cattle, primarily because of manner of management. In the western range herds in particular, salmonellosis is seldom seen until animals are segregated by age groups for transport to market.

Symptoms

Salmonella infections in all species of mammals are characterized by fever, recumbency, and gastrointestinal upsets. The clinical infection may be acute or chronic.

Acute salmonellosis in swine affects primarily young animals from 3 weeks to 6 months of age. The most common signs of infection are obvious debility and depression, refusal to eat, and fever increases to 104 to 106 F with a rapid rate of respiration. Some animals may not demonstrate diarrhea, although this is usually a predominant feature of this disease. In field cases the animal shows a rough, staring hair coat, a rapid loss of weight and dehydration due to persistent diarrhea. Some animals die in 2 to 4 days; others may survive and either recover or pass into the chronic phase, during which their continued growth rate is relatively slow.

In the chronic phase in swine, survivors of the acute type develop very slowly. They may have a persistent diarrhea which is yellow in color, semiliquid in consistency with an offensive odor. They have moderate fever and may stand with tucked-up abdomen and eat sparsely. If forced to move, the animals will groan, grunt and squeal with reluctance. They may either lose weight rapidly or gain poorly. Some have persistent respiratory distress and may not live longer than several weeks, although some consistently shed the bacteria until they reach advanced age in rather poor, thin condition.

Acute salmonellosis in calves occurs suddenly, with a fever of 105 to 108 F. Diarrhea is evident on the second day of infection. Dehydration, weakness, and loss of appetite appear in most affected calves by the third day. In the severe acute cases, the feces frequently are watery in consistency, yellowish in color and fetid in odor. The calves show depression, dehydration, and rapid loss of weight; death occurs in 3 to 7 days, depending upon the severity of the symptoms.

In a milking herd, symptoms progress rapidly with a drastic drop in milk production, severe diarrhea, dehydration and extreme lassitude. Temperatures are usually elevated above 105 F but seldom persist for more than two days before dropping to a lower level, although higher than normal. Pregnant cows may abort and death may occur in 2 to 4 days depending upon the severity of the symptoms.

In the chronic phase, the clinical form is usually seen in calves where pneumonia and arthritis may complicate the picture. Sporadic outbreaks are seen only in older cattle. Subclinical salmonellosis may be seen in bovines of all ages, however. Adult animals recovering from the acute clinical disease tend to excrete the organisms in their feces for a considerable length of time. It has been noted that *Salmonella dublin* infections tend to persist for particularly long periods, *Salmonella typhimurium* for shorter periods and other species for only a few days. Calves usually do not remain carriers after recovery. Salmonellae are excreted in the milk of lactating cows only in the febrile stage of the disease.

In general, the signs observed in an outbreak of salmonellosis in any mammals resemble those of acute septicemic disease. Milder forms of the infection accompanied by indefinite signs do occur, and it is quite possible that some animals become carriers of the disease without showing any visible signs.

Pathology

After ingestion, the microorganisms rapidly invade the body; they have been found on slaughter in the lungs, lymph nodes and blood of infected animals. In the intestine, bacteria proliferate and cause severe injury to the mucosa. Necrosis of epithelial cells and erosion of blood vessels cause hemorrhaging into the intestinal lumen. Irritation to the intestine provokes diarrhea early in the course of the disease. Some bacteria may penetrate the blood vessels to produce septicemia and foci of infection in the liver, spleen and lymph nodes. After a short course, death may result from dehydration, hemorrhaging, intoxication, and septicemia. Postmortem lesions in swine usually include bright red mucosa of the stomach, covered with a thin film of tenacious mucus. Some necrosis is always present. The most consistent postmortem lesion is a severe gastroenteritis. The spleen is enlarged, dark blue, and firm and swollen. There may be hemorrhages in the renal cortex, on the heart, and on the mucous membranes of the intestinal tract. The contents of the intestinal tract will be fluid and may contain blood. In cases of severe intestinal hemorrhaging, anemia is present. All animal tissues may be dehydrated.

Diagnosis

In the field, the diagnosis of salmonellosis is based primarily on herd history, prior vaccination status, and clinical signs. Profuse diarrhea with blood in the feces is highly significant. In cattle, one of the premonitory signs is failure to respond to treatment for other conditions resembling this disease. A laboratory confirmation may be obtained by isolation and identification of salmonellae from fecal samples and from lymph nodes of animals which have died in the herd or flock. If an animal or aborted fetus is infected with *Salmonella*, the organisms are easy to isolate.

Treatment

Several commercially available bacterins may be used to protect livestock against a specific species of *Salmonella*. However, most bacterins are of questionable efficiency and care should be taken not to rely entirely upon such prophylaxis. Mixed bacterins are available which confer a degree of resistance against infections by the organisms represented in the formula. The degree of resistance, however, is enhanced by a series of injections at two- to three-week intervals; usually, about three injections are required. Increased sensitivity to antigens may be a problem with repeated injections, however, and care should be taken to prevent anaphylactic shock or to treat it if it occurs.

Prevention

Preventive measures are important. The primary consideration in preventing salmonellosis is adequate sanitation. Livestock should be maintained in clean lots and pastures should be rotated to prevent a buildup of fecal material containing pathogenic bacteria. The introduction of infected animals into a herd or flock should be avoided at all costs. Calves should be segregated during the growing period by age group, as the most common manner of spreading the disease is mixing young animals with older animals which are inapparent spreaders of the bacteria.

Other diseases causing primary infection and lowering resistance should be prevented where possible.

Modern methods of sanitation, proper nutrition, and good management should be exercised. Such practices will allow the operator to maintain the health and vigor of his animals. When proper immunization methods are available, animals should be vaccinated on a routine basis.

In an effort to control the contamination of indigenous foodstuffs which may have a bearing on transmission of salmonellosis, either to livestock or to humans, an eradication and testing program has been initiated by the U.S. Department of Agriculture in cooperation with the various states. The program has been set forth in a set of regulations entitled "Uniform Methods and Rules for the Elimination of Salmonella in Animal By-Products Intended for Use in Animal Feeds." It is recommended by the U.S. Animal Health Association, and became effective January 8, 1969. A copy of the regulations may be obtained from state or federal regulatory veterinarians or agricultural extension agents.

27
Bovine Rhinotracheitis

INFECTIOUS bovine rhinotracheitis, or rednose, is a virus disease of cattle, goats, and wild deer, characterized by intense inflammation of the upper respiratory tract, the eyes, and the reproductive tract. Rednose is an acute, contagious infection that may be an important cause of abortion in both dairy and beef cattle. When it is complicated by secondary bacterial invaders, bronchopneumonia often results.

Rednose was recognized as a clinical entity in 1950, in dairies and feedlots in the western part of the United States. Since that time, the disease has been diagnosed in all parts of North America. Subsequently, the disease, in one or more of its forms, has been recognized and the virus isolated from cattle in all parts of the world except South America. While the disease persisted at a low incidence in dairies, it became so common in the great feedlots of Colorado and California that it has attracted more attention than any other disease of feedlot cattle. This attention has led to the rapid discovery of the cause of the disease and the development of an effective vaccine.

In early reports, the disease was characterized by an acute inflammation of the upper respiratory tract. Noticeable clinical signs were fiery red nose, copious nasal discharge, polypnea with open-mouth breathing and fever.

Etiology

Infectious bovine rhinotracheitis is caused by a filterable virus. The virus is fairly stable in a slightly alkaline environment at very low temperatures, but is less stable at room temperatures and will not remain viable for more than three days.

The virus is readily isolated from the nasal and ocular fluids of infected cattle, but rarely from blood. The virus may also be found in the tissues of aborted fetuses, in the placenta and vulval secretions of cows which abort, and in the brain of calves with encephalitis.

It may also be found on the penis and prepuce of range bulls. Apparently healthy cattle may harbor the virus in the respiratory tract for several months, and so serve as healthy carriers of the disease.

There are four serotypes of the virus but all are equally pathogenic. The disease may occur in cattle of all ages and both sexes, at any time, but the greatest incidence is found in the fall when range cattle are concentrated in feedlots.

Transmission

The virus is primarily transmitted directly, by infected droplets spread by coughing animals and by contact with infected secretions from the nose, eyes, and vulva. Secondarily, the infection is spread indirectly by contaminated examination instruments. The virus may invade the placenta and developing fetus by way of the maternal circulation, and consequently either abortion or death and resorption of the fetus about 60 days after infection may occur. Young nursing calves may contract the infection from the dams and develop symptoms of encephalitis.

The usual method of spreading the virus to the vulva of cows and penis and prepuce of bulls is venereal. Within 36 to 48 hours following infection, clinical signs begin to appear.

All ages and all breeds of cattle are susceptible to the virus, although range cattle seldom develop clinical signs of the disease until they are confined in fairly large groups. The incidence is highest and the course most severe in feedlot cattle, as the virus becomes more virulent by passage through many susceptible animals.

Factors Influencing Susceptibility

Upon primary infection with the respiratory form of rednose, the incidence of the disease and the virulence of the infection are both low in the first few animals in an affected herd. However, virulence is enhanced by continual passage through a herd. The respiratory form of the disease is most prevalent in large concentrations of animals, while the genital infection is more often seen in smaller breeding herds where passage is not swift or continuous enough to enhance virulence. A mild infection may occur in heifers before breeding age, making them immune to all forms of the disease; if they subsequently breed with infected bulls, however, they may become carriers and shedders of the virus.

Symptoms

Rednose can exist in a mild or inapparent form. The incubation period is usually 5 to 7 days, but even in infected feedlots 30 to 60 days may pass before clinical signs are observed in most animals. The temperature is usually high, with typical readings from 104 to 107 F. This is accompanied by a clear serous nasal discharge which may, on rare occasions, contain flecks of blood.

This discharge later becomes mucopurulent and tends to be tenacious, hanging in strands from a fiery-red or encrusted muzzle. It is accompanied by depression, lack of appetite, and labored breathing due to accumulations of serofibrinous exudate in the trachea, sinuses and turbinates. Coughing is a prominent symptom, often accompanied by a heaving action, with the tongue protruded. Primary pneumonia is not usually present, although at times secondary bronchial pneumonia develops. Morbidity in infected herds may range from 25 to 100 percent; however, mortality is usually low, ranging from 0 to 5 percent.

Lacrimation due to conjunctivitis is commonly present, and close observation will reveal edema and small granular proliferations on the conjunctiva. The ocular exudate may go from serous to mucopurulent to purulent. Either one or both eyes may be involved. On occasion, a thin film of fibrous exudate de-

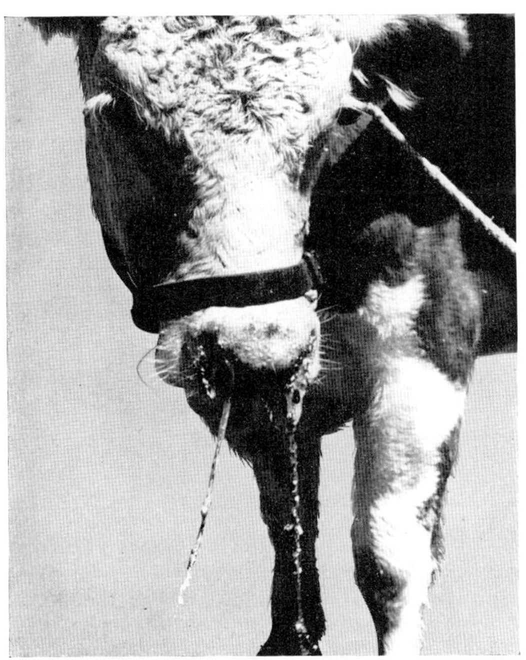

FIG. 17. Typical appearance of cattle suffering from rednose. (From Gibbons, W. J.: *Clinical Diagnosis of Diseases of Large Animals.* Philadelphia, Lea & Febiger, 1966.)

velops on the lids and, when removed, reveals a granular, reddened conjunctiva. In some outbreaks inflammation with clouding of the cornea may develop.

Corneal involvement appears to be an extension of the conjunctivitis, a fact which helps distinguish this form from infectious bovine keratitis, a condition beginning with ulceration of the center of the cornea. Eye lesions in observed outbreaks are usually healing at the end of the clinical outbreak. It is well to remember that, in rednose, there can be not only a conjunctivitis but a keratitis, although the keratitis is usually secondary to the conjunctivitis.

In heifers, another form of the disease is characterized by pustular vulvovaginitis. Clinically, there are circumscribed areas of inflammation, with the development of pustules, a fibrinous pseudomembrane, and a yellowish exudate visible on the vaginal floor or the vulvar tuft.

In steers, the virus has been known to produce dermatitis in the anal, perineal and tail-head regions and exudative lesions on the penis and prepuce.

Confirmed outbreaks of infectious bovine rhinotracheitis abortion have occurred. The virus was isolated from the placenta and from liver, spleen, kidneys, lungs, heart, blood and pleural fluid from aborted fetuses.

In one such outbreak none of the animals had been previously vaccinated. An infectious bovine rhinotracheitis respiratory and conjunctivitis outbreak had occurred a few months previously in other cattle on this farm, and this was evidently the virus source in the outbreak. The abortions occurred at about six months of pregnancy and the only common lesion noted was a perirenal hemorrhage in the fetus. The infectious bovine rhinotracheitis virus has been isolated from fetuses aborted as a result of vaccination, but this is not routinely produced by either the intramuscular or intranasal routes of inoculation.

Experimentally, abortions can be produced at any stage of pregnancy and ordinarily occur 3 to 5 weeks after infection. Some confirmed actual field abortions have occurred before any antibodies were detectable in the dams. This situation has also been noted in abortions after vaccination; the virus was isolated from the fetus and must have invaded the fetus before circulating antibodies developed. Fetuses aborted as a result of vaccination are normal and not decomposed, indicating that fetal death and abortion occur close together. Although the clinical entities induced by infectious bovine rhinotracheitis are of economic importance, the abortion syndrome appears to be increasingly significant as more is learned about the genital form of the disease.

In addition to abortion, there is a marked drop in milk production when lactating cows are infected. In some outbreaks, diarrhea is an important and common clinical finding.

Although encephalitic infectious bovine rhinotracheitis does not appear to be common, it does occur. In Australia in 1962, the virus was isolated from the brains of cattle showing encephalitis.

Diagnosis

History and symptoms, helpful in differentiating this disease from shipping fever or parainfluenza-3, are as follows:

Infectious bovine rhinotracheitis may occur independently of stress, movement, or transportation. A severe pupillary conjunctivitis with purulent exudate is indicative of infection with the disease. Unless secondarily complicated, there is no pneumonia. The uncomplicated form involves only the upper respiratory tract. Diarrhea, although observed, is not a common clinical finding, whereas it is often associated with the shipping-fever syndrome. All ages of cattle are affected, whereas shipping fever and parainfluenza are more common in cattle under one year of age. Clinically, the nasal and oral mucous membranes are markedly reddened in infectious bovine rhinotracheitis.

Pathology

Postmortem lesions of rednose are those of acute respiratory infection, with marked reddening of the oral, nasal and tracheal mucosa. Hemorrhagic or purulent exudate with frothing is noted in the nose and trachea and, occasionally, in the large bronchi. Obstruction of the respiratory tract with edema and exudate often causes death by suffocation.

Many small hemorrhages are noted in the upper respiratory mucosa. Mucosal edema is common; regional lymph nodes are enlarged. The virus may be isolated from lacrimal, nasal and vulvar secretions. In instances of abortion, the virus can usually be recovered from the fetus. Identification of the virus can be made by reciprocal cross-neutralization studies or serological tissue-culture inhibition studies. The disease can be readily reproduced in susceptible calves.

Treatment

Treatment does not alter the clinical course of the virus infection but it is beneficial in controlling the secondary bacterial invaders and in shortening the course of the disease. Attenuated modified live-virus infectious bovine rhinotracheitis vaccines, used singly and in combination with other virus vaccines, are available for prophylaxis and control. Immunity produced by the vaccines appears to last at least one year.

The use of vaccines is not recommended in pregnant animals or very young calves. However, on some farms with endemic problems due to infectious bovine rhinotracheitis, vaccines have been used on day-old calves with apparent good results and with no reaction.

The vaccination program for the herd should be considered carefully, since the vaccine can induce abortion. Incidence of abortion may be greatest when vaccination occurs during the sixth, seventh, or eighth month of gestation. (Conceivably, abortion due to the virus may occur at any stage of gestation, since the critical effect of the virus is exerted primarily on the fetus. However, most abortions under field conditions seem to occur at the fourth to seventh month of pregnancy.)

Abortion may be accompanied by retention of an edematous placenta in which cotyledons usually are blanched and degenerated by a generalized necrotizing placentitis. Traction may be required to remove the membranes.

Most veterinarians believe that the vaccine may be used in fresh cattle shipped directly to another farm and may be administered with safety at the time of unloading. Vaccination during an outbreak is indicated for the control of the disease, and some veterinarians have reported therapeutic results from the intramuscular or intravenous administration of the vaccine to animals sick with infectious bovine rhinotracheitis.

Because of the infectivity and rapid spread of this infection, vaccination of all animals in a feedlot is recommended. Evidence is available to show that virus transmission from vaccinates to nonvaccinates does not occur under ordinary farm conditions, but that the virus is rapidly spread when cattle are congregated in close confinement.

28 Bovine Virus Diarrhea

BOVINE virus diarrhea is an acute or chronic contagious and infectious disease of cattle characterized by fever, nasal discharge, coughing, profuse watery diarrhea, rapid dehydration and emaciation.

There has been confusion in distinguishing among infectious bovine rhinotracheitis, mucosal disease, and virus diarrhea in herd infections. Recent investigations utilizing tissue culture and cross-protection tests have revealed that the rhinotracheitis is a separate entity, and that the other two are either the same or so closely related as to be indistinguishable serologically.

Bovine virus diarrhea was first described in New York in 1946 and since that time, by serological survey, has been found to be widespread through all countries where cattle are produced. Up to 56 percent of adult cattle have antibodies to this virus, and the author experienced difficulties in finding baby calves, either dairy or beef, without demonstrable antibodies.

Etiology

Bovine virus diarrhea is caused by one of several strains of a virus. All strains are serologically and immunologically related, although some are cytopathogenic while others are not, and there are varied manifestations of the disease for each strain of the virus. The causative agent will proprogate in cell cultures of sheep, goats, cattle, and embryonating egg.

Bovine virus diarrhea occurs at all times of the year. It principally affects young cattle from 8 months to 2 years of age, of both dairy and beef breeds, although it has also been observed in aged cattle. A few cases on record indicate, by clinical manifestations and by the demonstration of ascending bovine virus diarrhea antibody titers on paired serum samples, that the disease can occur in baby calves 1 to 4 weeks of age. There is a strong antigenic relationship between this virus and the viruses of mucosal disease and of hog cholera.

Transmission

The mode of transmission is thought to be direct contact from infected to susceptible cattle, but the exact method of transfer is not known. The virus may be transmitted indirectly by contaminated feed, water, and bedding, and by contact with fecal matter during the stage of viremia. The disease often appears in a herd after the addition of replacement cattle, or after subjection to the stress of shipment. Subacute symptoms will appear in one or two animals, followed in a week or ten days by a fulminating outbreak in the herd.

Symptoms

Bovine virus diarrhea is characterized by a chain of symptoms initially of a respiratory nature: serous or mucous nasal discharge, labored breathing, coughing, and elevated temperatures. In addition, an affected animal usually appears gaunt, due to decreased feed consumption and diarrhea. Acute laminitis occurs occasionally. In dairy cattle, a reduction in milk production, and abortions in some animals, may be found. Bovine virus diarrhea has a course of several days in adult dairy cattle. The course in feedlot cattle, on an individual basis, is usually from 10 days to 2 or 3 weeks in acute outbreaks, and from 4 to 6 weeks on a lot basis. Chronic cases extend over a period of months and affected cattle are finally sold or eventually die.

While the morbidity is generally high, the mortality is low. The loss is primarily economic because of weight loss, prolonged feeding periods, chronic sickness, abortions, loss of milk production, proprietary drug costs, and fees for veterinary diagnostic laboratory services.

The onset often is sudden, with temperatures ranging from 104 to 106 F. Since cattle that appear well may have a high fever, it is advisable to check the temperatures of several animals in the herd. Depression is moderate to severe, respirations and pulse are rapid. Affected cattle have almost no appetite; however, they drink large amounts of water.

Moderate to severe nasal discharge occurs shortly after onset and may be accompanied by a low throaty unproductive cough. The nasal discharge is serous at first, but in chronic cases may become mucopurulent and, in severe cases, can cover the entire muzzle. The nasal mucosa may show marked hyperemia, and it is at this stage that the disease may be confused with infectious bovine rhinotracheitis or even shipping fever. In some outbreaks there may be many subclinical cases.

Excessive lacrimation is sometimes seen and may be followed by a progressive corneal opacity. Oral lesions, in some cases, are found early in the course of the disease. They usually are uneven round or shallow erosions, but may consist only of areas of congestion. They are most common on the dental pad, inner surface of the lips, and buccal mucosa. Similar lesions are sometimes found on the muzzle and in the nares.

Lameness, apparently caused by laminitis, is seen in the severe cases, and is characterized by a peculiar stance. The soreness causes many cattle to lie down more than usual. In severe cases the tissues around the coronary band of the feet are severely reddened.

During the early febrile stage the feces are hard and dry, and may be covered with mucus and a few flecks of blood. Diarrhea may occur in about 10 percent of cases. When present, it begins after the peak of the febrile response has passed, and may continue intermittently for 4 to 6 weeks or even longer. The feces are watery and fetid, containing many bubbles and long strings of mucus; they vary from yellowish to slate gray and later, when more erythrocytes are present, red. Since diarrhea occurs so inconsistently in affected cattle, the term virus diarrhea may be considered somewhat a misnomer.

Dehydration is severe, and some affected

animals lose considerable body weight. The eyes are dull and sunken, and the skin becomes dry and scurfy. The skin changes are particularly severe on the neck.

A few younger animals may show convulsions prior to death. Death is most likely to occur early in the course of the disease. In severely affected cattle that recover, convalescence is protracted and often causes as much or more economic loss as does death. The course of the disease is milder in small calves and in older animals. In these cases, mild respiratory involvement and diarrhea may lead to unthriftiness, and temperatures may not rise above 102 to 103.5 F.

There are three distinct forms of bovine virus diarrhea. The *inapparent* form is evidenced by mild symptoms and slightly elevated temperature, although, due to the diphasic temperature pattern, the clinical examination may reveal a temperature from 102 to 107 F without serious complications.

The *acute or severe* form is sudden in onset and involves an entire herd with the full gamut of symptoms.

The *chronic* form is likely to be an extension of the inapparent form. It is characterized by rough hair coat, poor condition, persistent nasal discharge, failure to gain, and lameness.

Pathology

Lesions occur primarily in the alimentary tract and adjacent lymphatic tissues; they are hemorrhages, inflammation, edema, and shallow irregular erosions of the mucosal lining. Oral lesions occur in only a small percentage of diseased cattle. Ulcerative lesions are extensive throughout the gastrointestinal tract and in the buccal cavity. Consistently, inflammation, edema, hemorrhages, and ulcers, in various stages of formation and repair, are found in the abomasum. Occasionally, there are erosions on the pillars of the rumen. Usually there is a catarrhal enteritis with some erosions of the lining, and often subserous edema around the small intestine. The lymph glands adjacent to the gastrointestinal tract may be enlarged and edematous.

Diagnosis

A presumptive diagnosis can be made from clinical evidence and postmortem lesions. A definitive diagnosis can be made by isolating the virus from nasal discharges and blood during the acute febrile phase, before circulating antibodies are formed. The virus can also be isolated from the spleen and mesenteric lymph glands.

The most practical means by which to arrive at a definitive diagnosis is serological. Cross-protection or serum neutralization studies can be made with paired-serum samples. The first or acute blood samples should be taken when the sick animal is first observed. A second or convalescent blood sample should be taken 2 to 3 weeks later and processed the same way. Ideally, there will be no bovine virus diarrhea antibodies in the first serum sample, whereas the second will contain demonstrable antibodies.

It is not unusual for cattle vaccinated against infectious bovine rhinotracheitis to undergo an attack of bovine virus diarrhea. This causes the owner and/or the veterinarian to think they are experiencing an infectious bovine rhinotracheitis immunity failure. At times, both diseases have been found to be active not only in the same lot of cattle but in the same animal.

The one disease most difficult to differentiate and most often confused with bovine virus diarrhea (BVD) is infectious bovine rhinotracheitis (IBR). Clinically, IBR is a respiratory disease in feedlot cattle, whereas BVD is an enteric disease. Laminitis, frequently seen in BVD, is not a part of IBR. The suppurative, palpebral conjunctivitis of IBR does not involve the eyeball, whereas that of BVD occasionally does. Corneal opacity with keratitis, seen in BVD, is not seen in IBR conjunctivitis on a lot basis.

Treatment and Control

Because of its virus origin, there is no specific treatment for bovine virus diarrhea. Symptomatic treatment seems to be of little value. Supportive treatment combating dehydration, electrolyte loss, and the effects of anorexia is of some value in severe cases. Feed should be materially reduced, and cattle should be taken off succulent feeds that tend to cause soft feces.

An effective modified live-virus vaccine is available and may be used prophylactically. All replacement cattle should be kept in quarantine and vaccinated at least two weeks before being mixed with other cattle. In feedlots, all cattle should be vaccinated upon arrival. Vaccination immunity lasts for one year and annual vaccination is recommended. Recovery from the clinical symptoms of the disease provides some degree of immunity, but its duration is unknown.

29
Tuberculosis

Tuberculosis is a chronic infectious disease caused by several pathogenic species of the genus *Mycobacterium.* It is usually characterized by the formation of nodular swellings, called tubercles. Tuberculosis is a disease with serious public-health implications, as man has been infected by animals of many species. Technically, tuberculosis cannot be considered a strategic disease, in the usual sense of this text, because there is no vaccine acceptable in this country to protect susceptible animals. The BCG vaccine is available and used in Europe. However, regulatory officials in this country do not consider the protection adequate and have not permitted its use in the United States.

Historically, tuberculosis is one of the oldest diseases of known record. Recent examination of Egyptian mummies show lesions in the lungs of individuals who died during the far reaches of the past. Legislative enactments concerning the destruction of affected animals and forbidding the use of the flesh date back into the Middle Ages. In the sixteenth century, the disease was considered identical with syphilis in man. In consequence, stringent laws were enacted which made the destruction of tuberculous cattle compulsory. In the eighteenth century, this erroneous conception of the nature of the disease was abandoned and all restrictions against the use of tuberculous animals for meat were removed. Since that time, however, the communicable nature of tuberculosis has been established by many investigators, and the tide of opinion has again turned in favor of eradicating the disease from this country.

Although the disease was well known, it was not until 1882 that the tubercle bacillus, the actual cause of tuberculosis, was isolated; as a consequence, tuberculin (a diagnostic aid in determining the spread of the disease) was manufactured in 1890. In 1898 the human and bovine strains were differentiated by their growth characteristics and pathogenicity.

Geographically, tuberculosis is found wherever livestock are maintained in crowded conditions. The disease is prevalent in cattle, swine, sheep, humans, wild herbivores, and even domestic pets, in most countries of the world. Tuberculosis tends to be more common in temperate to cold climates because of winter housing of animals during unfavorable weather; in close quarters aerosol transmission of the disease is enhanced.

Etiology

The microorganisms which cause tuberculosis in all species of animals, including man, are related culturally and morphologically. Although they are significantly different they have one characteristic in common, that is, all pathogenic species of the genus *Mycobacterium* are acid-fast in their staining properties. The microorganisms appear as slender rods; they are gram-positive by the usual stains but are distinguished by differential staining techniques from other gram-positive bacteria. Each of the three types of *Mycobacterium* has growth characteristics of diagnostic importance. However, colonies of the microorganisms grow on diagnostic media at a very slow rate.

The mycobacteria causing tuberculosis are often called tubercle bacilli because of their appearance and the characteristic lesion which develops around pockets of infection within the animal's body. Although the pathogenic tubercle bacilli are relatively susceptible to heat and to destruction by normal pasteurization temperatures, they can withstand drying for a considerable length of time. They remain viable in the presence of putrefaction and are unaffected by cold weather.

Three types of pathogenic tubercle bacilli are recognized: human, bovine, and avian; the microorganisms are classified as *Mycobacterium tuberculosis, Mycobacterium bovis,* and *Mycobacterium avium,* respectively. All three types produce naturally acquired disease in host species other than their own. The human type is most specific, since it rarely produces progressive disease in animals lower than primates. The avian type is the only one of consequence in birds, but it is also pathogenic for swine and sheep, though natural infection in sheep is very rare. The bovine type is the most universal, since it can also cause progressive disease in man, horses, sheep, goats, swine, dogs, cats, and a wide variety of wild animals. It is possible to produce local and sometimes general infections with all three types of *Mycobacterium* in a range of host species.

Transmission

Bacteria are usually spread from herd to herd and flock to flock by infected animals. The microorganisms may be spread from animal to animal by direct contact or by contaminated feed, water and equipment. Among cattle, bacteria are spread by aerosol droplets and dust which are breathed into lungs, and by feed and water contaminated with infected feces. Within contaminated manure accumulations, pathogenic mycobacteria may survive for many years. Calves may be infected by drinking raw milk from cows actively excreting the microorganisms in the milk.

Tuberculosis is not usually spread from hog to hog; however, pigs may get the disease from nursing a sow with an infected udder. Swine, because of their feeding habits, may be exposed to all three types of bacilli, particularly those picked up from the feces of infected cattle. Therefore, in swine the primary site of infection is the intestinal tract while in the bovine it is the lung and upper respiratory system.

The avian type is primarily seen in the intestinal tract of chickens which have picked it up from the droppings of infected chickens on the same property. The human type is transmitted from cattle and swine to humans through infective milk and poorly cooked meat, by aerosols or droplets coughed up by infected animals, and by bacteria-laden dust in areas of heavy livestock concentration. Droplet or aerosol infection, in humans, is more prevalent than digestive infection.

Factors Influencing Susceptibility

Since tuberculosis is a chronic problem, age has little influence on susceptibility to the disease (except of course that aged animals have more opportunity to come into contact with the infection than young animals). There is no difference in susceptibility by sex or by body condition, although animals in poor condition are usually debilitated by some other syndrome predisposing to lowered resistance to other pathogenic microorganisms. Feeding facilities and methods do have a bearing on the transmission of tuberculosis. The lack of cleanliness associated with poor feeding and drinking facilities is dangerous from the standpoint of spreading. Unpasteurized milk and dairy products are also sources of infection for young animals. Housing has a definite influence on susceptibility of the disease, as crowding in poorly sanitized facilities during inclement weather is conducive to spread by droplet infection. Poor lighting favors the perpetuation of the bacilli.

Season, climate and weather have little relationship to susceptibility to tuberculosis in livestock.

Symptoms

The clinical signs, frequently seen in cattle in the United States before the tuberculosis eradication program began, are now rare.

Infected cattle may undergo a gradual loss of weight and condition. Cattle with tuberculosis of the lungs may develop a chronic hacking cough. The lymph nodes are frequently involved and appear as enlargements on the throat and shoulder which may be palpated in living animals. Seriously affected animals may have trouble breathing. Diarrhea may develop if the infection extends to the intestine. Cattle with advanced tuberculosis have a rough hair coat and are generally unthrifty in appearance, have a soft persistent cough, and usually seem reluctant to move.

Symptoms vary depending upon the type and virulence of the microorganism, the resistance of the affected animal, and the part of the body in which the microorganism becomes localized.

Cattle, even in prime condition, may be severely affected and spread the bacilli even though exhibiting none of the external signs associated with the disease. Tubercles, pockets of infection walled off by thick fibrous bands of scar tissue, called nodules, may be formed where infective organisms localize in any tissue or organ. Under favorable conditions these walled-off pockets of tubercle bacilli break down, expelling virulent microorganisms into a bronchus or a body cavity. From a bronchus they then pass into the trachea, from which they may be expelled by coughing or reswallowed and passed out in the feces.

Other animals may inhale the bacilli directly into the lungs and become infected. Probably more often, the bacilli are picked up with food or drinking water; when swallowed, they may pass unchanged through the intestine. Manure and saliva containing the microorganisms may contaminate the hay, or small streams or stagnant pools, which may then shelter the viable microorganisms for a considerable length of time. Hogs following infected cattle in the feedlot and feeding on undigested grain in the droppings are particularly susceptible to the intestinal type of infection. Calves may become infected at a single nursing if the dam has tuberculosis of the udder. All of these potentials for spread are important when an eradication program is considered.

Because of the insidious nature of the disease and the variability of the lesions produced, the observable symptoms are different not only in the different species of animals but also in different individuals of the same species. In most cases of tuberculosis in cattle and swine, symptoms are either entirely lacking or are so vague and obscure as to be of no material assistance in the recognition of the disease. Small lesions in the lymph nodes may produce no notable symptoms, and even extensive lesions, particularly in the abdominal viscera, may be characterized by a complete lack of clinical symptoms. General symptoms—weakness, loss of appetite, emaciation, and low-grade fever—may occur if the disease is progressive.

Due to the chronic nature of tuberculosis in all domestic animals, the disease may be present with no signs visible to the naked eye. However, because of the development of bacilli in obscure places within the body, animals may reveal the disease when being tested with tuberculin. Because bacilli grow slowly and produce visible lesions only after a considerable length of time, antibodies may be demonstrated by the allergic intradermal skin test with tuberculin before lesions have become apparent. The tuberculin test is extremely sensitive and will reveal infection in an animal or herd before visible lesions are noted either upon external examination or on internal examination of a reacting animal at slaughter.

Tuberculosis in swine is most often caused by the avian type of mycobacterium. Most infected swine do not develop visible external signs of the disease because they are sent to slaughter at a young age. In some older hogs, however, tuberculosis may cause gradual loss of weight and condition, enlarged joints, and lameness in one or more legs. The lesions often remain localized in lymph glands of the head or in the intestines throughout life.

Pathology

Microorganisms are taken into the body with feed, water, or dust; in cattle such microorganisms usually lodge in the lungs. The bacteria are then ingested by leukocytes and multiply within these cells. The leukocytes containing the bacteria then localize in lymph nodes, from which they spread to other local lymph nodes or primary body tissues throughout the body. The lymphocytes are destroyed by the mycobacteria and, as dead cells, they stimulate the accumulation of epithelioid cells which ingest the leukocytes and bacteria. The bacilli are not destroyed but multiply within these cells and apparently produce a toxic substance which destroys adjoining cells. This produces an area of caseous necrosis and the beginning of a tubercle. The animal's body defenses may arrest the disease by effectively encircling the invading organisms in a tough, fibrous capsule, forming a tubercle.

Infection of the udder causes nodular, circumscribed, or diffuse swellings which develop slowly without producing pain. The supramammary lymph nodes are usually enlarged. Calves are frequently infected during the first few hours or days of life when nursing a tuberculous dam. In the past, many pail-fed calves were infected by ingestion of unpasteurized, skimmed milk from diseased cows. Calves infrequently contract tuberculosis as a result of intrauterine infection.

The bovine strain frequently produces lesions of the lungs and regional lymph nodes. Multiple lesions of varying sizes may involve the pleura and peritoneum. Numerous small lesions are referred to as miliary tuberculosis, and syndromes characterized by larger lesions involving the serous membranes are called "pearl disease." When the bloodstream is invaded by tubercle bacilli from a local lesion, tubercles develop in the major organs. This acute form of generalization, or miliary tuberculosis, is usually rapidly fatal. If small numbers of bacilli enter the bloodstream from the primary tubercle, one or more isolated lesions may be formed in other organs. These generalized lesions may become encapsulated and remain small for long periods of time, causing no detectable symptoms; however, if stress leads to a breakdown of either the small or the primary lesion and the release of large numbers of viable bacilli, massive destruction of tissues may lead to death. The primary lesion of tuberculosis is the tubercle, a firm, yellow, encapsulated nodule. In the bovine, the nodule is thick, dense, and commonly calcified.

Diagnosis

The clinical lesions of tuberculosis are usually not noted until the disease has reached an advanced stage. By that time, most individuals have become shedders of tubercle bacilli and are a menace to other animals in the herd or flock, and to humans. The most important tool or technique in the diagnosis of tuberculosis is the tuberculin test. The test is based upon the fact that the invading tubercle bacilli make the body sensitive to the products of those bacteria. Tuberculin is prepared for the express purpose of detecting animals affected with tuberculosis. When it is injected into the skin of the caudal fold (under the tail), a swelling will occur at the site within 72 hours if the animal is tubercular. (Injection in the loose skin of the head of the tail is approved and recommended for the tuberculosis eradication program.) The test must be administered by veterinarians trained to recognize and interpret the results.

All cattle injected with tuberculin should be identified with a metal tag in the right ear. All reactors to the tuberculin test are branded on the left jaw with the letter T, and identified by an eartag in the left ear. Reactor cattle must be sent to slaughter without delay.

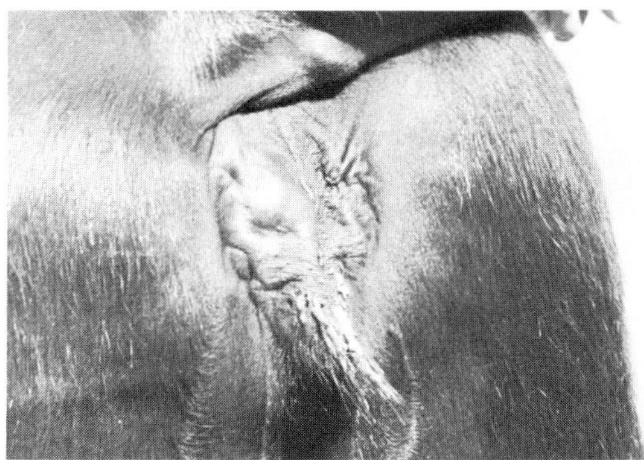

FIG. 18. A positive tuberculosis reactor. Note the swelling in the caudal fold of the tail, denoting an allergic response to tuberculin.

Prevention

Because there are no satisfactory vaccines or bacterins for prevention of tuberculosis in livestock in the United States, the prevention of the disease depends upon testing and eradication. Tuberculosis can be prevented only if animals are not exposed to the disease-producing bacteria. It is not always possible to protect animals completely, but good management and sanitation can reduce the chances of infection.

Prevention of the disease in swine depends upon the control and eradication of tuberculosis in cattle and poultry.

The test and slaughter program recommended by the U.S. Department of Agriculture and supported by the various states is the most efficacious means of eradicating tuberculosis from livestock. The rules and regulations concerning the state-federal cooperative eradication program may be obtained from local veterinarians, or from state and federal regulatory officials. In order to maintain a "Tuberculosis-Free Accredited" herd, and to profit from the benefits of such herd status, close attention must be given to "Uniform Methods and Rules for the Establishment and Maintenance of Tuberculosis-Free Accredited Herds of Cattle, Modified Accredited Areas, and Areas Accredited Free of Bovine Tuberculosis in the Domestic Bovine." As the eradication program progresses, significant changes are made from time to time in the regulations, which are applicable to all cattle entering into interstate movement, and to all commercial dairy herds.

30
Vesicular Stomatitis

VESICULAR stomatitis is a virus disease of cattle, swine, and sometimes horses, characterized by inflammation of the tongue, the mucosa of the mouth, the coronary band of the hoof, and the formation of thin-walled vesicles containing clear or yellowish serous fluid. The disease may be transmitted to humans. Public-health significance is related to the development of a systemic reaction and mouth lesions among susceptible laboratory personnel, veterinarians, and farmers when exposed to the virus.

Geographically, vesicular stomatitis is considered to be confined to the western hemisphere. However, during periods of great movement of cattle and horses, the disease has spread to Europe; its current significance in Europe is unknown. Within the United States, vesicular stomatitis is primarily found in the southeastern part of the United States, although it has spread in the past through the cattle-raising areas of the middle west. Since it is prevalent where the climate is temperate, there are areas in the United States where the disease is endemic at all times during the year.

Historically, the disease was first described in horses during World War I, and subsequently in horses shipped to Europe during that period of time. It was first described in cattle in 1926 and in swine in 1943.

Etiology

Vesicular stomatitis is caused by a virus. The host range includes sheep, dogs, deer, bobcats, many rodents, and cold-blooded animals. The virus may be propagated in tissue culture in the laboratory and on chicken embryos. However, since vesicular stomatitis in cattle and swine is clinically indistinguishable from foot-and-mouth disease and vesicular exanthema, a differential diagnosis is of great importance.

Two types of the virus are described in the United States: the Indiana type and the New Jersey type. Each of these is immunologically different from the other; however, the New Jersey type is considered more prevalent and possibly more virulent than the Indiana type.

The virus, found in abundance in the clear, vesicular fluid and the vesicular covering, is most infective at the time the vesicles rupture or shortly thereafter. It may be found in the blood during the febrile stage of the disease and for a short period afterward. However, once the blisters or vesicles have burst, the virus is no longer recoverable from the blood.

The virus remains active for several days at body temperatures, but is rapidly killed by direct sunlight. It is also susceptible to solutions of formalin, cresylic-acid soaps and hypochlorite, as is foot-and-mouth disease virus.

Transmission

Transmission of vesicular stomatitis virus is by direct contact with saliva, or material contaminated by saliva, of infected animals, and by the vesicular fluid expressed from ruptured vesicles. Mechanical transmission by insects has been demonstrated in the laboratory and, because infections usually vanish with the first frost, insect vectors have been incriminated as a means of transmission of the virus. Abrasions of the mouth, feet, or teats facilitate successful establishment and growth of the virus found on feed materials. Crowding of animals tends to lead to a spread of vesicular stomatitis; however, the disease is seen more frequently among animals on pasture than in those crowded into feedlots.

Factors Influencing Susceptibility

The incidence of vesicular stomatitis in all livestock appears to be greater during the warm summer than during the winter. Infection ceases with the first frost, lending credence to the assumption that an insect vector is the source of spread and the reservoir over the winter months. Age appears to be associated with susceptibility in cattle, as few cases appear in cattle less than one year of age. However, in swine the disease occurs in suckling pigs as well as in older animals. There appears to be no age susceptibility influence in horses.

Feeding on plants with acrid substance on the leaves (clover, rape and similar roughages) may produce slight irritation or abrasions in the mouth; these facilitate the entrance of viruses which may be on the pasture plants or in feed material or drinking troughs.

Symptoms

The incubation period for the virus appears to be 2 to 5 days, during which the temperatures may rise to 105 F; however, once the vesicles have formed and ruptured, the temperature decreases rapidly. The first symptoms noted in dairy cattle are a loss of milk secretion and a beginning of loss of condition. Examination of the animal at this time reveals lesions in the mouth varying from very small to pea size. When a small vesicle ruptures, others may rapidly develop around the site and coalesce to involve a considerable portion or the entire surface of the tongue or lips. These lesions cause pain resulting in loss of appetite, lowered milk secretion, and loss of condition. The lesions may cover the entire surface of the teats, or may occur as isolated vesicles on one or more teats. Lesions may also appear in the interdigital spaces between the claws, but are usually confined to only one foot. In swine, the vesicular lesions may appear on the snout and on the coronary band around the foot. Lesions on teats and feet do not occur as frequently as in other vesicular diseases. In the average herd afflicted with vesicular stomatitis, the morbidity rate will be approximately 50 percent; however, if blood samples are taken for laboratory diagnosis, 100 percent of the animals in the herd may show antibodies indicative of a frank or inapparent infection.

The lesions appearing on the mouth, tongue, gums, lips, and even extending to the nostrils on cattle and swine appear first as small macules, or raised pimples, which de-

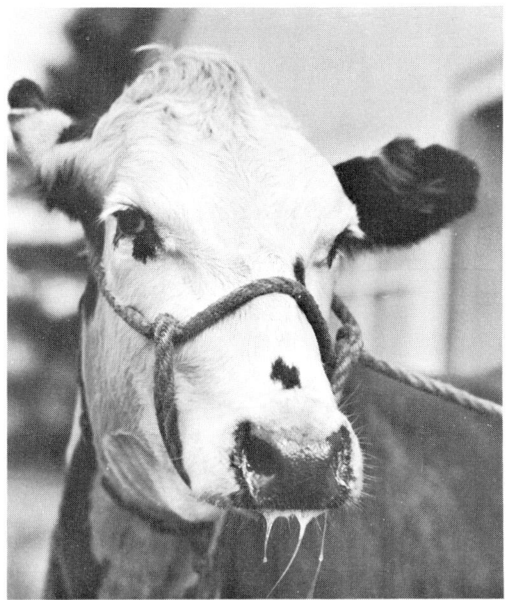

FIG. 19. Typical appearance of vesicular stomatitis in a cow 48 hours after experimental inoculation with the virus.

velop quickly into full-blown vesicles. The vesicles are filled with a straw-colored clear fluid in which the virus is propagating rapidly and which may serve as a source of contamination for other animals. Once the vesicles have ruptured, the site heals quickly; however, there may be time for entry of secondary invaders, causing additional ulceration and pain. Vesicles on the tongue usually rupture and leave a denuded area which may be extensive, sometimes including the entire epithelium of the upper surface, with bluish discoloration; this can lead to secondary bacterial invasion.

Pathology

The virus gains entry through abrasions in the mouth, around the coronary band of the hoof, or on the teat surfaces, with production of macules, vesicles, and erosions following the rupture of the vesicles. After invasion, the virus enters the lower level of the skin, attacks epithelial cells, and grows rapidly. In a few hours many cells are injured and the viral particles are released; the virus then invades other cells closer to the surface of the skin, and the resulting vesicles are formed. The virus appears in the blood during this stage of the disease, but the infective stage decreases after the vesicles have ruptured. Within 3 to 4 days the virus can no longer be demonstrated in either the blood or the saliva.

Diagnosis

The clinical diagnosis of vesicular stomatitis is based upon the occurrence of typical oral, foot, or mammary lesions in adult cattle and swine during warm months in a known enzootic area. Because of the similarity of this disease to foot-and-mouth disease and vesicular exanthema, great care must be exercised in arriving at a positive diagnosis. Whenever there is a question, expert veterinary assistance and laboratory confirmation must be obtained.

Treatment

In the past commercial vaccines have been available to combat this disease on a herd basis. However, because the disease is reportable in most states, and because eradication methods have been successful, vaccines are no longer necessary. Should an outbreak occur, vaccines to combat the ravages of the disease in endemic areas could be readily obtained.

Prevention

Prevention is based primarily on good management procedures, that is, a strict quarantine and the banning of shipment of animals for a minimum of 30 days after all evidence of an infection has passed. Recov-

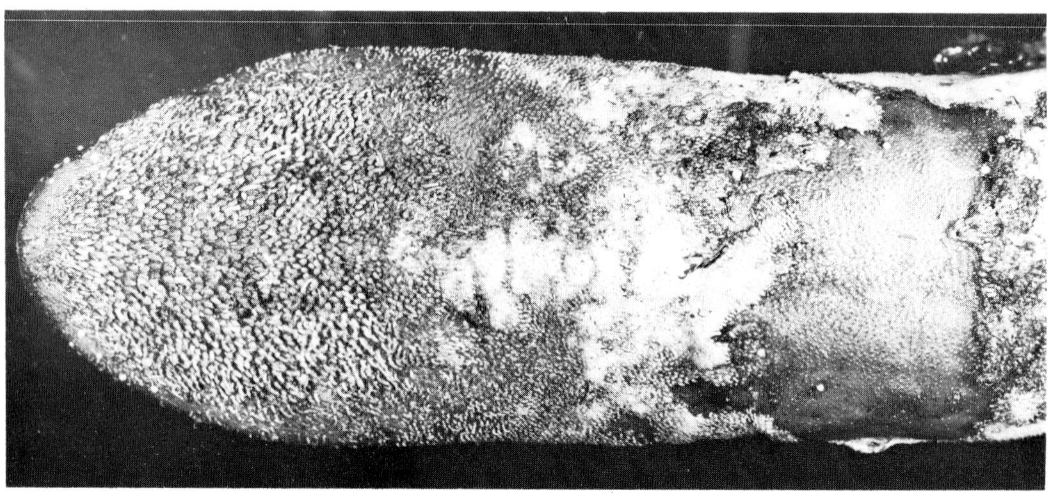

FIG. 20. Bovine tongue showing denuded area resulting from vesicular stomatitis. (From Jensen, R., and Mackey, D. R.: *Diseases of Feedlot Cattle.* Ed. 2, Philadelphia, Lea & Febiger, 1971.)

ered animals are immune for 2 to 3 months; however, no cross immunity exists with other vesicular diseases, or from one type of vesicular stomatitis virus to another type. It thus becomes necessary to segregate all infected animals and to use separate feeding equipment and material when the disease has been diagnosed. Even though strict quarantine is seldom applied, owners of diseased cattle should avoid direct or indirect exposure of other feedlots or farms. Flying and crawling insects should be controlled and palliative treatment of the complicated vesicles should be initiated.

31
Vibriosis

VIBRIOSIS in cattle is an infectious disease of the genital tract, caused by *Vibrio fetus* and characterized by infertility and occasional abortion. It is spread by breeding and is considered the most important cause of infertility in cattle.

Vibriosis also occurs in sheep, causing an infection of the bloodstream which results in abortion. In sheep, the disease apparently is spread by contact with aborted fetuses or contaminated food and water rather than by breeding.

Vibriosis is worldwide in distribution and was first described in this country in 1918. Due to the overshadowing importance of brucellosis at that time, and to the difficulty in culturing the vibriosis organism, research progressed slowly. In 1940, however, it was established that vibrio infection caused abortion and impaired breeding efficiency in affected herds. A few years later scientists proved that venereal transmission resulted in delayed conception and irregular estrual cycles.

Etiology

Bovine vibriosis is caused by the bacterium *Vibrio fetus,* bovine strain. Isolated cultures have a short comma shape but change to long, spiral-shaped filaments when cultivated artificially. Heat, light, and drying destroy *Vibrio fetus,* but the sheep strain can survive in soil, hay and manure for several days.

There are at least 21 species of the genus Vibrio, of which only four are known to cause disease: *V. fetus, V. cholerae, V. jejuni,* and *V. metchnikovii.*

Transmission

Bovine vibriosis is usually transmitted through breeding, although it may be spread by artificial insemination with infected semen, and by using contaminated instruments for examination. Naturally spread, it manifests itself primarily as temporary infertility with conception delayed 2 to 8 months. Some females have been known to carry the infection for at least 20 months. A few bulls become permanently infected, but all bulls may mechanically carry and spread infection.

Cattle of all ages seem to be susceptible, and spread is rapid in recently infected herds. Older animals usually throw off the infection eventually. Virgin heifers become infected upon exposure and maintain herd infection. Thus the disease may remain a herd problem for years, with replacement animals, bulls or carrier cows acting as reservoirs of infection. The infection rate in susceptible cows may approach 100 percent. Where cattle commonly mix on summer ranges, or where infected cows or bulls have access to clean herds during the breeding season, the spread of disease is inevitable; clean bulls and virgin heifers are infected by carriers.

Factors Influencing Susceptibility

Vibriosis was formerly a serious cause of temporary infertility in the east and midwest but is now effectively controlled by artificial insemination. Currently the disease is widespread in range herds of beef cattle in the west, where artificial insemination is not practiced.

The disease may be spread among bulls never used for natural service by mechanical transmission through contact with teaser animals, flies, or contaminated equipment.

Symptoms

The usual effect of vibriosis is temporary infertility. At times 16 services, with an average of five, have been necessary to obtain a detectable pregnancy. In a field outbreak of vibriosis, few cows conceived on the first service from an infected bull. A low spring calving rate may be the first real evidence of the disease, and the calving period may be extended over the entire year.

The other prominent symptom is the irregularity of the estrual cycle, which may range from 10 to 60 days. The long cycles occur as infection interrupts conception. The fetus is aborted or resorbed and a new cycle begins. If the fetus is expelled, it is often so small that it is overlooked and the abortion is undetected. Any endometritis, vaginitis and cervicitis sometimes produced may also be overlooked. Abortion rates of 4 to 29 percent have been reported. The abortions may occur at any stage of the gestation period but most are in the fifth and sixth months.

Vibriosis has no direct disabling effect on bulls; however, in infected herds with recurring estrus, bulls may become thin and emaciated through excessive breeding.

Pathology

Vibriosis is a venereal disease spread from infected bulls to noninfected cows. The bacteria are deposited with the semen in the genital tract of the susceptible female. The vibrios multiply and cause the death of the embryo in the first few weeks after fertilization. This is not followed by any signs of disease except the heifer's return to estrus. The infertility caused by vibriosis is temporary and eventually all animals recover. Some will conceive as early as two months after exposure, but some remain infected for as long as nine months. Six months after initial exposure about 75 percent have been found to be pregnant if the bulls were left with the cows. After recovery from the infection, cows have a measure of convalescent immunity to reinfection.

Most bulls are infected transiently, but are capable of spreading the infection for weeks after breeding an infected animal. Some bulls are permanently infected, and carry the disease for years. It appears, however, that cows carrying the infection are as important as bulls in maintaining the disease from year to year in the herd. Carrier cows may give birth to normal calves in spite of infection.

Diagnosis

The presence of vibriosis may be suspected from the reproductive history and symptoms within the herd, but laboratory confirmation is desirable. The history may include introduction of animals from herds where vibriosis or infertility is known to exist. Clinical tests to confirm a positive diagnosis of vibriosis include:

1. *Vaginal mucus agglutination test.* Vaginal mucus is absorbed on a sterile tampon. Then, in the laboratory, the mucus is extracted in saline and the agglutination test is performed.
2. *Isolation of Vibrio organisms from the bull.* This is difficult since the organisms in semen or preputial washings are usually overgrown with contaminants. On the average only one sample in five from known infected bulls is positive. In some instances 15 consecutive samples have been required to find the organism.
3. *Isolation of Vibrio from the female genital tract.* Vaginal or cervical mucus is removed with a sterile pipette and the organism is isolated by bacteriological methods. This is the most reliable procedure. (The organism can also be isolated from the stomach of an aborted fetus.)
4. *Transmission test.* Suspect bulls are bred to virgin heifers. Then the heifers are subjected to culturing techniques to recover and identify the organism.

Control

Control measures may be instituted in noninfected herds by restricting replacements to virgin animals from known free herds. In infected herds, control may be accomplished by breeding a second herd of virgin animals to eventually replace the infected herd. (The replacement of infected cows in a year-round breeding program is inadvisable since it is expensive and impractical.)

Another method of control in infected herds is artificial insemination; this does not eliminate the disease but will control further spread.

Usually the most practical and economical method of prevention and control is herd immunization with bacterin. A commercially produced *Vibrio fetus* adjuvant bacterin, after three years of extensive use in herds in all parts of this country and abroad, has been proved to be so effective that pregnancy rates of 90 percent or higher have resulted in almost all infected herds treated with the bacterin.

Properly, the bacterin is used 30 to 120 days before breeding and consequent possible exposure to vibriosis. Experiments have shown that active immunity is similar to convalescent immunity, and that both decrease with time. It is economically sound to revaccinate annually to maintain a maximal level of immunity. Cows vaccinated 12 months prior to heavy exposure to vibriosis were only 56 percent pregnant, while those bred to infected bulls following vaccination had a 70 percent pregnancy rate when rebred to infected bulls the second year. Infection and bacterin immunity complement each other, but infection cannot be depended on since most bulls lose the infection between breeding seasons. It is not necessary or desirable to vaccinate bulls, for vaccinated bulls can continue to spread the disease mechanically. Pregnant animals can be vaccinated. Revaccination may be done at the usual weaning time, when the cows are being handled, without loss of efficiency.

The most important cause of infertility in cattle can, thus, be controlled effectively by vaccination. The cost is low enough that many ranchers with clean herds are using vaccination to protect them from accidental infection from infected herds in the vicinity.

PART 3

Selected Tactical Diseases

32
Pinkeye

PINKEYE is an acute infectious disease of cattle, sheep and sometimes other animals, characterized by marked inflammation of the tissues of the eye and often designated by the synonyms *infectious bovine keratitis* and *infectious conjunctivitis.* It has been recognized since 1889 and is believed to be caused by a bacterium, *Moraxella bovis,* and an unclassified virus. The disease is widespread throughout the United States, especially among range and feedlot cattle. It is encountered in nearly half of all beef cattle herds and affects about 3 percent of all beef cattle.

Pinkeye is known to occur all over the world and may appear at all seasons. It is most commonly seen in summer months, although there are reports of its occurrence during colder months, especially when the ground is covered with snow. It is always more prevalent when cattle are on the range without protection from intense light and especially during the seasons when flies are most active. Pinkeye affects animals of all ages, but animals under two years seem to be most susceptible. Sheep and goats may also be affected, but this should not be confused with virus pinkeye. The bacterium *Colesiota conjunctivae* is the usual cause of pinkeye in sheep.

The severity of the disease and its yearly drain on the cattle industry are of great economic importance.

Etiology

The disease has a complicated and unsettled etiology. It is generally believed to be caused by *Moraxella bovis* and by a virus, either of which may act separately; both organisms are found in discharges from the eyes and noses of infected animals in which the primary lesions are confined to the cornea and conjunctiva. Some investigators have indicated that the Moraxella microorganism is the cause of infectious keratitis of cattle, but others believe that this has not definitely been established even though it is usually present in acute cases. Inability to agree on the role of *Moraxella bovis* in pinkeye may be due to lack of uniformity in the types studied. It is possible that the differences may be accounted for by bacterial variation. *Moraxella bovis* is a short, plump rod, usually occurring in pairs and short chains, nonmotile, aerobic, gram-negative, killed at 140 F in 5 minutes. Other bacteria are frequently isolated from infected cattle, and they are streptococci and staphylococci species. Both *M. bovis* and the virus have been studied separately and in pure form. Both have the ability to produce ocular lesions.

Factors Influencing Susceptibility

Cattle of all ages and both sexes are susceptible but pinkeye is more severe and frequent in those under two years of age. Dust, wind, bright sunlight, insects (especially flies), poor nutrition, vitamin A deficiency, and other conditions causing injury to the eye are usually predisposing causes. Cattle with non-pigmented faces, such as Herefords and Shorthorns, are severely affected.

Transmission

It is possible that cattle recovered from the disease may be able to spread the infection for several months after all symptoms have disappeared. Once the outbreak has started, microorganisms are rapidly spread by flies that cluster alternately around the eyes of infected and healthy animals. The disease is believed to be carried through the winter in a chronic form by carrier animals, and seems to spread slightly before the arrival of flies. Secretions from the eyes have been demonstrated to contain *M. bovis* several months after apparently complete recovery. Pinkeye may also be transmitted by direct contact, and possibly by infected dust. Because nasal secretions of infected animals contain the causative agents, aerosols may be sprayed by coughing and sneezing. Common water troughs and feeding equipment also provide opportunities for spread. Introduction of carrier animals into susceptible herds is a frequent method of initiating the disease within a herd.

Symptoms

Pinkeye is characterized by inflammation of the cornea, accompanied by nasal discharge, lacrimation and copious ocular discharge which streams down the cheeks. The cornea turns a cloudy, opaque white and eventually the eyelids close. In this condition animals display extreme discomfort, and a sharp drop in milk production results. Affected animals behave as "loners," suffer injuries because of temporary blindness, and require special handling. In extreme cases permanent blindness occurs, greatly decreasing the value of the animal.

The incubation period is 3 to 5 days and the average outbreak lasts about three weeks. Young animals are most seriously affected, and some older animals seem to retain considerable resistance after one attack, although

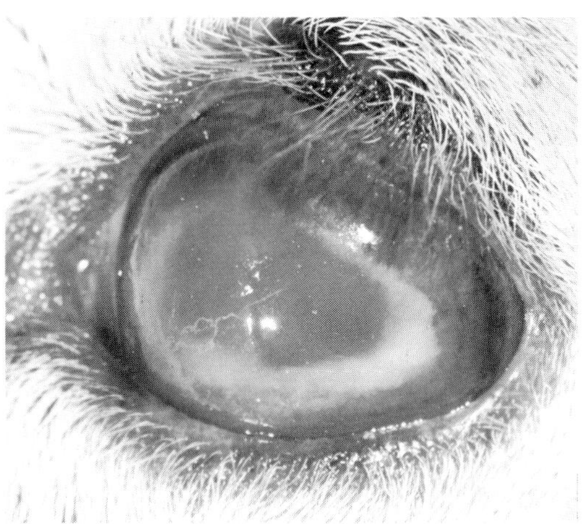

FIG. 21. Corneal opacity characteristic of pinkeye in cattle. (From Jensen, R., and Mackey, D. R.: *Diseases of Feedlot Cattle.* Ed. 2, Philadelphia, Lea & Febiger, 1971.)

they are not completely immune. Ulcers may form in severe cases on the front of one or both eyes near the pupil, and if progress is unchecked they may cause blindness and even loss of the eye. The attack may also be marked by slight digestive upset. Most animals completely recover from the disease.

Pathology

Rapid passage of the microorganism causing pinkeye through a succession of susceptible animals causes an increase in virulence. Once the causative agents localize in the eye, they cause injury to the epithelial cells of the conjunctiva and bring about circulatory disturbances accompanied by swelling and congestion. The cornea becomes edematous, with thickening, clouding and opacity. Within a few days small ulcers form on the cornea; these may regress or coalesce to form larger ulcers and penetrate into the deeper layers, resulting in loss of aqueous humor and lens. If regression does not occur, secondary pathogens gain entry through the cornea. In most cases, however, the infection is controlled before perforation of the cornea occurs and the eye heals rapidly, usually with a residual scar of varying opacity.

Diagnosis

Diagnosis is usually based on the typical symptoms and the appearance of the lesions. The disease may sometimes be confused with irritations due to dust and wind, foreign bodies in the eye, or injuries by weed stems; however, there is of course no spreading from the latter conditions. Laboratory isolation of *M. bovis* and/or the virus will confirm the diagnosis of pinkeye.

Prevention

There are no specific vaccines, bacterins, or serums that will prevent the disease.

Good management is the most effective and practical measure of control. Affected animals should be placed in dark quarters to avoid the irritation of flies and direct sunlight. Upon the advice of a veterinarian, an infected animal may be isolated and treated with antibiotics. (If dark quarters are not available for isolation, infected animals should be moved to distant pastures.)

Newly purchased animals should be kept isolated for at least 60 days before mingling with disease-free animals. Because flies spread the disease, spraying the herd with fly repellents and insecticides at regular intervals will help reduce the number of animals affected. Healthy animals should be checked daily for symptoms that would indicate the spread of the infection.

33 Mastitis

MASTITIS, an important disease of lactating females, is a disease complex in which bacterial infections, trauma and faulty managerial practices play important roles. The disease has been studied extensively from etiological and management standpoints, and methods of diagnosis, therapy and control have been thoroughly investigated. The actual pathological processes occurring in the inflamed mammary gland have received less attention, however.

Several pathogenic agents are commonly involved in mastitis. The most important are streptococci, staphylococci, fungi, and, occasionally, gas-producing bacteria. Contributing causes are bruises, cuts, cold weather, and rough handling.

Mastitis is a disease that may occur in all types of mammals, although it is of greatest economic importance in dairy cows and goats. It is the most serious disease of dairy cows and is to be found wherever they are raised. The incidence of the disease has increased over the years in direct proportion to the increased production of milk by dairy cows. Mastitis may thus be considered a consequence of progress.

Etiology

The primary cause of mastitis in the past has been *Streptococcus agalactiae,* associated with some type of trauma. In recent years, however, *Staphylococcus aureus* has been incriminated in about 50 percent of mastitis cases. Occasionally, the disease may be caused by coliform bacteria and by gas-producing bacteria.

Fungi and molds have been isolated from cases of mastitis, but only rarely.

Because mastitis is complex, complete elimination may be an unrealistic goal. Good, sound preventive measures will go a long way toward controlling the condition. There are no short cuts to prevention, and good management is essential.

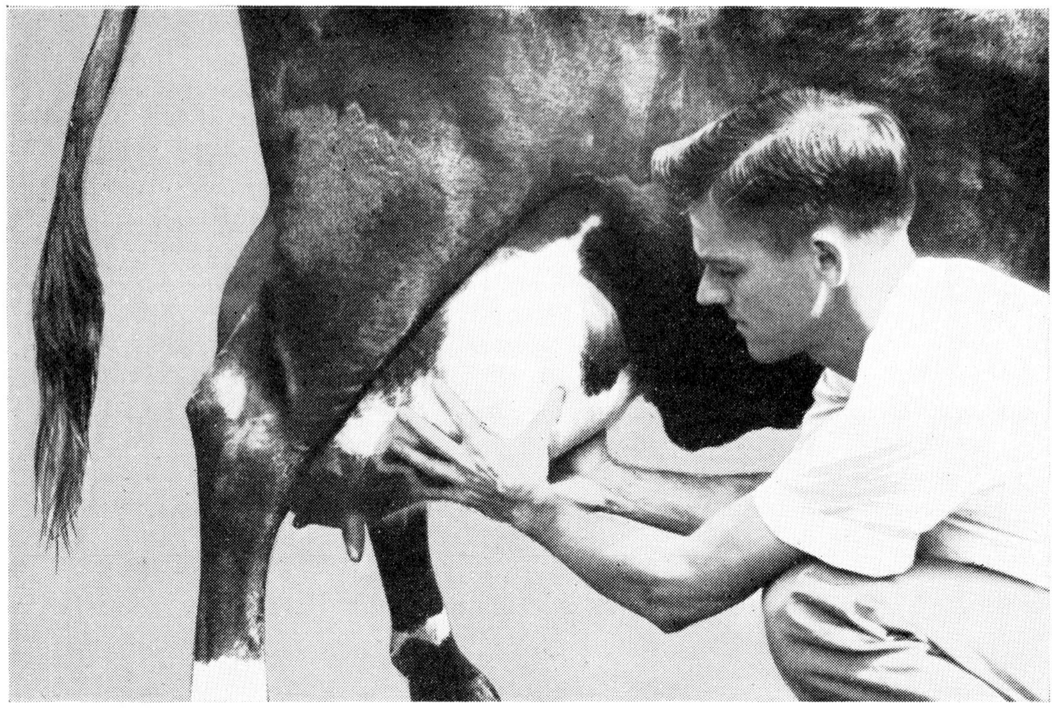

FIG. 22. Palpating the udder for mastitis. (From Gibbons, W. J.: *Clinical Diagnosis of Diseases of Large Animals.* Philadelphia, Lea & Febiger, 1966.)

Factors Influencing Susceptibility

Clinical mastitis is usually associated with some type of trauma—accidents in the barn, barnyard, or pasture that may bruise or injure the udder. Injury is important in itself as a cause of poor milk, but of greater importance as a means of providing a focus for the development of pathogenic bacteria.

Other predisposing factors include: the size of the streak canal and the condition of the sphincter muscle, completeness of milking, rough handling of the udder during milking, pressure on the teat cups, and chilling of the udder.

The tightness of the spincter muscle and the size of the streak canal can prevent the invasion of bacteria into the mammary gland, where they would find a suitable medium for growth. Milk remaining on the tips of the teats may harbor pathogenic organisms which will invade an enlarged streak canal.

Incomplete milking causes stress to delicate secretory tissue and directly affects milk production while, secondarily, the stress-damaged area provides a focus for pathogenic microorganisms. Teat cups remaining too long on the udder, excessive negative pressure on the milking machine, and rough hand milking all lead to trauma of the udder. One of the most common causes of mastitis in the winter is chilling of the udder while the animal is standing in cold, muddy water, or lying on the snow or on cold concrete.

Transmission

Sources of infection for mastitis are microorganisms found in the natural environment.

Causative bacteria may live on the body of cows and may be inapparent invaders of the udder, awaiting proper conditions in which to reproduce and cause inflammation. Flies may transmit the causative bacteria, as may the milker. It may be assumed, however, that the principal mode of transmission is through mismanagement of the milking herd. Good management is essential if the disease is to be controlled, and is the key to prevention.

Symptoms

There are several types of mastitis, each with a slightly different set of symptoms: acute, chronic, coliform, and gangrenous mastitis.

Acute Mastitis

This is sudden in onset and very obvious. The udder is enlarged, hot to the touch, and tender. One or more quarters may be inflamed but the infection is most often confined to only one. Milk removed from the infected quarter will either appear thick and flaky or thin and watery. The affected cow will be reluctant to move, and will usually have a fever. Prompt treatment by a veterinarian will lead to rather dramatic recovery without undue loss of production. If not treated promptly, the quarter may be permanently damaged and milk production lowered or lost.

Coliform Mastitis

Here the onset of symptoms is rapid, the temperature may be high, and the cow may appear unsteady on her feet. The milk is usually thin, watery, and brownish in color. Unless treated promptly, the quarter or quarters may be damaged and will not remain productive. However, if treated in time, the infected quarter will return to production at the next lactation.

Chronic Mastitis

Intermittent symptoms consist of repeated mild mammary swellings, periodic clots in the milk, mild anorexia, and fever. Chronic mastitis seems to be related to age and may appear in latent, subclinical, and mild forms in many cows in a herd.

Gangrenous Mastitis

In the clinical stages of this infection the udder will be cold to the touch, bluish in color, with a definite line of demarkation between inflamed and healthy tissue. The inflamed tissue will be nerveless, and if cut will release bubbles of gas in the serum. Chronic streptococcal mastitis is usually followed by atrophy of the quarter, while severe chronic staphylococcal mastitis results in swelling and fibrosis, leaving a firm, enlarged quarter. Gangrenous mastitis may, on the other hand, result in the loss of the teat through vasoconstriction.

Prevention

Proper management includes particular attention to the milking procedure, operation of and working condition of milking equipment, feeding and care of the herd, sanitation, and maintenance of health records for each lactating animal.

Health records, in conjunction with readily available aids such as the strip cup and the California mastitis test paddle, will reveal cows with abnormal milk. Such knowledge will be of value in arranging the milking order of the herd to prevent the spread of infection. All cows having udder irritation or abnormal milk should be regarded as possible sources of infection to other cows and should be milked last; if several cows are bothered with mastitis, a separate milking machine should be reserved for them. To restrict the spread of infection, the milking order would be:

heifers, uninfected cows, suspected cows, infected cows. Individual shedders of microorganisms should be separated, kept under observation, and treated.

Scrupulous cleanliness of barns and lounging areas will reduce the numbers of infectious microorganisms causing mastitis, but will not eliminate them. It is particularly important to replace infected cows with healthy ones and to prevent calves from sucking each other. A regular routine of such preventive measures will take less time and effort than individual attention to infected cows. A good preventive program should keep to a minimum the number of cows requiring special attention and handling.

Recent research by the U.S. Department of Agriculture has shown that mastitis can be reduced by teat-dipping after milking, thus reducing the numbers of bacteria on the udders. This may be related to the susceptibility of the teat opening to an invasion of pathogens immediately after milking, when the sphincter muscle at the opening of the streak canal is stretched and partially relaxed. Teat-dipping helps wash away and kill these organisms, and also removes from the teat end any milk in which potential mastitis microorganisms could grow and multiply.

Although teat-dipping will not affect the amount of infection already in the udders of a herd of dairy cows, if properly carried out it will reduce the number of new infections. However, it is not a substitute for sound milking and management practices, but merely a step in a good milking routine that can limit the incidence of mastitis.

34
Ketosis

KETOSIS is a metabolic disease of lactating cows caused by an imbalance between nutritive intake and nutritive requirements. The disease occurs within a few days or weeks after calving. It is characterized by low blood-glucose levels, depletion of liver-glucose stores, mobilization of body proteins as amino acids, mobilization and utilization of fat-storage depots of the body, and infiltration of the liver, associated with increased production of ketone bodies in the blood and urine.

An accurate appraisal of the economic loss caused by ketosis is difficult, because the disease is not associated with high mortality. Observations from widely separated areas indicate that clinical ketosis is responsible for a heavy loss in milk production. It also is of considerable importance to the beef cattle industry, as it occurs frequently in the heavier milking cows of the beef breeds. Ketosis in cattle occurs in practically every country in which dairying is practiced. However, only a few cases occur in those areas where modern selection and production management practices are ignored. Therefore, it would appear that ketosis is a disease associated with high production of both calves and milk.

Ketosis may occur at all ages but it is most common during the years of greatest production, that is, after the second or third lactation. Therefore, it is associated with age and sex of dairy animals.

Etiology

Although there are several predisposing factors associated with ketosis, the exact etiology is not known. A complex of factors can be associated with this metabolic condition. It may be said with certainty, however, that interactions between the diet and endocrine glands in cattle are mechanisms of development of the disease. Certain aspects of ruminant physiology and nutrition predispose the lactating dairy cow to ketosis. Metabolic dependence upon rumen microorganisms and the excessive demands of heavy lactation are principal contributing factors. Competition by the mammary gland for energy products leads to a metabolic breakdown. When the major energy mechanism is blocked, the ruminant is unable effectively to utilize certain substances produced by digestion, among them ketone bodies (or acids). It is apparent then that the incidence of clinical ketosis can be minimized by bringing nutrient consumption into line with physiological needs, particularly in the critical pre- and postpartum periods.

One school of thought regards the disease primarily as a carbohydrate deficiency, associated with a defect in carbohydrate metabolism. Another theory is that the disease is basically a temporary adrenal insufficiency.

The carbohydrate-deficiency hypothesis is based on the observation that, of the various forms of carbohydrate ingested by the ruminant, little is absorbed as glucose. If this is so, the lactating cow receives little or no carbohydrate beyond that required for the synthesis of the lactose secreted in the milk. The metabolic-defect theory is supported by the fact that ketosis occurs when the dietary intake of carbohydrate or its precursors is inadequate. As only a few lactating cows develop ketosis, there is obviously some deviation in the metabolism of affected animals. This metabolic defect remains undiscovered, but since the endocrine glands influence the function of the various biochemical pathways, it might well be due to some endocrine imbalance.

When all available evidence is evaluated, it is difficult to escape the conclusion that carbohydrate deficiency and not adrenal insufficiency is of major importance in the etiology of ketosis in cattle. Any evidence of adrenal insufficiency, instead of weakening it, appears to support and strengthen the carbohydrate-deficiency concept.

Factors Influencing Susceptibility

At the time of calving and lactation, an animal's nutritive and metabolic requirements are increased about 100 percent—partly because of the loss of sugar, proteins, and fat in the milk and partly because of the increased metabolic work associated with the production and secretion of milk. If the dietary intake is adequate, the animal remains normal. If the diet is too poor to maintain approximate normal levels of blood glucose and liver glycogen, an imbalance in metabolism occurs.

This upset is indicated by anorexia, hypoglycemia, and depletion of liver glycogen. In response to these disturbances, compensatory metabolic adjustments are initiated in an attempt to correct the imbalance. When the blood-glucose level is low, the carbohydrate stores in the liver tend to become depleted in an attempt to maintain the level of blood glucose and, in turn, the carbohydrate requirements of other tissues. Ketosis tends to develop under these conditions.

There are several classifications of ketosis, all of which have similar symptoms although slight variations do occur. *Primary ketosis* indicates a simple imbalance between nutritive intake and nutritive requirements of lactating animals. *Secondary ketosis* may occur in varying intensities in lactating or nonlactating cattle, and includes cases in which the metabolic disturbance is precipitated or aggravated by infections, exposure, foreign bodies in the rumen, traumatic gastritis, peritonitis, mastitis, cystic ovaries, vaginitis, displacement of the abomasum, indigestion and starvation.

Ketosis may also be classified as lactation ketosis, digestive ketosis, or nervous ketosis, depending upon the premonitory symptoms. The first two types are similar in their manifestations. Nervous ketosis is evidenced by a derangement of the nervous system brought about by the temporary malnutrition of the brain caused by low blood glucose. The condition can be described as a semiconscious state indicating a depression of the cortical nerve centers of the brain.

Symptoms

The symptoms and signs of ketosis usually appear 1 to 28 days following calving, especially in high-producing cows. All animals with uncomplicated ketosis do not evidence the same symptoms; low blood glucose causes a variety of symptoms even among animals of the same species. These include extreme nervousness, convulsions and lethargy resulting ultimately in coma, lack of appetite, and constipation with hard mucus-covered feces retained in the rectum. There may be a striking picture of depression accompanied by rapid weight loss, drop in milk production, staggering gait, and finally paralysis, with cattle lying with their heads tucked into the flank, in which case the disease resembles milk fever.

The body temperature and the respiratory and pulse rate are usually normal except in the nervous type, or when the ketosis is complicated by other conditions. However, as the severity of the condition varies directly with the degree of nutrient imbalance, it is possible for animals to show shallow and increased respiration accompanied by a strong acetone odor of the breath. Grinding of the teeth and some salivation may also occur.

Nervous symptoms may appear in a small number of cases of ketosis, in which event the animals are extremely excited and have been known to exhibit symptoms often attributed to rabies. Cows often push against the wall or stanchion, manifest unusual movements, and may even attack the handler. They will usually hold their heads in a lowered position and will appear as if blind. Lowered blood-glucose levels and high ketone levels in blood and urine are always present. Unless laboratory tests are made, the blood ketone levels will be difficult to demonstrate. However, simple chemical tests can be conducted on small samples of urine in the field; color changes indicate the level of ketone bodies in the urine.

Postmortem lesions of animals that have died as a result of fulminating ketosis are rather indistinct. Few changes may be seen grossly, except that the liver may show a diffuse yellow color due to fatty infiltration. This liver change plus the history of the animal prior to death present a presumptive diagnosis of ketosis.

Prevention

Ketosis, with or without complications, increases the metabolic requirements roughly proportionately to the magnitude of the combined stresses associated with lactation and other disturbances.

Diet during pregnancy or lactation can increase or reduce the chances of ketosis. If the diet consists entirely of roughage, fermentation in the rumen favors production of acetic acid; this cannot be converted to glucose but can form ketones. However, if the diet contains a high ratio of grains and concentrates, rumen fermentation favors production of propionic acid, which can be converted to glucose.

Animals susceptible to ketosis should be maintained on a relatively high energy intake before calving, and the level should be increased substantially after parturition. To limit the degree of stress, precautions should be taken to avoid marked changes in the environment of the animal during the parturient period.

35
Toxemia of Pregnancy

TOXEMIA of pregnancy is a metabolic disease of sheep resembling ketosis in cattle. The disease is characterized by nervous involvement brought on by low blood sugar and depletion of liver glycogen.

Pregnancy toxemia occurs primarily among ewes in the last few weeks of gestation. Ewes carrying twins or triplets are particularly liable to the disease, although wethers and rams on starvation diets may develop the symptoms.

This disease is frequently found in range flocks where severe climatic conditions restrict grazing, and where sheep are maintained at a poor level of nutrition for the latter part of pregnancy. Therefore, the disease is found worldwide.

Etiology

The knowledge of the etiology and pathogenesis of this disease is not complete. From critical observations, however, it is apparently associated with stress and nutrition level. The primary cause of the toxemia is poor nutrition in late pregnancy. Ewes in good condition carrying twins are more susceptible than ewes carrying a single lamb or those in poor condition. The usual course of events follows a pattern: Ewes well fed at the beginning of pregnancy become overfat, suffer a setback in nutrition followed by a period of stress, and then die. Ewes on a high plane of nutrition will die quickly if forced to consume a poor-quality diet, or to starve for a few days because of severe weather or mismanagement.

Symptoms

Affected ewes are not easily detected in the early stages of the disease. If the flock is driven, however, they tend to fall behind, and, if closely examined, may exhibit a stilted gait with the head held high and often a slight tremor of the muscles of the face and lips. Later they become dull, appear blind although the eyes seem normal, and stand sleepily in one position with the head drooped, inattentive to their surroundings. Finally, they lie down, often with the head resting in the flank, and are unable to stand when assisted to their feet. Unconsciousness follows, and death occurs in 1 to 5 days.

Affected ewes generally show little or no change in level of blood calcium and do not respond to treatment by injections of calcium. The level of blood sugar is reduced and ketones are present in the blood and urine in abnormal quantities. Similar changes can be caused in normal pregnant ewes by starving them for a time, and conditions which cause a setback late in pregnancy are likely to cause an outbreak. Malnutrition during the later stages of pregnancy, especially if associated with cold wet weather, is a predisposing cause for losses in lean seasons.

Ewes left undisturbed on good grazing may die of pregnancy toxemia, but in such cases some unknown factor has caused them to lose appetite, and consequently weight, in spite of the abundant feed.

At postmortem examination the only striking feature (aside from the usual presence of two lambs in the uterus) is that the liver is soft and fatty and yellow to grayish-red in color.

Diagnosis

Pregnancy toxemia is easily confused with milk fever or hypocalcemia. Many ewes are lost each season under the impression that they are suffering from pregnancy toxemia, whereas they are in fact suffering from milk fever and could be saved by injections of calcium. With milk fever the symptoms occur just before or just after lambing; the course of the illness is short and death occurs within 24 hours.

Treatment

Once well-marked symptoms have developed, the chance of recovery with any treatment known at present is very slight. Occasionally, in early stages of the disease, good results are obtained by drenching with molasses; however, in other outbreaks this treatment appears to have no effect.

Once toxemia is discovered, immediate steps should be taken to prevent more cases from developing. The flock should be given the best and most palatable feed available; if young nutritious hay is available, they should feed on it an hour or two every day. If the disease develops in a flock on good feed and in high condition, gentle exercise each day is beneficial; they should be taken at an easy pace for about two miles a day, and allowed to graze as they go. Ewes and lambs should be removed as they drop to facilitate handling the remainder. If individual ewes are of high value, the veterinarian may remove the lambs by cesarean section; if near term, the lambs as well as the dam may survive.

Prevention

Since treatment of pregnancy disease is of little value in the advanced stages, prevention is the best policy. It matters little if ewes lose weight slightly just after the mating period, but from the second month of pregnancy onward they should be kept in good condition, increasing in weight. During the last five or six weeks of pregnancy the lamb in the uterus achieves 80 percent of its total growth, and the ewe is also preparing for milk production when the lamb is born. The strain on the mother's resources is thus great, especially if she is carrying more than one lamb. Anything which lowers nutrition level at this time must be avoided as far as possible.

Give ewes the best feed and shelter available, and a good and easily accessible water supply. If it is necessary to yard them during this period, furnish good nutritious diet with as little delay as possible. Do not change suddenly from one type of feed to another, but make the change gradually over a period of a few days. Failure to do this has frequently precipitated outbreaks.

In dry seasons when natural feed is scarce, begin supplementary feeding of the breeding flock while there is still plenty of roughage in the fields. The supplemental feed should be rich in easily digestible protein. Where natural protein-rich fodders, such as legumes, are available, a cereal supplement of corn, oats or wheat may be fed. Alfalfa hay of good quality cannot be excelled.

It is impossible to recommend the quantity of supplement to feed under every condition. Overstocking, severe winter or summer conditions, and unseasonable cold wet weather may upset the most careful plans. To allow for this, adequate reserves of hay or silage, or both, should be carried from year to year.

Obesity should be prevented early in pregnancy but an adequate, nutritious diet is particularly important during the last six weeks.

36

Bloat

BLOAT, or tympanites, is a specific disease of ruminants causing an annual loss to producers of millions of dollars. It is characterized by retention of gas in the rumen, with consequent overextension of the abdomen from pressures produced within the rumen.

The rumen, a diverticulum of the esophagus, is essentially a large fermentation vat, in which different types of microorganisms actively break down the coarse fibrous material consumed by cattle and sheep. In the process of fermentation, gas is produced. To relieve the pressure caused by this normal production of gas, ruminants eructate or belch. Whenever an event or series of events restricts the ruminant's ability to eructate, gas pressures reach abnormal amounts in the rumen leading to overdistension, discomfort and even death.

Bloat occurs in all domestic ruminants, but is most common in cattle. It is particularly important in dairy cattle grazed on a year-round basis, especially on pastures rich in alfalfa or the clovers. Bloat is not considered of economic importance in sheep in other countries, but is a serious economic aspect of sheep husbandry in the western United States.

Although pasture bloat may occur at any time, the incidence is highest in wet summers on rapidly growing clover-dominant pastures. Bloat occurs less often in animals in feedlots and barns.

Etiology

Many complex factors have been implicated at one time or another as contributing to bloat in ruminants, and there are many different methods of classifying this condition; this discussion will classify the disease by nature of probable cause, that is, physical bloat, biochemical bloat, and hereditary bloat.

HEREDITARY BLOAT

This is commonly seen in dwarf cattle, and dwarf calves are habitual bloaters. A few of these individuals have been studied and it has been found that anatomical defects natural to the animals interfere with the eructation process. Some families or strains seem to be more susceptible than others, and in this light the condition appears to be inherited; however, the exact nature is undetermined and the bloat may be due to an accumulation of factors on a given farm or property which may predispose to the disease.

Physical Bloat

This is a result of interference with the eructation reflex, which hinders the passage of gas. Any type of obstruction in the esophagus—foreign bodies, abscesses, adhesions, or gastritis—may predispose to this condition. Overfilling of the rumen with feed and moisture to such an extent that the cardial orifice is obstructed, preventing the release of gas pressure, will also lead to bloat.

Physical bloat may be caused by such solid objects as corncobs, turnips, apples, potatoes, or peaches, which commonly lodge in the esophagus and prevent eructation. External pressure on the esophagus by enlarged mediastinal lymph nodes, interference with cardial innervation, as in indigestion and diaphragmatic hernia (occurring sporadically in young calves) are further examples.

Biochemical Bloat

The overproduction of gas by microorganisms within the rumen, or anything of a chemical nature which has to do with destruction of the reflex action of the eructation process, will lead to bloat. Overfeeding, damage to the right ventral branch of the vagus nerve, drugs and poisonous plants which bring about hypomotility of the rumen, and alkalosis which may cause paralysis of the rumen are all factors which have been implicated.

It should be clearly understood, however, that all types of bloat have one thing in common: the bloat results from a failure to get rid of fermentation gases as rapidly as they are formed. Overproduction of gas per se is not the important factor, since normal animals can eliminate more gas than normally produced under bloating conditions.

Factors Influencing Susceptibility

The occurrence of bloat varies with the region and the type of management on a particular property. The season of the year is important with dairy cattle. Pasture bloat is most common in the spring and early summer when cattle are grazing on succulent legumes such as alfalfa and clover. In the feedlots, however, bloat is seen in the late summer and early fall when cattle are brought in from pasture and fed fresh young hay. Alfalfa hay harvested in the fast-growing stage is particularly conducive to bloat.

Bloat is directly related to the consumption of diets high in legumes and concentrates. There appears to be no correlation between amount and rate of consumption of the forages. However, rations high in starch and protein are conducive to the production of excessive amounts of gas by the slime-producing bacteria residing in the rumen. A secondary factor is that animals put out to pasture on succulent feed often overgraze, producing a moisture level in the rumen so high that it covers the cardial orifice of the esophagus and prevents the escape of gas.

Any circumstance which leads to an increase of alkalosis in the rumen may lead to paralysis of the rumen itself. It has been found that the administration of alkali, either per os or intravenously, causes this condition; although reflex mechanisms are not eliminated, they are greatly weakened by the chemical.

Mechanical injury, or obstruction of the esophagus, or the reticulitis that results from ingesting hardware, are factors frequently leading to bloat. Abnormal growths in any area which may put pressure upon the esophagus may lead to restriction of eructation and to bloat. However, the importance of such abnormalities appears to be minor.

Drugs and toxic factors produced by rumen microorganisms have been implicated as agents which reduce rumen motility and may interfere with eructation. Therefore, it can be seen that ingestion of legumes, which stimulate rumen microorganisms, may result in bloat at one time or another. Other factors, for example, overfilling of the stomach, may also be important in legume bloat. The relative importance of these factors is unknown, but it is presumed to be minor compared to excess production of bubbles by the slime-producing bacteria within the rumen following consumption of legumes.

The bloat caused by legumes is primarily characterized by the production of froth; there is then very little free gas within the rumen. Gas bubbles trapped in the ingesta create a situation resembling sticky foam which does not allow the escape of the gas. Cows dying of bloat invariably have froth in the rumen. However, the rumen contents of animals dead several hours frequently contain only free gas, since the froth breaks down after death.

Symptoms

Antemortem signs observed in bloated cattle include: gaseous extension of the left flank and the abdomen, uneasiness as indicated by stamping of the feet, frequent urination and defecation, extension of the head and neck, labored breathing, slight protrusion of the tongue, and finally collapse and death without a struggle.

Death from bloat has been thought to be due to mechanical interference with circulation and respiration from overdistension of the rumen. Biochemical alterations of plasma due to the abnormal absorption of carbon dioxide and other noxious gases produced in the rumen have also been implicated. Normally, carbon dioxide and methane gases are innocuous but under pressure may be forced into the capillary circulation, thus causing intoxication.

Pathology

The most prominent sign is distension of the rumen; however, this may be seen as a natural postmortem phenomenon in all ruminants, as gas continues to be produced after death.

Generalized symptoms include extreme congestion of the lymphoid tissue of the head and neck, with absence of congestion in the muscles and lymph nodes of the hindquarters. Extensive hemorrhages into the mucosa of the trachea and, in the rumen, congestion of large areas of the ventral sacs may be found. Edema of connective tissue is not associated with lesions of muscle tissue. The rumen is filled to maximum capacity and overextended; it usually contains a mixture of feed and stable foam. The upper plain contains a mass of free gas, but foam and feed fill the cardia. There is an absence of blood in the vessels and organs of the abdomen and the thoracic cavity, including the heart, although peripheral blood vessels are congested.

Diagnosis

The diagnosis of bloat is based upon typical clinical signs and upon the finding of froth in the rumens of dead animals suspected of bloat.

Treatment and Prevention

Bloat may be caused by one or more of a series of complicating conditions predisposing a ruminant animal to excess gas production and the inability to relieve this condition by eructation. Because no single entity causes bloat in domestic animals, the condition must be controlled by careful application of modern management practices. However, these are subject to many inexplicable failures and therefore only guarded recommendations may be made. In general, procedures to attempt to control bloat include provision of adequate minerals, salt, and water in the diet (a nonbloating type of diet, obviously). Secondly, nonbloaters should be selected for breeding, and all dwarf animals should be eliminated from the breeding herd.

Pasturing should be controlled so that hungry animals will not overfeed on growing legumes. Wherever possible, animals grazing on legume pastures should be restricted to as much feed as they will consume in one day, requiring them to graze thoroughly. If possible, and wherever bloating becomes a problem in a given field, it may be well to spray the field with light mineral oils or peanut oil to reduce the frothy bloating. In some instances antibiotics may be added to the feed on high-concentrate diets; however, this provides only minimal protection and rapidly induces changes in the rumen flora. It may sometimes be efficacious to add surface-active agents such as detergents to ruminant feeds. It must be remembered, however, that this practice may be harmful to ruminant microorganisms and may cause irritation to the mucosa of the digestive tract. If at all possible straight legume pastures should be avoided. If animals are turned out on fast-growing young legume pastures, dry forage should be provided before they are allowed to graze.

When it becomes necessary to change feeds, it is important to change slowly to prevent overeating. Where green alfalfa is fed it is best to chop it and mix it with straw so that the fresh alfalfa will not layer in the rumen, forcing the moisture level above the cardial orifice. Cattle will overeat when put on succulent pasture after a period of dry feeding.

When bloating does occur, treatment must be initiated immediately as animals suffering from bloat may die within one hour. The method of treatment varies with the degree of distension. If time permits, a stomach tube can be passed into the rumen to expel some of the gas. In more severe cases, however, a trocar can be passed into the rumen through the left paralumbar fossa to relieve the distension; however, this should be attempted only when death is imminent. A handful of common laundry detergent into the mouth often brings about a reflex eructation, providing some relief for nonfrothy bloat and helping to lower the surface tension of froth, allowing the gas to consolidate into one large bubble. To prevent recurrences once bloat has been primarily relieved, stand animals with front quarters elevated, and if necessary apply a stomach tube or a stick across the mouth to provide an open passageway for the relief of gas.

The recent development of medicated salts which may be left in fields and barns for free-choice consumption by ruminants has indicated that some measure of control may be possible. These products have been successful in limited trials and may prove to be a means of preventing bloat in the future.

37
Foot Rot

FOOT ROT, or infectious ovine pododermatitis, is a chronic, contagious, nonsuppurative disease of the feet of sheep and goats. It is characterized by progressive necrosis of the deep layers of the epidermis, separating the horn from the soft tissues and resulting in lameness.

Historically, foot rot has been recognized and mentioned in the literature of Europe for several hundred years. The disease has been known in America since the arrival of the first sheep, but it was not until 1904 that scientists in the United States Department of Agriculture discovered the causative microorganisms.

Geographically, the disease is worldwide, but the incidence varies appreciably and is most common in those areas where heavy stocking is practiced and where rainfall is abundant.

Etiology

The disease is caused by two distinctly different bacteria; it will not exist if only one is present. Both of these organisms are anaerobes, that is, they will live and grow only in the absence of air. This fact is important in understanding the prevention and treatment of the disease. Of the two, *Sphaerophorus nodosus,* a strict parasite that will not live more than a week away from an infected foot, is the primary cause, but *Spirochaeta penortha* must also be present to produce the disease.

The incubation period for foot rot is 7 to 14 days. Therefore, purchased or borrowed animals should be kept under quarantine for 2 to 3 weeks before being allowed to mingle with noninfected sheep.

The causative microorganisms live and are carried in the dead tissue trapped in overgrown and neglected feet of sheep and goats. Moist, lowland pastures are conducive to rapid overgrowth of the hoof and lack of normal hoof wear, and are therefore often associated with the disease. However, the disease cannot exist unless the specific bacteria are present.

One or several feet may be affected. Both claws on the affected foot are usually involved. An injury or wound is usually the point of entry of infection, but by the time the disease is recognized this is seldom apparent.

Transmission

In almost all cases the disease is introduced into a flock through the purchase or borrowing of infected animals. The disease spreads within a flock as a result of infection picked up on pasture, in wet areas around water tanks and water holes, and in filthy pens contaminated by the feet of infected sheep. The infection does not survive long in the presence of air. Pastures that have been free of sheep for 2 to 3 weeks may be considered clean and safe to use.

Foot rot is potentially economically serious in sheep, especially in the larger flocks. The reason for this is twofold: (1) the tremendous amount of time and labor required to eradicate the disease, and (2) the losses in breeding flock and market lambs during the treatment and eradication period.

Contagious foot rot is a specific disease of sheep and goats, and is not acquired from contact or association with other species of farm animals. It is totally different from, and should not be confused with, foot rot in cattle.

Factors Influencing Susceptibility

Sheep and goats of all ages, sexes, and breeds are susceptible. Certain breeds have, at times, been claimed to have natural resistance to the disease, but these claims have not been substantiated by field observation or research.

Symptoms

The first and most obvious symptom is lameness, commencing with a mild inflammation between the claws. As the infection progresses, it causes a break in the skin of the junction with the horn, and spreads rapidly under the horn tissue to the sole.

In the early stages of an outbreak, one or more individuals will show an area of tenderness, reddening and puffiness between the toes and on the heels. The foot may feel warmer than normal. The infected areas of the foot then become grayish, and, if the dead tissue is trimmed away, a cheesy, yellowish-gray material with a characteristic foul odor will be found. The infection spreads into cracks and pockets, and the sole and horny hoof become separated from the normal soft-hoof structures. If both front feet are involved, sheep are often seen eating and moving around on their knees.

Foot rot has been reported in lambs as early as the sixth day. Needless to say, such lambs and sheep will be unthrifty and subject to malnutrition and disease. Death loss from foot rot is rare, but does occur from complications arising as a result of the initial foot-rot problem.

Foot rot does not usually start in the lambs. It is a ewe-flock problem that subsequently spreads to the lambs.

Diagnosis

Foot rot may be diagnosed by clinical signs, flock history, and environment. The causative microorganisms may be demonstrated, although care must be exercised in the interpretation. Lameness and a foul smell are strongly suggestive of the disease.

If the flock has not had foot rot and there have been no flock additions within the past 10 to 14 days, the lameness is probably not due to foot rot. If the lameness is due to foot rot, neither the foot nor the joints are swollen, because the horny portion of the hoof, and not the soft tissue above the coronary band, is involved. In typical contagious foot rot, there is not an abundance of moist, oozing, foul-smelling discharge.

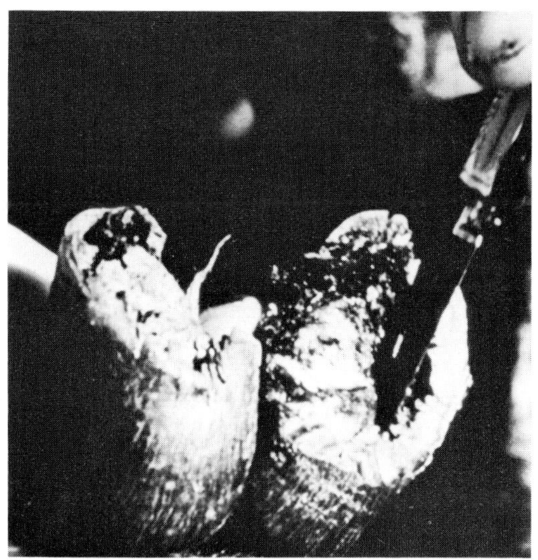

FIG. 23. Hidden pockets of infection in foot of sheep with foot rot. (Courtesy USDA.)

All sheep have an interungulate or biflex gland between the toes on each foot. If this gland becomes plugged, infected, injured, or otherwise irritated, it may cause lameness. The ability to squeeze a grayish, cheesy mass of material from this gland should not be regarded as a sign of contagious foot rot, however; it is perfectly normal.

Prevention and Control

Preventive measures for the control of foot rot are based upon good practical animal husbandry. Eliminate those factors that predispose to the disease and prevent exposure. Preventive measures should be initiated in the dry season and include elimination of potential mud holes, inspection and trimming of feet of all animals including rams, application of an approved foot bath, and proper quarantine for all additions to a flock, including those returned from shows, fairs, and sales barns.

The feet on each sheep on the farm or in the flock must be trimmed thoroughly and completely. All pockets, cracks, and crevices should be trimmed and healthy tissue exposed to the air. Once this is done, any good disinfectant will accomplish the remainder of the task. Do not attempt to spot-check sheep that are lame. Foot rot is a flock problem and must be treated on a flock basis. Every animal must be examined, the feet trimmed, and infected animals removed from the flock.

Because the organisms which cause the disease live only in the absence of air, it should be apparent that the first and most vital step in the control and treatment of this disease is regular feet trimming. By removing all dead and abnormal tissue, air is permitted to get to all parts of the normal foot and the infecting organisms, if present, can no longer survive.

There is no self cure or recovery of untreated sheep. Likewise, sheep that have been treated and are cured are not immune to future infection. However, if an affected flock is thoroughly and adequately treated and the infection is eliminated, the disease will not recur unless introduced into the flock by the addition of infected animals.

The complete control and eventual eradication of foot rot in sheep depends upon accurate diagnosis, prompt and complete compliance with the recommended procedures, and cooperation among producers, veterinarians, feedlot operators, sellers, and carriers.

38
Foot Abscess

FOOT ABSCESS is a sporadic condition of sheep caused by *Sphaerophorous necrophorus* (the microorganism found in foot rot of cattle). The infection involves soft tissue and causes severe lameness and swelling above the hoof. When an infection is unattended, it spreads and joints often become involved. Noticeable abscesses will form and drain, seeding the soil with viable microorganisms. Foot abscess causes more pus and drainage than foot rot. The separation of sole and hoof wall from soft tissue seen in contagious foot rot will not be noted. Often only one foot or one claw on a foot may be involved, and the infection will not spread. Foot abscesses treated prior to joint involvement will respond to antibiotics, thereby further distinguishing this condition from contagious foot rot.

Unlike foot rot, foot abscess is not a contagious disease. It can arise when and where the conditions are suitable, whether or not there have been previous cases. Therefore, eradication is not possible. Lambs and yearlings are rarely infected but older sheep are more susceptible.

Etiology

Foot abscess of sheep is caused by *Sphaerophorous necrophorus,* a saphrophytic bacterium which lives in the soil and propagates rapidly in manure. The bacteria enter the soft tissues through injuries to the skin of the foot or trauma to the tissue between the claws. Outbreaks affecting a large number of animals in a flock can occur only when predisposing factors are present. These include an environment in which the feet stay wet and in which the bacteria will live, and injury that may provide entry to the hoof or to the skin between the claws. Such trauma may result from briars, wire cuts, and the abrasive action of pebbles in muddy soil.

Symptoms

Foot abscesses cause acute lameness. The first sign may be an ulcer between the claws. The infection may then penetrate into deeper structures of the foot involving tendons, ligaments and even joints and when this happens abscesses form and drain. When only one claw is involved, the hoof may appear normal but feel hot to the touch. Severely infected sheep may be so lame that they will be unable to forage and will die of starvation or other complications.

In any form of foot abscess, whether spreading under the horn or involving deeper structures, a good deal of swelling occurs and pus is usually discharged.

When abscesses form they may discharge for several weeks or months. Occasionally when infection spreads, sheep may die from generalized septicemia. In most cases, however, the condition subsides and heals spontaneously but slowly, leaving perhaps a slight deformity of the foot.

Treatment

In cases of lameness in the early stages, when the infection is hidden under the horn, the claws should be pinched with fingers or pliers to elicit a flinching response. By careful paring through the horn at the tender spot, the pressure can be released and drainage provided. The pared foot may then be dipped in disinfectant. Unless the infection has already penetrated the deeper tissues, most cases will respond well to such treatment.

Once the deeper tissues are involved, external treatment is of little use. Sheep have remarkable natural powers of recovery and many will recover if left alone, provided they are removed to clean, dry quarters. As a foot-abscess outbreak may be at its worst when ewes are about to lamb, or during lambing, handling and treatment may be out of the question. The number of deaths in untreated sheep is small; losses are due to deterioration in condition, reduced milk supply in lactating ewes, and a break in the wool.

There is no proved method of preventing foot abscess. Trimming the feet and passing the sheep through an approved foot bath probably have preventive value if performed just before or immediately after the early break in the weather. Strict sanitation of holding yards, avoidance of low wet areas, and isolation and prompt treatment of lame sheep are the most effective control measures.

39
Edema Disease

EDEMA disease, or gut edema, is an acute disease of young swine characterized by sudden onset, incoordination, and swelling of various tissues of the body.

The most susceptible period is weaning time or shortly thereafter, and appears to be related to such stress factors as the radical change in feeding at this time, castration, and vaccination against other diseases. The most typical manifestation, and the most useful diagnostically, is a staggering gait which is considered to be a toxic manifestation.

Although edema disease in pigs was first described in North Ireland in 1938, its wide distribution and economic importance have been recognized only recently. Currently the disease has been diagnosed in the United States, Canada, South Africa and most countries in Europe, and there is reason to believe that it probably exists in many other countries where it is either undiagnosed or confused with some other condition. In some areas of the United States this is considered to be one of the major pig diseases, responsible for more deaths of weaned pigs than any other disease.

Edema disease typically affects pigs 8 to 16 weeks of age, and within 7 to 10 days after weaning. The rapid increase in incidence of edema disease during the past few years may be explained partially by the growing practice of adding a concentrated supplement to the grain fed to pigs. The fast growth of the pig and the higher protein level of the feed, therefore, may be two important factors to consider when dealing with outbreaks of edema disease.

Etiology

The attention of several investigators has been directed to the disease because of its economic importance and its considerable academic interest. Efforts have been made to determine the specific cause of the disease so that it might be controlled by prophylactic means. For a long time the etiology has remained obscure and numerous possibilities have been suggested. One theory is that the disease may be a specific toxemia either originating in the digestive tract or from the ingestion of a preformed toxin. The symptoms and lesions of edema disease have been produced experimentally by the supernatant fluid from centrifuged intestinal contents of affected animals, and by saline extracts of the same material. This observation provides evidence that a specific enterotoxemia originating in the intestines can cause the disease.

Because of the predominance of hemolytic *Escherichia coli* in the intestinal contents of affected animals, a relationship between the organism and the disease has been postulated. The rapidly growing *E. coli* organisms invade the intestinal epithelium, and their endotoxins are absorbed into the systemic circulation. The endotoxins could therefore exert a damaging influence on the nervous and vascular systems, and thereby produce characteristic symptoms and lesions of the disease.

Symptoms

The disease can be severe, with a mortality of 50 to 70 percent. Sometimes the course is rapid, and many pigs may be found dead without having shown previous signs of illness. In many outbreaks, mild diarrhea occurs 24 to 36 hours before any other symptoms are noticed. In most cases, however, typical nervous symptoms associated with toxemia are present. Such disturbances usually are manifested by locomotor ataxia affecting either the front or rear limbs, or all four limbs. Thus a staggering gait is one of the most frequently observed symptoms of the disease. Partial or complete paralysis and stupor usually occur in the final stage. At no time during the course of the disease is there any elevation of temperature.

Edema in various sites is a characteristic finding useful in diagnosis. Edema of the eyelids, the ears, and the face occurs commonly. When a postmortem examination is made soon after death a remarkable amount of edematous fluid frequently is found in the gastric or intestinal submucosa and the colonic mesentery. The stomach, which usually is full of food, has a wall thickened from the accumulation of edematous exudate. The lymph nodes may be grossly swollen from congestion and edema. The gallbladder, perirenal areas, lungs, subcutaneous tissues and the nervous system also may be markedly edematous.

However, edema is not observed grossly as consistently as are incoordination, paralysis and severe dyspnea; it is only one manifestation of toxemia and may not always be present. The most characteristic symptom, and the one by which the disease is most frequently recognized, is the staggering gait.

Prevention

Every attempt to induce active or passive immunity in pigs thus far has failed.

No suitable prophylactic bacterin or vaccine is available. Therefore, one should bear in mind that hygienic and dietary measures appear to be important. The radical changes in diet and other stresses routinely imposed on growing pigs at weaning should be eliminated where possible. Feeding changes can lead to fatal consequences. A transitional diet at weaning can establish a new balance without causing rapid changes in intestinal flora which might encourage the development of the microorganisms suspected in this disease. Good management is the best prevention.

40
Hypomagnesemia

HYPOMAGNESEMIA, or grass tetany, is a metabolic disease of sheep and cattle of any age or condition, particularly beef cattle grazing on low-quality feed and subjected to climatic stress. The disease is most common, however, in lactating cows and ewes grazing on lush grass pastures in the spring.

Grass tetany is characterized by low blood-serum magnesium. However, it appears to be a mineral imbalance involving not only magnesium but also calcium and phosphorus. The disease occurs in Europe, Australia, New Zealand, North America, and other parts of the world where advanced animal husbandry and pasture methods are employed. The incidence varies from property to property, according to the type of management exercised, and this may account for the erroneous belief that the condition is of genetic origin.

Etiology

The exact cause and the resulting pathogenesis of grass tetany are not well understood, although several predisposing factors have been associated with the disease. A syndrome of rapidly developing symptoms during the first few days after being turned out on grass pasture in the spring, especially in dairy cows, has been implicated. The grass alone is not the whole cause of the disease, however, as stalled cows also develop the symptoms.

Hypomagnesemia occurs in mature cattle, usually over four years of age, when they have been maintained on low nutrition and then subjected to stress such as cold, inclement weather, parturition, or movement. Agronomists have demonstrated that grasses grow quickly following a cold spell, and that rapidly growing grasses are low in magnesium. In the early spring, too, in mixed pastures, grasses grow more quickly than legumes, and the latter normally contain more magnesium than grasses. In addition, the early, rapidly growing grasses are high in nitrogen, especially if the fields have been fertilized. All of these factors contribute to lowered magnesium consumption and utilization.

Livestock grazed on wheat and other cereal grains, especially crested wheat grass, which provide a high intake of potassium develop a relative hypomagnesemia leading to clinical symptoms. Although other grasses are undoubtedly capable of causing grass tetany, crested wheat may be incriminated most frequently because it develops early in the spring and is ready for grazing before most other grasses.

Grass tetany appears to be more a result of low utilization of magnesium consumed than of low intake of magnesium. The fact that many pastures producing grass tetany have marginal levels of magnesium, with respect to animal requirements, compounds the problem and accelerates the development of the deficiency.

Symptoms

Symptoms of grass tetany are excitement, incoordination, loss of appetite, viciousness, staggering and falling, muscle twitching, anxious wild look, grinding of teeth, unusual salivation, general muscle contractions, labored breathing, and pounding heart beat, usually followed by convulsions and death.

There are two apparent types of grass tetany, acute and chronic. The acute type is characterized by sudden onset of clinical symptoms. The animal may be found dead shortly after being turned out to graze on lush grass, or, if observed, may suddenly appear frenzied, stagger, fall down into a convulsion and either die or recover, only to repeat the performance at short intervals until death occurs. In less acute cases the seizures may be two or three days apart but progress dramatically unless treated.

The chronic type can be diagnosed only by an examination of blood which reveals a lowering level of magnesium. However, the acute symptoms may develop at any time such an animal becomes stressed. During the chronic period animals may lose weight but clinical symptoms of hyperexcitability will not occur unless the serum magnesium levels drop below 1.0 mg per 100 ml. A drop in serum calcium is usually associated with the drop in magnesium. Cows affected by the chronic type of hypomagnesemia will continue to eat and lactate, although milk production will decrease.

Increased heart rate and loudness of heart sounds are diagnostic features of both types.

Hypomagnesemia may occur in calves maintained on a milk diet for 3 or 4 months. The condition is characterized by tetany and the same clinical symptoms seen in adults. An additional predisposing factor in calves may be scours, or hypermotility of the intestinal tract, through which ingesta pass so quickly that magnesium and calcium are poorly absorbed.

Prevention

Good management is essential in preventing this disease. Cows and ewes should be protected from the elements and maintained on a nutritious diet, especially during the last part of pregnancy.

The University of Illinois Extension Service recommends that ". . . herds with a current or recent history of grass tetany be fed supplemental magnesium. This is such an acute disease in many herds that affected animals may not recover even when calcium-magnesium gluconate is administered promptly after the animal becomes tetanic. Feeding grade magnesium oxide (MgO) is recommended as an economical product in which the Mg is readily available. Current recommendations are directed toward ensuring an intake of ½ to 1 ounce per cow per day from late fall until the spring pastures have "hardened." Emphasis must be placed upon the daily intake since body stores of magnesium are not readily available. The MgO may be fed with grain or on silage. In herds fed only hay or pasture, 10 to 15 percent MgO may be mixed with loose salt. If greater percentages are used, the salt intake may be depressed. In order for this method to be effective in preventing clinical grass tetany it is essential that the MgO-salt mixture be (1) the only source of salt, (2) always readily available, and (3) consumed by each animal daily.

"It is helpful to administer 2 ounces of MgO in a capsule to cows that are treated intravenously and also to feed cows MgO in grain or silage for 2 weeks or more to help prevent relapses."

41
Water Belly

WATER BELLY, or urolithiasis, is a noninfectious disease of cattle, sheep, and swine caused by the formation or lodging of concretions within the urinary tract. Urinary calculi are commonly found in feedlot cattle and sheep, and are of greatest economic importance in feeder animals. In domestic animals, the condition may be found in either sex; the greatest clinical incidence is in steers and wethers, although bulls, rams, and females may also be affected.

Water belly is most frequently seen in feedlot cattle and sheep during the winter months, on full feed, in semiarid parts of the country where the mineral content of the water is high, and where animals are maintained on a heavily supplemented diet. In particular, feeds with high levels of calcium and phosphorus, such as legumes and cereal grains, and root fodders, such as beets, potatoes, and turnips, tend to lower the urine pH and induce the precipitation of ionic salts. Bacterial cells in the bladder, or desquamated epithelial or blood cells, may serve as nuclei for the deposition of dissolved salts when the urine pH changes. Excessive crystalline salt concentration occurs with inadequate water intake, high mineral intake, or associated urinary infections. Once deposition of salts around a nucleus has begun, the resulting calculus may serve as the framework for further deposition, and consequently calculi may increase to large size if undisturbed in the bladder. Most calculi, however, are small, varying in size from that of a grain of sand to that of a pea.

In females, the small gravel readily passes through the relatively large, short, unrestricted urethra and does not usually cause damage. Calculi remaining in the bladder, however, may increase in size appreciably and may eventually occlude the lumen of the urethra where it leaves the bladder.

In males, the calculi usually lodge at the sigmoid flexure of the penis, where further deposition, with inflammation and occlusion of the urethra, takes place. When males are castrated too early, the penis remains in an infantile condition and may not allow small gravel to pass with the normal urine. Estrogenic hormones in the feed of fattening steers may also predispose to the retention of calculi in the urethra.

Etiology

Water belly is caused by obstruction by concretions in the urinary tract, including the kidneys, ureters, bladder, and urethra. The contributing factors are complex but appear to be related to a deficiency of chloride and sulfate ions in the urine.

Symptoms

The symptoms of water belly, or urolithiasis, may vary in severity and appearance according to the location of occluding calculi. Animals suffering from advanced symptoms of this condition will appear depressed and will exhibit edema of the belly wall. If calculi form in the hilus of the kidney, there may be no signs of discomfort, especially if only one side is involved, as the opposite kidney will compensate for the loss of kidney function. If, however, a ureter becomes blocked, the animal will exhibit intermittent pain. If the calculi lodge in the urethra, there will be restlessness, reluctance to move, pain in the abdominal region, and depression. The temperature will be elevated. The animal will stamp its feet and strike at the abdomen. Affected animals will walk with a straddling gait, and will stretch and attempt to urinate frequently with little or no success. An accumulation of fine gravel may be deposited on the preputial hairs and the tail head will be held high. If the urethra is palpated over the ischiatic arch, it will be enlarged and pulsating, and if the bladder is palpated via the anus, it will be distended and tense.

With complete urethral obstruction, the animal will be unable to pass any urine; this leads to distension of the bladder and the abdomen. If not relieved, the bladder will rupture and the subcutaneous tissues of the lower abdomen will be infiltrated with urine, hence the name "water belly." Rupture of the bladder will relieve the pain associated with this condition, but the distension of the abdomen with urine leads to uremia and eventually death.

At autopsy, the principal findings are calculi occluding either the bladder outlet or the urethra, usually at the sigmoid flexure. The tissue around the site of the obstruction, and extending back toward the bladder, will be inflamed, necrotic, and hemorrhagic. In case of rupture there will be a noticeable rent in the bladder. The abdominal cavity will contain considerable blood-tinged urine, and the lower abdominal wall will be swollen and infiltrated with urine. After rupture of the bladder, the carcass cannot be used for human consumption as the meat will emit a strong odor of urine when cooked.

Prevention

The only treatment for water belly is surgical removal of the offending occlusion before the bladder ruptures. After the frank symptoms appear little can be done; therefore, prevention is the most economic course of action. Some investigators have suggested that the disease may be prevented by adding salt in an amount up to 4 percent of the dry matter of the ration. This would cause the animal to drink considerable water, if available, and thus tend to dilute the crystalline salts and wash them out with the urine. Others have recommended that the calcium and phosphorus ration be held to a 1 : 1 ratio and that adequate mineral-free water be available at all times. It is also suggested that castration be avoided until some genital development has taken place.

In consideration of preventive measures against urolithiasis, strict attention to diet must be emphasized. Rations high in sorghum grains, cottonseed hulls and meal, and molasses are conducive to the formation of cal-

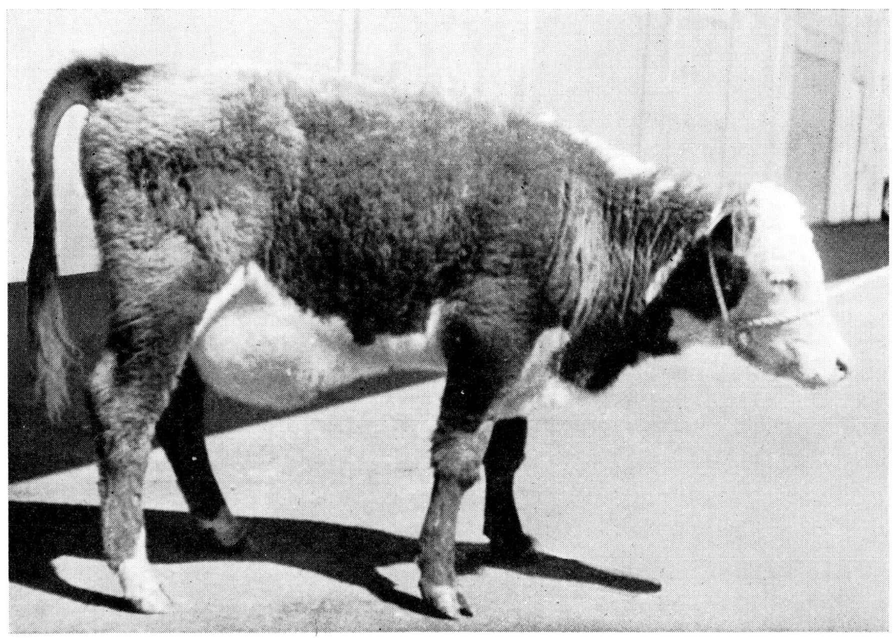

FIG. 24. Distension of sheath and subcutaneous abdomen due to rupture of urethra. Note elevation of tail head. (From Gibbons, W. J.: *Clinical Diagnosis of Diseases of Large Animals.* Philadelphia, Lea & Febiger, 1966.)

culi. In most semiarid areas where livestock are fattened in feedlots, the water usually is high in calcium and magnesium salts, which predispose to the formation of calculi. It has been shown that, under such circumstances, the use of ammonium chloride in the drinking water or in the diet will protect cattle and sheep from urinary calculi. Ammonium chloride added to the diet at a rate of $1\frac{1}{2}$ oz per steer, or $\frac{1}{4}$ oz for lambs, will reduce the incidence of water belly to a low level. Calculi that form in lambs after treatment are small and usually pass easily in the urine. Calculi are seldom formed in steers after treatment.

Ammonium chloride is the best supplement found, to date, for lambs and cattle. Research will have to be conducted on other susceptible animals to determine whether this supplement will reduce the incidence of urinary calculi universally.

PART 4

Exotic Diseases

42
African Horse Sickness

AFRICAN horse sickness is one of the major infectious diseases with which stockmen in Africa have to contend. Recent outbreaks in the Middle East, Asia, and Europe have made it a disease of worldwide significance.

African horse sickness is an old disease. References to it were made in parts of Africa as early as the second century A.D. Evidence that the virus existed in an unidentified reservoir host became apparent when the first horses to exist in the area of the Cape of Good Hope were afflicted in epidemic proportions. The worst outbreak on record was that of 1854, when some 70,000 horses out of 160,000 in the Cape of Good Hope were reported to have died of the disease. More recently, severe outbreaks have occurred in 1914, 1918, 1923, 1940, 1946, and 1953.

African horse sickness appears capable of existing permanently in any area of the world where the principal insect vector, *Culicoides,* is found. It has been reported that 36 horses died, 220 were destroyed and 20,000 vaccinated in southern Spain in the summer of 1966 because of African horse sickness. That was the first recorded appearance of the disease in Europe. Ten thousand animals have died during subsequent outbreaks in Morocco and 250,000 have been vaccinated. United States quarantine officials and veterinarians are constantly on the alert to prevent the introduction of African horse sickness into this country.

A seasonal, insect-borne virus disease enzootic to Africa, it is noted chiefly for the high mortality (up to 90 percent) it causes in horses. The principal vector is a species of tiny gnats, the *Culicoides.* The virus is harbored in an unknown reservoir host even in the absence of any of the equine species.

The disease has been known to occur in dogs fed meat from infected horses. There is no other public health significance; African horse sickness does not affect humans.

Etiology

The causative agent of African horse sickness is a viscerotropic virus found in the blood, tissue fluids, serous exudates, and various internal organs of equines. It is found in the blood from the onset of the febrile reaction. The virus attaches itself to the cells and cannot be separated from them. Forty-two strains of the virus, round in shape, all about 50 mμ in size, have been identified and placed into nine antigenic groups. The virus is moderately resistant to drying and heating but, stored in a refrigerator without preservatives, it will retain infectivity for many months.

The natural occurrence of African horse sickness in the enzootic areas of Africa is seasonal, appearing usually in the late summer and disappearing after the first frost. In most instances the outbreaks are preceded by abnormally high rainfall, which apparently creates highly favorable conditions for the development of the insect vector of the virus reservoir. As a general rule, the relatively lower-lying parts of a given area are most severely infected.

Factors Influencing Susceptibility

The equine is the only animal naturally affected by this virus. Mules are considerably less susceptible than horses, and infection is extremely rare in donkeys. Experimentally, horses can be readily infected by small injections of virulent blood, tissue emulsions or bronchial secretions. African horse sickness is not directly contagious; therefore, affected animals placed in stables with susceptible horses do not cause outbreaks of the disease. All available evidence points to biting flies as the natural vectors, but thus far only the *Culicoides* gnat has been widely incriminated. In areas of enzootic infection, horses protected from *Culicoides* do not contract the disease.

All horses are susceptible regardless of age, condition, or previous experience with the disease. Because of the various types of virus, a horse may recover from one type only to become ill with another. Usually the second attack is milder than the first.

Transmission

Horses do not retain the virus for more than thirty days after recovery from the clinical manifestations of the disease, and there is no evidence that recovered animals play any part in the carry-over of the infection from season to season. It appears that the virus is maintained during the winter in a reservoir host confined to the recognized area of distribution of the disease. Extensive transmission experiments from a variety of wild animals, birds, and amphibians caught at random in areas of enzootic African horse sickness all produced negative results. However, the disease was transmitted experimentally to a horse by the bites of *Aedes aegypti* mosquitoes which had been fed a virus suspension. A nonvaccinated yearling horse, obtained from an insect-proof stable, was exposed to ten mosquitoes during a 7-hour period. Nine of the mosquitoes bit the horse. Six days later fever was present and swelling of the eyelids was evident. The horse died 18 days after exposure.

The *Culicoides* gnat has worldwide distribution, yet the disease occurs principally in Africa. Horses from South Africa introduced into Madagascar did not precipitate an outbreak of the disease, although the *Culicoides* gnat is present on that island. The fact that African horse sickness has occurred in horses introduced into areas where horses, mules, and donkeys have been excluded for many years also points to the virus being maintained in some nonequine host. The infection in the horse seems to be purely a matter of choice. Once the first case occurs, horse-to-horse transmission readily results. Infected animals moved into areas free of African horse sickness easily provide a focus for transmission of the disease through native gnat vectors.

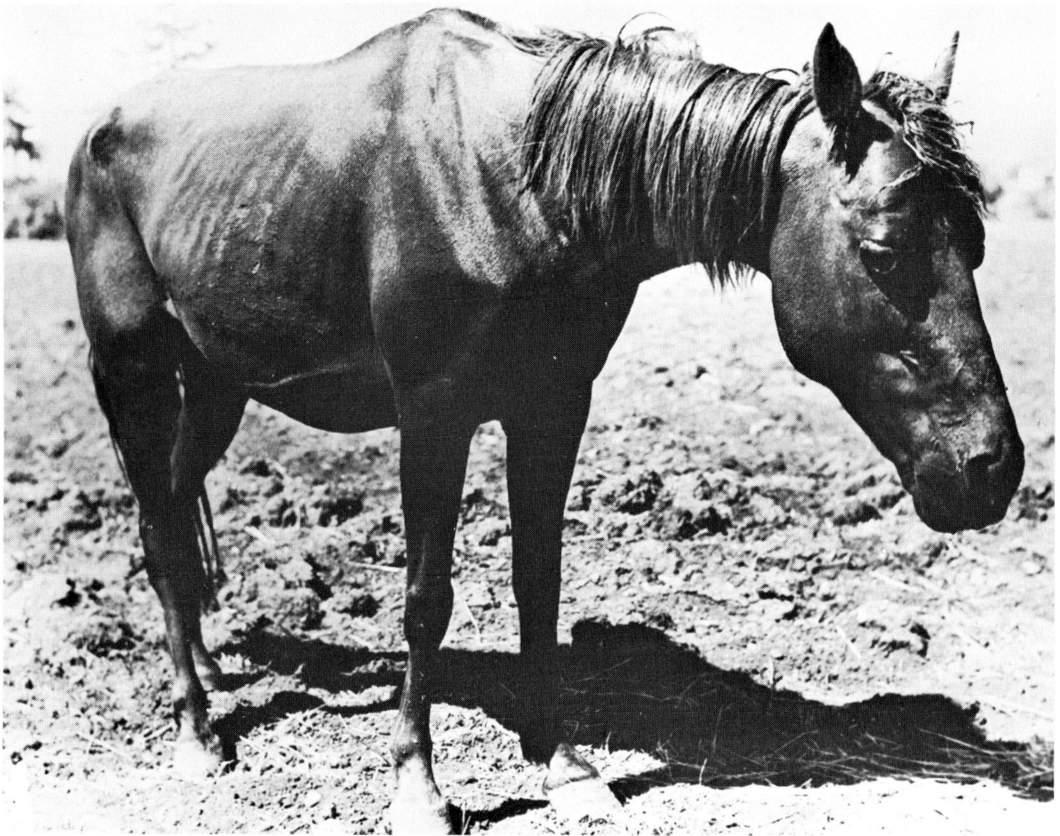

FIG. 25. General appearance of horse suffering from African horse sickness.

Symptoms

The symptoms of African horse sickness are variable, because there are four forms of the disease. The incubation period is generally 5 to 7 days, though it may be shorter or longer. An intermittent fever reaching 104 to 106 F 24 to 72 hours after onset is common in all forms.

Pulmonary or Acute Form

This is commonly seen in current virulent outbreaks. Distinct signs of respiratory difficulty appear within 3 to 4 days of infection with a temperature rise to 105 to 106 F. The appetite remains good even after severe coughing develops. As the disease progresses, the animal is seized by fits of coughing and may discharge large quantities of yellowish serous fluid and froth. It stands with head and neck distended and ears drooped, and sweats severely. Finally, it may choke, then sway, stagger and fall. The voluminous discharge of fluid indicates that the animal drowns in its own fluids. In rare cases less severe symptoms occur; the animal recovers but experiences difficulty in breathing for some time after the other signs disappear.

Cardiac Form

This is the subacute form of the disease. The incubation period may be as long as three weeks. The rise in temperature generally occurs more slowly and persists for a longer period than in the pulmonary form. The most evident symptoms are distinct swellings of the temporal fossae (area above the eyes), edema of the eyelids and lips. Hemorrhages may also develop on the eye membranes. In fatal cases, there are distinct signs of heart failure; the heart sac may be partially filled with fluid. The recovery rate from the cardiac form is higher than from the pulmonary form.

Mixed Form

This results from infection by mixed strains of the virus. Horses contracting this form are those immunized with a polyvalent vaccine and unusually susceptible to it. Signs typical of the two forms above are common, and the animal shows combined lesions upon postmortem examination. The death rate is variable.

Horse Sickness Fever

A mild form of the disease, the incubation period varies from five days to a month and symptoms are slight. The only indications of infection may be a brief rise in temperature to 105 F, slight conjunctivitis, an accelerated pulse, some loss of appetite, and slightly labored breathing. This form is generally seen in horses undergoing immunization, and recovery is usually rapid.

Diagnosis

In the severe forms of the disease the course is rarely longer than five days, since the animal dies by that time. In milder forms the course may be several weeks.

With current outbreaks of African horse sickness in the Middle East, Europe, and parts of Asia, locale can no longer be relied upon as a factor in diagnosis. In enzootic areas, familiarity with the gross symptoms and lesions makes quick diagnosis possible. However, because of the many virus strains and the various forms of the disease, a confirming laboratory diagnosis is essential. This is usually done by serum neutralization tests and is similar in principle to the toxin-antitoxin reaction.

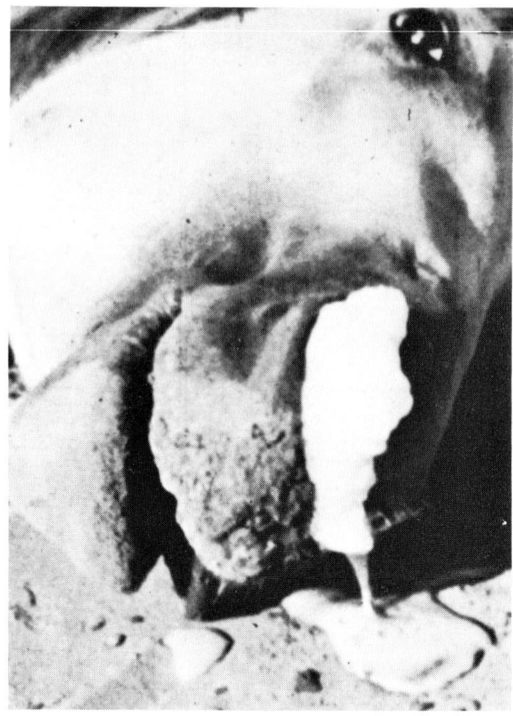

FIG. 26. After choking, staggering, and falling, a dying horse discharges a great volume of frothy material from its nostrils and mouth. (Courtesy USDA.)

Treatment and Control

As might be expected, no form of specific therapy has been successful in the treatment of African horse sickness. Upon recognition of the disease infected animals should be slaughtered and buried.

Prophylactic immunization has been accepted as an indispensable aid to control African horse sickness. A polyvalent vaccine made from the nine separate virus serotypes found in Africa and the Middle East has been found to provide passive protection for a limited time. The immunity is not permanent, and exposed animals should be vaccinated annually before the horse sickness season.

Vaccine is produced by intracerebral passage through mice. With serial passage in this species, neurotropic adaptation of the virus occurs. (Virus adapts itself to nervous tissue.) By the 100th passage, the virus becomes attenuated to the point where it may be injected into horses with almost complete safety. Immune mares convey a passive immunity to their foals, protecting them until after weaning.

In addition to vaccination, susceptible animals should be protected from nocturnal biting insects by stabling and insecticides, and by grazing on high-lying pastures away from rivers, streams, or wet ground. It is good control practice to treat ponds, lakes, slow-moving water and other breeding places of gnats in an affected area.

Movement of animals from known areas of infection should be restricted. The extensive spread of the disease in the Middle East and Asia since 1959 provides evidence of the problems involved in confinement. There is little possibility of intercontinental introduction of the disease through shipments of horses vaccinated and quarantined before and after shipment in insect-proof stables. However, because of the speed of modern means of transportation, the infected vector may be transmitted by airplane; this is probably the way the infection reached the Middle East.

Since the present experience in Asia and Europe indicates that the disease cannot readily be eradicated even by intensive application of effective vaccination, the solution to control lies in the identification of the unknown virus reservoir. While this may not simplify control of the disease in enzootic areas, it may be of extreme value in preventing its spread into countries at present free of African horse sickness.

43

African Swine Fever

AFRICAN swine fever is a highly contagious peracute disease of domestic swine, characterized by fever, pronounced hemorrhages of the lymphatic glands, kidneys, and mucosa of the alimentary tract, marked cyanosis of areas on the skin, and mortality approaching 100 percent. Clinically African swine fever resembles acute hog cholera, but it is an immunologically distinct entity. It is the most deadly of all foreign diseases of swine.

Etiology

The causal agent is an exceptionally resistant filterable virus. Infective blood stored at ordinary room temperature remained virulent after 18 months, and when stored in a coldroom (4 to 5 C) was still active after six years. The bush pig and warthog can harbor the virus, but usually manifest no objective symptoms. Viremia is a consistent feature of this disease and all tissues, organs, and excreta contain the virus.

In South Africa outbreaks of swine fever were recorded during the period 1903 to 1935. In East Africa in areas where contact with other domestic pigs could be definitely excluded, it was determined that the African virus differed from the virus of classical hog cholera. Wild pigs were incriminated as inapparent carriers from which domestic pigs obtained the infection. Researchers were also able to infect susceptible pigs by inoculating blood collected from a number of apparently healthy warthogs. However, blood obtained from warthogs in other areas proved to be noninfective.

Prior to 1957, African swine fever was confined to continental Africa. In that year the disease appeared in Portugal, and in 1964 in France. By 1967 the disease had spread to Italy, causing a serious threat to swine in the rest of Europe and other swine-raising areas of the world.

Transmission

Wild boars or bush pigs and warthogs serve as reservoirs in Africa. Contact of domestic swine with wild pigs harboring the virus may initiate the disease. Once the disease is established in domestic swine it spreads rapidly by contact.

Urine and feces from infected hogs contain the virus in sufficient amount to infect susceptible hogs. The virus can be spread mechanically by caretakers and others who pass from infected premises without taking proper measures of disinfection. Meat from infected animals contains the virus and, as in hog cholera, the feeding of raw garbage may spread the disease. In South Africa infected pigs were deliberately slaughtered and carcasses sent to bacon factories; this bacon was the source of sporadic outbreaks of disease for some considerable period. Attempts to transmit this disease by lice and fleas have been unsuccessful, although Spanish scientists have found that it may be transmitted by a tick.

In a few cases where swine have survived this disease there is evidence that they may act as carriers for as long as 10 months after recovery. Investigators have failed to demonstrate that contact of susceptible hogs with warthogs with blood harboring the virus resulted in infection of the hogs. For this reason the theory has been advanced that infection may be transmitted from warthogs to pigs by an insect vector or by pigs actually eating carcasses of virus-carrying wild pigs.

Symptoms

Unless the herd is under close observation, the first indication of the disease may be the discovery of one or two dead pigs. On close observation, the first symptom is a marked rise in temperature to 104 to 108 F. About 24 hours prior to death sick animals become dull and listless, refuse to eat, and may be found lying huddled in a corner and disinclined to move. On being made to rise, they exhibit a swaying movement and weakness of the hindquarters. The hindquarter weakness is less prevalent and less severe than in American hog cholera. Cyanosis of the skin on the ears, snout, abdomen, and legs is usually pronounced. In about 40 percent of the cases there is enough pulmonary involvement to cause labored respirations and associated heart rate markedly accelerated to 180 per minute and irregular. Pregnant sows usually abort. Some strains may produce a mucopurulent discharge from the eyes and a mucous discharge from the nostrils. Constipation is frequently present although diarrhea, usually bloody, may develop. Death generally occurs on the fourth to seventh day after the onset of symptoms and is preceded by a marked drop in temperature. For about 24 hours before death, an infected animal is comatose, lying on its side with stretched-out legs and closed eyes, and grunting only feebly when stirred. The disease is so highly contagious that, in a few days after the first case is noticed, most swine in the herd have become infected and show a rise of temperature. Nevertheless, in Africa the virus coming from the warthog or wild pig frequently appears to take some time to attain high virulence. Thus, a common history of outbreak shows an isolated death, followed a week or so later by one or two more deaths, and then after a further interval by many cases with rapid spread.

The incubation period is usually 4 to 7 days when exposure is by contact with infected pigs.

Pathology

The outstanding lesions are hemorrhages, thrombosis, infarction, hyalinization, and necrosis of the internal organs. These changes are caused by damage done by the virus to the endothelial cells of the small blood vessels, for which it seems to have a predilection.

The skin almost invariably has a patchy or diffuse purplish color and, more rarely, single or multiple irregular, dark red, hemorrhagic patches distributed on the abdomen, head and limbs.

On opening the carcass one may be startled

by the degree of hemorrhage seen. The internal lymph glands may be deep bluish-black due to extravasation of blood into the reticular spaces and lymph sinuses. The hemorrhage is often so extensive that the glands appear as blood clots. The lungs may be cyanotic and in some cases edemic, often dark and swollen to as much as twice the normal size. The liver is engorged and irregular dark patches of hemorrhage are often seen through the capsule. Engorgement of the blood vessels of the gallbladder is common. The so-called turkey-egg kidney of hog cholera is not common in African swine fever, where there is a tendency for parenchymal and pelvic hemorrhage rather than subcapsular petechiae.

Hyperemia, severe even to the point of giving rise to hemorrhage, is fairly consistent in the mucosa of the stomach. The stomach is usually full of food. The changes in the small intestine vary from normal appearance to severe hyperemia with hemorrhagic or even diphtheritic enteritis. There is often marked edema in the walls of the cecum, spiral colon and the mesentery of these organs, giving a gelatinous appearance. A hemorrhagic inflammation of the rectum is characteristic. However, it should be pointed out that the lesions encountered in African swine fever may vary considerably, and animals may die of this disease without showing any obvious gross lesions.

Diagnosis

In Africa a diagnosis can be made when characteristic symptoms and lesions occur in swine that have had possible contact with wild pigs.

It is obvious that African swine fever so closely resembles hog cholera in this country that a clinical or pathological differentiation is extremely difficult. A presumptive diagnosis can be based on gross pathology—the marked severity of the lesions of African swine fever, especially the hemorrhagic lymph glands and vascular engorgement of the mesentery, and particularly in swine that have been vaccinated against hog cholera.

At present, the only conclusive method of diagnosis is the production of the disease, under strict isolation, by inoculating susceptible swine (including cholera-immune and hyperimmunized pigs) with suspect material such as blood or spleen taken from a recently dead animal. Swine immune and even hyperimmune to hog cholera are susceptible to African swine fever, and this fact is of value in making a differential diagnosis. A laboratory test is available but is time consuming, as it is based upon growing the virus on swine leukocyte cultures.

Control

African swine fever is undoubtedly the most serious of the exotic diseases insofar as the swine industries of the United States and Canada are concerned.

The best available methods of control are to slaughter all infected and exposed animals immediately, to dispose of all carcasses by burning or deep burial, to disinfect the infected premises, and to quarantine infected areas. In Africa, measures taken to prevent contact of domestic swine with wild pigs have resulted in a marked decrease in incidence of the disease.

44
Rinderpest

RINDERPEST, or cattle plague, is an acute, highly contagious, generalized virus disease, primarily of cattle and secondarily of sheep, goats and wild ruminants. The disease is characterized by a rapidly fatal, febrile course with inflammation and necrosis of the mucous membranes of the digestive tract leading to emaciation and profuse bloody diarrhea. Rinderpest has been found to infect wild and domesticated pigs, but horses, carnivorous animals and man are not susceptible.

Since ancient times, rinderpest has been the world's most devastating disease of cattle, and as such it has had a major influence on man's food supply. In many parts of the world, cattle plagues have been devastating from the fifth century until development of methods of disease control in the present century. It has been estimated that, before 1949, rinderpest was responsible for the loss of over 2,000,000 cattle and buffalo each year, and it is only through modern prophylactic measures, persistently pursued, that large-scale raising of cattle has today become profitable in much of Africa and in the Middle East and Asia.

In the literature, there are numerous mentions of scourges of rinderpest which wiped out cattle in many parts of the civilized world, following military campaigns of the past. More recently, commercial shipments of live animals from one part of the world to another have introduced the disease into many countries which were formerly free of it. The disease is not present in the western hemisphere nor in western Europe; however, this is only because stringent methods have been exercised to keep it out. In fact, one outbreak did occur in Brazil in 1921, but prompt methods of eradication were exercised and rinderpest has not appeared again in this part of the world. However, it is still enzootic in most of Africa, Asia, and the Middle East. In tropical Africa, it occurs in different degrees of severity. In eastern Europe, outbreaks continue to occur periodically although the disease has not been diagnosed in western Europe since 1920.

The persistent use of modern vaccines and drastic tests and slaughter procedures have eradicated rinderpest from the Philippine Islands, Australia, New Zealand and Japan.

Etiology

Rinderpest is caused by a relatively fragile virus ranging in size from 120 to 300 mμ. Although all field strains of virus have been reported immunologically similar, they vary widely in pathogenicity, lethality, ease of transmission, and host affinity. Prolonged passage of the virus in cattle may cause it to lose its capacity for natural transmission. Serial passage of some strains of the virus in goats, rabbits, chick embryos, and tissue cultures has lead to attenuation for cattle. Some of these attenuated strains have been widely used in vaccines. There also appears to be an immunological relationship between rinderpest virus and the viruses of measles and canine distemper. Because of the fragile nature of the virus, in a moist medium at room temperature it will lose its infectiveness within a matter of hours; it will, however, remain infectious for many days under refrigeration. If the virus is frozen, it will remain infectious for a considerable length of time. Strong alkalis, acids and the common disinfectants will destroy the virus.

In the infected animals, however, the virus is extremely virulent and may be found in large quantities in blood, tissue fluids, secretions, and excretions; it is also present in meat from slaughtered animals.

Factors Influencing Susceptibility

In enzootic areas where most mature cattle acquire some degree of immunity, many cases are mild and inapparent. Because of this degree of resistance or immunity acquired through generations of exposure in enzootic areas, the disease is most often seen in young animals. Sex is of no importance in the transmission or incidence of the disease, but good condition appears to make animals more resistant. There is no relationship of the disease to either season, climate, or weather. The appearance of rinderpest in sheep and goats is relatively rare but there have been instances of the infection appearing in swine. Reports of outbreaks are rather common in certain native breeds of swine in the Far East. The disease, however, has not been reported among African wild swine or hogs. In enzootic areas, native cattle—exposed to rinderpest for generations—are generally more resistant than newly imported breeds. Contrary to the rule, however, a few native breeds in enzootic areas have remained very susceptible to the disease.

Transmission

Rinderpest is usually transmitted by direct contact between infected and susceptible ruminants, and the movement of infected animals is primarily responsible for the spread of the disease. The ingestion of virus-contaminated feed or water may transmit the disease, but, based upon experimental transmissions, the chances of transmission are much more likely by way of the respiratory tract from the inhalation of virus-laden aerosols from infected animals. There is evidence that on rare occasions a recovered animal may continue to harbor and excrete the virus for several weeks after the first development of the disease; however, immune carriers are not considered to be a prevalent factor in transmission.

The major means of transmission has been considered to be droplet infection onto the conjunctiva, internal nares, and respiratory tract; however, it has been experimentally shown that infective material placed upon the external nares, lips, mouth and esophagus and the first three stomachs rarely produces the disease.

The mechanical transmission of rinderpest by biting insects appears possible but there is no evidence in the literature that insects are involved in the natural transmission of the disease. With some virulent strains of rinderpest, virus may be disseminated by an infected animal one or two days before it shows signs of apparent illness. The dissemination of virus prior to apparent illness poses a major control problem for animals kept in congested sales yards or while in transit. All tissues and excretions from infected animals should be considered infectious throughout the period of clinical illness.

Symptoms

In general, three forms of the disease may be described: (1) typically acute, (2) subacute, occurring mostly in countries where the disease is enzootic, and (3) peracute. Various atypical forms of the disease are sometimes seen. Many of the unusual features are due to complications caused by concurrent or superimposed virus infections. Rinderpest can be so highly contagious that, when cattle infected with a virulent strain of bovine virus are allowed to mingle with susceptible cattle, the morbidity may approach 100 percent and, among highly susceptible cattle, mortality may reach 90 percent. Recovery confers a permanent immunity, and the development of immune carriers able to disperse the disease to susceptible cattle has not been reported. A temporary maternal immunity is observed to protect the calves of immune dams for the first several months of life. When this maternal immunity is present, it proportionately lessens the effectiveness of vaccination.

Although the method of transmission of the disease is direct, the rinderpest virus enters the body primarily through the digestive tract and passes to the bloodstream where it propagates rapidly. It is transmitted then to the mucous membranes of the digestive tract for which it seems to possess a degree of selectivity. In any case, the virus enters the capillary epithelium, causing an inflammatory process accompanied by early necrosis of epithelial cells; these erode, causing the serious bloody diarrhea which is one of the common symptoms of the disease. In natural outbreaks, the period of incubation varies from 3 to 9 days, except in countries where the disease is enzootic when it may be somewhat longer. Artificial infection by inoculation results in a rather short incubation period of 40 to 60 hours.

Differences in strain virulence and in host susceptibility account for a wide range of clinical severity from inapparent to peracute cases. After natural infection and an incubation period of 3 to 15 days, the onset in cattle is typically marked by an abrupt rise in temperature of 104 to 105 F. Within 48 hours after the temperature rise, nasal and lacrimal discharges appear accompanied by depression, thirst and loss of appetite. The pulse and respiration are accelerated and milk secretion diminishes or ceases. The conjunctiva is deeply infected and copious lacrimation occurs. It has been reported that congestion of the vaginal mucosa usually precedes all other lesions. Similar lesions are found in the preputial mucosa of the male. Usually on the second or third day of fever, small gray papules (about the size of a pinhead) are usually found in small numbers on the gums, lips, and undersurfaces of the tongue. During the next 24 hours, vesicles form in these papules and rupture to form ulcers, and a fresh crop of papules develops. These oral lesions appear to induce excessive salivation as they increase in severity. The saliva, however, does not form the long, tenacious, mucoid strings common in foot-and-mouth disease.

The temperature reaches its peak by the third to fifth day, and diarrhea commonly starts with the drop in temperature to normal or subnormal levels. As the diarrhea increases in severity, it may become hemorrhagic and is associated with abdominal pain, accelerated respiration, occasional cough, severe dehydration, and emaciation followed by prostration and death. The feces, which were at first dry and covered with mucus, become soft and finally blackish, liquid, and often bloodstained. There may be twitching of superficial muscles, grinding of the teeth, and arching of the back. Animals show extreme depression with occasional periods of excitement. Not uncommonly, animals die in the second day of this phase; if not, diarrhea continues, and they become debilitated, remain recumbent, waste rapidly and finally die, usually between 4 and 8 days after the first appearance of fever.

In some cases, the respiratory tract is affected. A nasal discharge develops, later becoming purulent and bloodstained. There may be bronchial rales and coughing. Pregnant animals frequently abort.

In the *peracute* form of the disease, there is marked congestion of the mucosa and great acceleration of pulse and respiration, and death may occur before diarrhea has developed. This form is common in calves, which may die on the second or third day without showing typical buccal lesions.

The *subacute* form occurs primarily in animals in countries where the disease is enzootic. The clinical features are essentially the same as in the acute cases, although milder and more prolonged.

Atypical forms are sometimes seen. Sometimes cutaneous lesions develop in the form of red maculae, either separate or confluent on various parts of the body, most often where the skin is thin. They pass through papular and vesicle pustular stages, and may be followed by shedding of patches of epidermis.

In buffalo, camels, sheep and goats the clinical features vary from those seen in typical acute cases in cattle to a mild form which may not be fatal. In general, the disease in sheep and goats is much milder than in cattle. Swine, both domesticated and wild, show variable forms of the disease. Infection of adult hogs by ingestion or subcutaneous inoculation usually produces a hypothermia lasting several days without the development of any striking signs of illness, although the blood is infective. Young swine appear to show severe clinical disease more frequently after inoculation, with lesions in the buccal cavity, mucopurulent conjunctivitis, and diarrhea.

Pathology

As the virus has a particular affinity for the epithelial linings of the digestive tract and lymphoid tissues, the predominant postmortem signs seen in cattle which have died of rinderpest are related to these tissues and structures. The animals commonly show the effect of the severe diarrhea. They are dehydrated and emaciated, and the hair coat is rough and soiled. While in rare instances death may occur prior to the development of the characteristic lesions, if necropsies are conducted upon several animals in an outbreak, the composite picture will usually include the following changes.

The rinderpest virus has affinity for and is highly destructive of the lymphoid tissues. Grossly, the lymph nodes are soft, edematous, and moderately enlarged. Peyer's patches show the most marked gross evidence of lymphoid destruction. Being in an exposed location, composed of highly susceptible digestive-tract mucosae and lymphoid tissue, they usually become acutely inflamed; later, necrosis and erosion may leave raw craters at the site of the patches.

The epithelial lining of the mouth and digestive tract is highly vulnerable to the rinderpest virus. The initial lesions in the oral epithelium include formation and necrosis of a few papular-like lesions. The extension of this necrosis toward the surface indicates an increase in the size of the necrotic lesions. The first such lesions to be grossly evident occur on the intersurfaces of the lower lip, adjacent to the gum, on the cheeks, and on the ventral surfaces of the tongue. Later these erosions may enlarge and coalesce to involve most of the oral mucosa.

Gross lesions are only occasionally found in the rumen and reticulum, but hemorrhages and erosions are fairly frequent in the omasum.

There is extensive congestion and hemorrhage associated with the degeneration, necrosis, and erosion of the mucosae of the abomasum and the intestines. Erosions here leave a raw, bleeding surface. Edema, hemorrhage, and erosions of the mucosa of the gastric fundus are often found. The small intestine usually shows slight involvement except for frequent necrosis and erosion of the Peyer's patches.

The most frequent lesions are seen in the large intestine and involve the cecum, the cecocolic junction and the rectum. The upper respiratory passages may be congested, but most often the nasal mucosa is markedly hyperemic, showing some hemorrhages and covered more or less uniformly with mucopurulent exudate, accompanied by some ulceration. Similar lesions may also be found in the trachea. At the commencement of an outbreak, death may occur so rapidly that typical lesions are not apparent.

Diagnosis

The diagnosis of rinderpest in those countries where the disease is prevalent is based upon clinical features, or gross lesions, and a knowledge of the history of the disease in a given area. The clinical and gross pathological features of rinderpest, which are very much like those seen in virus diarrhea and mucosal diseases, require that particular emphasis be placed upon proper laboratory diagnosis when the disease is suspected to have occurred in a country normally free of rinderpest. A presumptive diagnosis must be confirmed by serological means, utilizing neutralization tests either in cattle or in tissue culture, or by cross-protection tests in cattle. A knowledge of the disease is essential to facilitate prompt recognition. Small areas of infection in otherwise rinderpest-free countries are customarily eliminated by strict quarantine and slaughter.

Control

Any regimen of control of rinderpest is based first of all upon proper sanitation and elimination of the virus. Because of the failure of the virus to survive for any length of time outside the animal body, sanitation and disinfection facilitate control of the disease. Clean quarters, well-ventilated and exposed to sunlight, and the proper application of thorough disinfection techniques will help prevent the spread of the disease.

In those areas where the disease is common, immunization techniques have been used. When the disease is too widespread for the costly measures of slaughter and quarantine, control can be achieved through vaccination and isolation. Two types of vaccines are commonly used: (1) a killed virus, and (2) an attenuated virus which has been passed through unusual hosts. The current use of attenuated vaccines has largely outmoded older vaccines, using modified live viruses and killed viruses. These attenuated vaccines are produced by serial passage through goats, rabbits, chick embryos, and also tissue cultures.

In the United States, the prevention of the entry of the disease is still the primary method of control and, should an outbreak occur, the drastic measures of tests, slaughter and disposal would be undertaken. Rinderpest has been designated a reportable disease by all state and federal authorities, and the federal government has placed an embargo on the importation of cattle from countries where the disease is known to exist.

45
Foot-and-Mouth Disease

FOOT-AND-MOUTH disease, also known as apthous fever and aftosa, is an acute, febrile, highly contagious disease of cloven-footed animals caused by a filterable virus. It is characterized by the formation of vesicles in the buccal mucous membrane, in the skin above the hoof and in the interdigital spaces. The first recorded outbreak of this disease was in Europe in 1544. In 1897, European scientists determined the cause. These investigators showed that bacteria-free lymph collected from infected animals could be used to transmit the infection. Later, in 1898, they proved that the causative agent of foot-and-mouth disease could be passed through filters which retained bacteria.

Foot-and-mouth disease occurs in most of the cattle-raising regions of the world. The disease has never obtained a foothold in Australia, New Zealand, and North America because those regions have long used drastic means of preventing it. There have been nine outbreaks in the United States, but each was successfully stamped out without excessive cost or extensive loss of cattle. The disease continues to be of great interest to animal disease-control authorities because of the great outbreak which occurred in Mexico between 1946 and 1954. In 1951–1952, a small outbreak in western Canada, very close to the international border, caused considerable concern in this country. Most of the North American outbreaks have been traced to contaminated products imported from other countries.

Etiology

The filterable virus causing foot-and-mouth disease is one of the smallest viruses known, being about 22 $m\mu$ in diameter and spherical in shape. There are seven types of the virus and at least 35 subtypes, all of which are antigenically distinct. Three types have thus far been reported from Africa while the others have been found in various parts of the world. Each of the seven types produces a disease picture comparable to the other six.

The virus appears to be quite sensitive to

heat and is removed from milk through standard pasteurization. When kept in an incubator at about 98 F the virus loses infectivity within 48 hours. At average room temperature it remains viable for 2 to 3 weeks. At ordinary refrigeration temperatures the virus usually remains infective for many months when properly buffered. When rapidly dried under vacuum at low temperatures, it remains viable for several years. The virus is more sensitive to acids than to alkalis and is resistant to alcohol, ether, chloroform, and other fat solvents. The cultivation of the virus is usually accomplished by the inoculation of scarified areas of the buccal mucosa and tongue of calves or by footpad inoculation of guinea pigs, and by tissue-culture techniques in the laboratory.

Transmission

Contact with infected animals, and especially the ingestion of contaminated food and water, are the principal means of transmission of the disease. Although indirect transmission may take place by contact with inanimate objects of various kinds, the spread of foot-and-mouth disease is primarily by and from infected animals. The virus may also be transmitted from infected animals' surroundings by people, horses, dogs, birds, flies, rats, and by inanimate articles such as harness, vehicles, brushes, and clothing which may be contaminated with saliva, urine, feces, milk and meat of infected animals.

Factors Influencing Susceptibility

Susceptibility to natural infection of this disease is almost exclusively limited to cloven-footed animals, domestic and wild. Cattle, hogs, sheep, and goats are most frequently affected in the order mentioned. Deer were seriously affected in an outbreak in California and naturally infected hedgehogs have been found in England. The virus does not persist in animals in the carrier state with any regularity, but the disease has recurred on farms up to a year following eradication procedures.

Carnivorous animals are resistant and solipeds are completely immune to this disease, although dogs and cats, especially young ones, are slightly susceptible to artificial infection. Young farm animals on a high level of nutrition are most easily and acutely infected. Purebred animals seem to be more susceptible than grade animals, and close housing and feeding are conducive to the spread of the disease. Debilitated animals frequently suffer more from secondary effects. The severity of the disease varies with the strain of the virus and the state of health of the herd.

Symptoms

The disease is characterized by depression, fever, and the appearance of vesicles filled with clear fluid in oral mucous membranes and portions of the skin. The virus multiplies only in the inner layers of epithelium, where it causes degenerative changes and separation of these layers from the more superficial cornified layer. This space then fills with fluid and thus forms vesicles. The vesicles generally appear on the mucous membranes of the mouth (tongue, cheeks, dental pad, and gums), on the skin of the muzzle, in the interdigital spaces, around the tops of the claws, and on the teats and occasionally the surface of the udder. Vesicles may also appear around the base of the horns and in the pharynx, larynx, trachea, esophagus, and wall of the rumen around the esophageal groove.

These pathological changes in the tissues produce a series of other symptoms such as an increase in body temperature, loss of appetite, lassitude, and profuse slobbering. Because chewing may be painful, the animal may eat little or not at all, and therefore lose condition and weight. Infected animals usually become lame and milk flow usually ceases. Abortion, mastitis, and sterility may also occur. The incubation period following natural exposure is 2 to 7 days. Within 24 to 48 hours after virus multiplication in the epithelium, the virus escapes into the bloodstream and is carried to all organs and tissues. This often results in the appearance of secondary vesicles in epithelium remote from the point of entry of the virus. Although the virus does not multiply in the blood or organs, it does produce degenerative changes in muscular tissues, particularly in the heart. Yellowish streaks and foci of parenchymatous degeneration are the manifestions of this damage.

Pathology

The vesicles in the mouth, 0.25 to 1.0 inches in diameter and circular, rupture within a few hours of the time they are formed, leaving large flaps of whitish, detached epithelium under which the tissues are raw and bleeding. Often, a large part of the tongue is denuded. Secondary bacterial infections of the denuded areas between the claws usually occur and result in deep necrosis of tissues and suppuration that frequently undermines the claws, causing them to be loosened from the soft tissues and eventually to be sloughed off. The mouth lesions usually heal within 1 to 3 days, but the foot lesions often persist much longer.

The virus reaches the epithelium in the region in which it localizes either by direct contact or by way of the bloodstream. Two to 7 days after the virus enters the epithelium, vesicles and erosions develop. The epithelial cells in the lesions begin to enlarge and undergo a liquefaction degeneration sometimes called hydropic degeneration. The intercellular bridges disappear, and the cells consequently become loosened from one another. Their nuclei become pyknotic. Separation of the epithelium is aided by the endematous fluid arising from the hyperemic vessels of the skin. Adjacent foci, thus filled with edema fluid arising from cells undergoing liquefaction degeneration, fuse to form small vesicles.

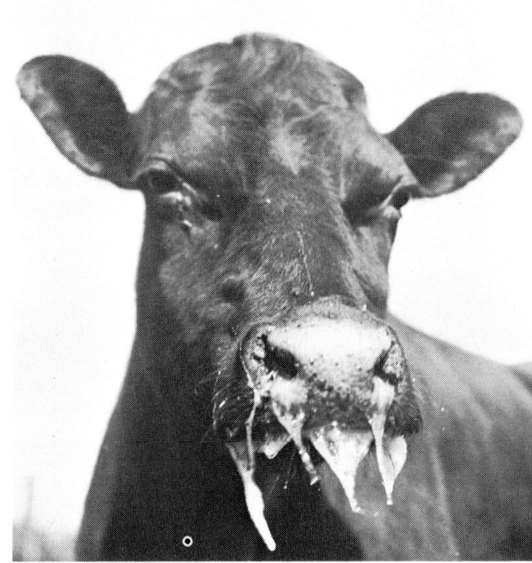

FIG. 27. Cow slobbering, an early sign of foot-and-mouth disease.

Small vesicles coalesce to form larger ones. Internal pressure within the vesicles becomes great and the superficial covering becomes increasingly thinner. This, plus softening due to excessive saliva, leads to rupture of vesicles.

Loss of epithelium is most common on the dorsal surface of the anterior part of the bovine tongue. The entire epithelium over the anterior area may be lost, leaving a raw, red surface which oozes blood. In addition to the virus, the vesicles contain necrotic epithelial cells, leukocytes, occasional erythrocytes and, in the late stages, bacteria. Lesions in the myocardium are most common in fatal cases of foot-and-mouth disease. The lesions, observed in the wall and septum of the left ventricle, but seldom in the atria, appear as small, grayish foci of irregular size, which may give the myocardium a somewhat striped appearance. In skeletal muscles, lesions similar to those in the myocardium may be observed. Sharply delineated areas of necrosis are seen grossly as gray foci of various sizes and microscopically as necrosis of muscle bundles associated with rather intense leukocytic infiltration.

Diagnosis

The characteristic appearance of vesicles in the mouth and on the feet of animals usually narrows the possibilities to two to three virus diseases. In the United States, three viruses must be differentiated in vesicular diseases of swine, and, in cattle, two viruses must be considered. The determination of susceptibility in three or four species of animals is the first step in positive diagnosis. Those species used in such a test and their susceptibility to the three viruses are presented in the table below.

TABLE 3.

Disease	Cattle	Swine	Horses	Guinea pigs
Foot-and-mouth	+++	++	−	++
Vesicular stomatitis	++	++	+++	++
Vesicular exanthema	−	+++	±	−

Differential filtration in the laboratory may aid in distinguishing foot-and-mouth disease and vesicular stomatitis viruses, since elementary bodies of the latter are about 10 times the size of the foot-and-mouth virus. The fact that vesicular stomatitis virus can be cultivated in chicken embryos and foot-and-mouth virus cannot is useful in diagnosis. It has been shown that the virus of foot-and-mouth disease will regularly produce typical lesions following intramuscular inoculation into a susceptible calf, while the intramuscular inoculation of vesicular stomatitis virus fails to do so. Cross-immunity or complement-fixation tests must be made to determine the strain of the virus causing an outbreak. In addition to vesicular stomatitis and vesicular exanthema, other diseases such as rinderpest, mucosal disease, bluetongue, cowpox, and contagious ecthyma in sheep are suggestive of foot-and-mouth disease at times.

Control

Foot-and-mouth disease is endemic in many countries of the world and the prognosis depends upon the severity of the disease. It generally has a benign character and in most cases the mortality is not high, seldom averaging more than 3 percent and often less than 1 percent. The death rate among young stock is higher than among adults and somewhat greater in young pigs than in calves. The death rate among sheep and goats is usually low. Prognosis is not of much concern in the United States because all exposed animals are slaughtered.

Formerly, there were only two important methods to control foot-and-mouth disease: (1) isolation, quarantine and disinfection of premises, and (2) slaughter and burial of infected and exposed animals. Slaughter, however, has seldom been used in countries subjected to epizootics, and many countries have come to depend largely on vaccines to control the disease. A complete eradication method consists of: complete isolation of the infected premises, prompt slaughter and proper disposal of infected animals, thorough cleansing and disinfection of premises and all equipment, immediate quarantine of an area of 5 to 50 miles around the infected premises, and periodic inspections coordinated among federal, state, and local authorities. Treatment alleviates the symptoms of the disease, but does not prevent the spread of infection and interferes with attempts to eradicate the disease. Treatment, therefore, has no place in an eradication program.

Natural immunity in cattle and swine is negligible, although some individuals have greater resistance than others. The new types of viruses and the variations among types may have resulted through the use of vaccines which imperfectly immunize animals, thus setting up within them the means for forcing variations in the field strains. Animals recovered from foot-and-mouth disease caused by a particular type of the virus generally are sufficiently resistant to that type to withstand additional exposure for 4 months to 1 year. They may, however, be immediately infected with one of the other types and exhibit typical symptoms of foot-and-mouth disease.

Susceptible animals may be given a measure of passive immunity to foot-and-mouth disease by injecting them with immune serum just before, or simultaneously with, exposure to the virus. Such protection is short-lived, lasting only 1 to 2 weeks, and often it is not sufficient to prevent clinical symptoms. Animals infected with foot-and-mouth disease may also get a so-called passive immunity by injection of material prepared from lymph, blood, or tissues containing the virus, treated chemically or by heating, in emergency situations. The resulting immunity, however, is of a limited character and the inoculations must be repeated frequently.

Of the vaccines used to control foot-and-mouth disease, the most commonly used is one developed in Germany just before World War II. Essentially it consists of the virus adsorbed on aluminum hydroxide, inactivated by formalin and incubated. Variations of the vaccine have been used in different parts of the world. Generally, the virus for the vaccine is derived from the tongue epithelium of artificially inoculated cattle, and anybody using vaccine must know the type of virus prevalent in the outbreak. Vaccines must be critically tested to prove that they do not produce the disease and do protect against it. There is also some evidence that hogs and sheep are not satisfactorily immunized with vaccine made with virus of bovine origin.

Human beings are only slightly susceptible to the virus of foot-and-mouth disease. There have been no recognized cases of human infections in any of the recent outbreaks of the disease in Mexico and Canada, but in the recent one in England several cases were diagnosed as countless people had close contact with active strains of the virus. Humans are usually affected by drinking milk from infected animals, and laboratory workers may be accidentally infected through handling the virus.

The symptoms in man are fever, vomiting, a sense of heat and dryness in the mouth, and the appearance of small vesicles on the lips, tongue, and cheeks. Lesions on the hands have also been described. The course of the disease is short, and there are no records of serious complications or deaths.

In the United States, treatment of foot-and-mouth disease is strictly forbidden. Under federal law, all infected and exposed animals must be slaughtered and the carcasses destroyed. The use of immune sera and vaccines is also expressly forbidden. The only acceptable procedure is complete eradication, even though drastic and costly.

46 Contagious Bovine Pleuropneumonia

CONTAGIOUS bovine pleuropneumonia is a specific disease of cattle caused by an exceedingly small microorganism, *Mycoplasma mucoides.* It is a highly infectious acute, subacute or chronic septicemia.

For many years the causative agent was believed to be a virus, since it passes through many of the filters which stop ordinary bacteria. The microorganism can, however, be grown on lifeless laboratory media, and by the use of special techniques it can be seen with a microscope. The agent is sensitive to drying and to other environmental influences. It is readily susceptible to disinfectants and does not survive outside the animal body in nature for more than a few hours.

This destructive disease of cattle is essentially a disease of dry countries although it occurs in all parts of the world except western Europe, the western hemisphere, and a few other smaller areas. It has been known for more than 200 years. In the early part of the nineteenth century the disease became widespread in Europe, and from there was disseminated to South Africa, Australia, and the United States in exported cattle. It was found in the United States in 1843, but has not occurred in this country since March of 1892. It presently occurs in parts of Asia, Africa, Australia, and Russia.

Transmission

Under natural conditions the disease is contracted by susceptible animals by droplet inhalation of the causal microorganisms produced by coughing of infected animals.

The infection may persist in the affected parts of the lungs of apparently recovered animals for a period of several months. Such animals remain a potential source of infection indefinitely. The virus may persist in encapsulated lesions for over 15 months, and latent carriers may harbor the infection for 2 to 3 years before they transmit the disease.

The incubation period is usually 3 to 6 weeks, but periods as short as 10 days or as long as 10 weeks between contact with infected animals and the first appearance of symptoms have been reported. The disease usually spreads slowly in an infected herd but occasionally it spreads quite rapidly.

Symptoms

Cases of contagious pleuropneumonia may be peracute, acute or subclinical. The peracute form, in which the pneumonia lasts but a few days, is uncommon. Cattle with this form may develop many of the signs described for acute infection, or they may have a severe form of pneumonia and die in from 1 to 3 weeks.

The acute form is the most frequently seen. In the early stages there is a rise in temperature, the animal appears dull, the coat is rough and there is disinclination to feed. Later, typical symptoms appear—a cough, at first dry and painful and subsequently moist, labored breathing, and grunting expiration. The animal stands with the elbows turned outward and the head extended to relieve pressure on the chest, almost invariably facing into the wind and with nostrils dilated. In the later stages there may be mucopurulent discharge from the nose and sometimes an edematous infiltration of the lower part of the chest. Flesh is lost rapidly and finally the animal lies down. Often the infection becomes encapsulated in the lungs and breaks out with acute signs during a period of stress.

Swellings at the joints are sometimes seen in young calves.

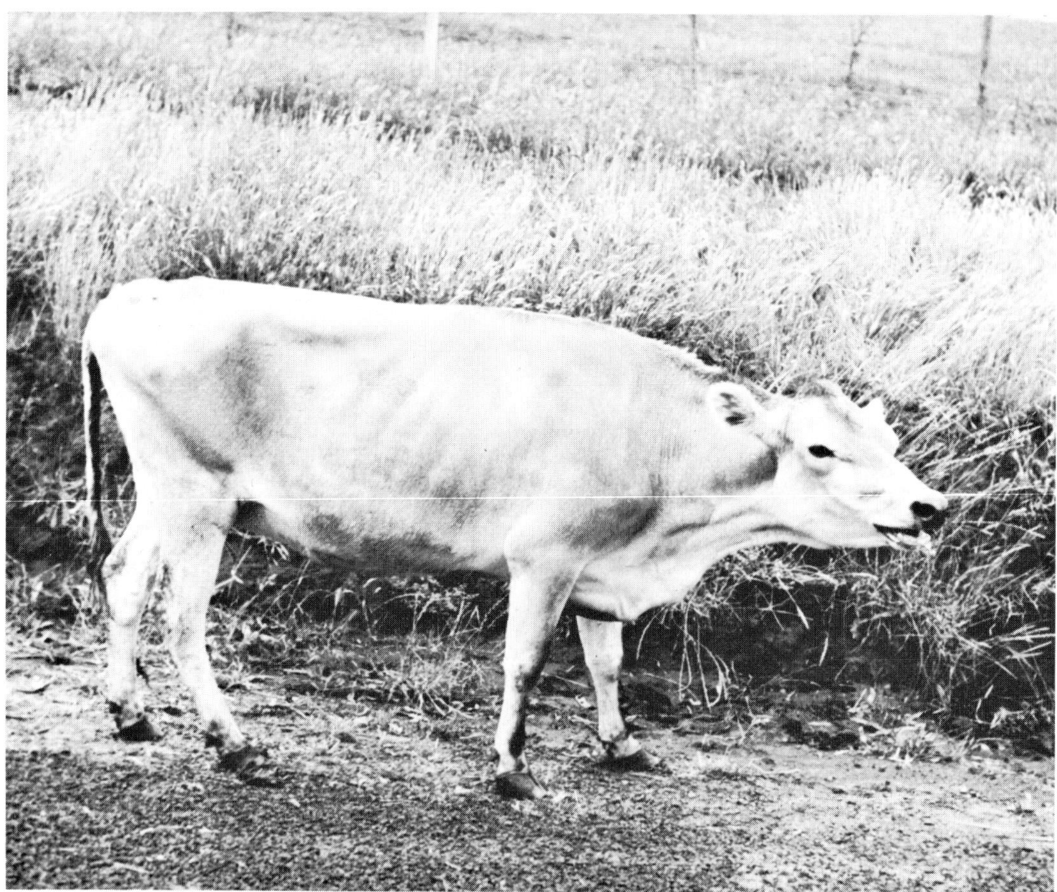

FIG. 28. Characteristic stance of contagious pleuropneumonia. Animal spreads front legs and hangs head to ease chest pain. (Courtesy USDA.)

In fatal cases death occurs 2 to 3 weeks after the onset of symptoms. Many infected animals make partial and eventually complete recovery. Recovery is favored by good grazing and favorable weather.

Pathology

Postmortem lesions depend upon the stage at which the animal dies or is killed and upon the type of infection. In thc ordinary acute case involvement is usually restricted to one lung. On opening the chest, the pleural cavity on the affected side is found to contain a varying quantity of straw-colored or reddish exudate in which are floating yellow flecks and strands of fibrin. The affected part of the lung is usually affixed to the chest wall by a yellow spongy mass of tissue.

The diseased lung tissue does not collapse but appears raised above the relatively more normal portions. It is solid, and the freshly cut surface has a marbled appearance, areas of pink, dark red and gray lung tissue being marked off by yellow streaks of varying width. Close examination of these streaks, which are the thickened tissue partitions separating the lobules of the lungs, shows a beaded appearance. The lymph spaces, round, oval or elongate in shape, are distended with lymph. On standing, a clear yellow exudate, which clots on exposure to the air, will exude from the cut surface.

At a later stage the interlobular tissue consists of firm connective tissue, while the lobules lying between are either dark gray or brown or, if they have become necrotic, sometimes yellow. Still later, in recovering animals, the affected portion of the lung is usually enclosed in a thick fibrous capsule. The encapsulated portion, which may vary in size from that of a pea to a large orange, represents a foreign body. Eventually, even this may be absorbed or become liquefied and appear as an abscess. In many old cases of pleuropneumonia the only evidence of past infection may be the thickened pleura and firm adhesions between lung and chest wall, together with thickening of the fibrous septa of the lung in the area adjacent to the adherent pleura.

Diagnosis

During life it is difficult to distinguish cases of contagious bovine pleuropneumonia from pneumonia and pleurisy of other origin. Postmortem, however, the naked-eye appearance of the lung lesions is usually sufficient to make a definite diagnosis.

A fairly satisfactory complement-fixation test is available, but, since it depends on the presence of immune bodies in the serum, it tends to pick out vaccinated animals as well as those recently recovered from infection and those in which infection still persists.

Control

It is conceivable that carrier animals might spread the disease. The most effective method of dealing with an outbreak is prompt isolation, quarantine and slaughter, possibly combined with the use of the complement-fixation test as an assessment of prevalence.

When bovine pleuropneumonia has been diagnosed, affected farms should be placed in strict quarantine and all cattle subjected to the complement-fixation test to gauge the extent of the discasc. In most cases slaughter of reactors is desirable, and this is certainly the quickest way to eliminate a confined outbreak. If this is not possible, quarantine restrictions must remain in force until the test shows all animals to be negative.

Vaccination may also be practiced in areas where the disease is enzootic. However, the variable susceptibility of different strains of cattle, the lack of immune response in significant numbers of vaccinates, and the frequent serious reaction to vaccination leaves some doubt as to the value of any of the numerous inactivated, living culture, or avianized vaccines as the sole method of eliminating the disease.

47
Lumpy Skin Disease

LUMPY skin disease is an acute, febrile, infectious disease of cattle characterized by the rapid appearance of skin nodules of varying size and extent, edema of one or more limbs, and swelling of superficial lymph glands.

The disease is caused by a virus thought to be transmitted by an insect vector. The blood from animals which subsequently proved to be infected with lumpy skin was distributed and used as anaplasmosis vaccine. Some cattle inoculated with this blood developed signs of lumpy skin, thus providing the first evidence of the infectiveness of the disease through inoculation. Investigators have observed the spread of this disease in an insect-proof stable and have reproduced the disease by subcutaneous injection of saliva from infected bovines. The incubation period is 4 to 14 days. The virus is present in the saliva for a limited period during the febrile reaction, in the blood from the second to tenth days, and in nodules from the third to fifteenth days. The virus has also been isolated from semen and nasal mucus.

Factors Influencing Susceptibility

In an outbreak in northern Rhodesia the disease was reported most prevalent during the summer rainy season, with most cases in low-lying areas and fewest on the hills. Severe epizootics have been recorded occasionally during weather when insect population is at its lowest number.

The disease is known to affect only cattle; all ages and breeds are susceptible, but the thin-skinned breeds particularly so. Calves may develop only slight infection or none at all.

Transmission

The disease has been transmitted experimentally by subcutaneous inoculations of blood and emulsions made from fresh nodules or from the spleen. Recovered animals harbor the virus only up to 22 days after signs appear. Virus has been found in the saliva of cattle at the height of the fever reaction. The disease has been observed to spread over long distances under conditions which would rule out all means of conveying the virus except insect vectors. Although proof is lacking, the circumstantial evidence is overwhelming that certain insects are transmitters of the disease.

Recovery from a typical reaction or an inapparent infection confers a solid immunity of 3 to 4 months.

Symptoms

The disease suddenly strikes individual cattle of any age, leaving others in the same herd unaffected. Usually the first sign is a high temperature (to 105 F) followed by the appearance of skin nodules in 7 to 10 days. Occasionally nodule formation precedes a noticeable pyrexia. There may also be lacrimation, nasal discharge and salivation. The animal may be disinclined to move and walk with a stiff, awkward gait. Frequently edema of the brisket, one or more limbs and the udder is seen, and the lymph nodes are commonly swollen markedly.

The characteristic lesion is a firm nodular swelling in the skin. These nodules may vary in number from single ones to many hundreds and they may vary from pea size to several inches in diameter. They are circumscribed and usually painful at first. Typically the center of the lesion dies and becomes dry; a few days later the necrotic core may fall out, leaving an ulcer underneath. However, in other cases the lesions may resolve rapidly and disappear, or they may become indurated and persist for a year or more. In more severe cases lesions may join to form large firm lumps which often become dry and separate from the skin, leaving suppurating sores

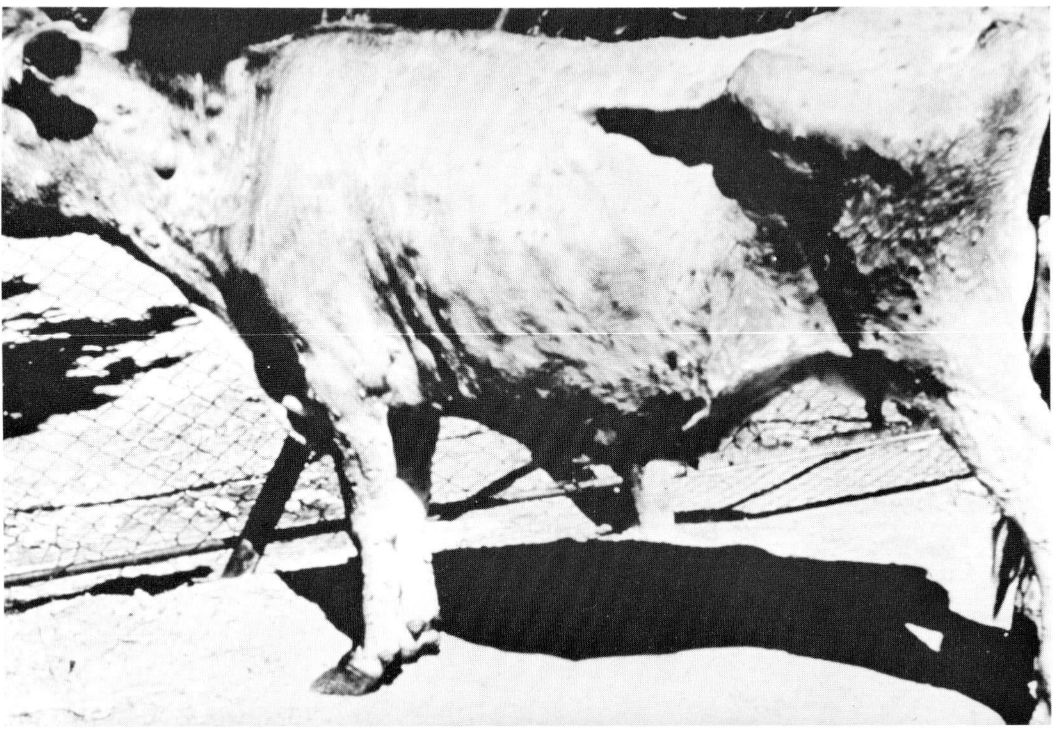

FIG. 29. Lumpy skin disease. Note the widely distributed lumps of varying sizes. (Courtesy USDA.)

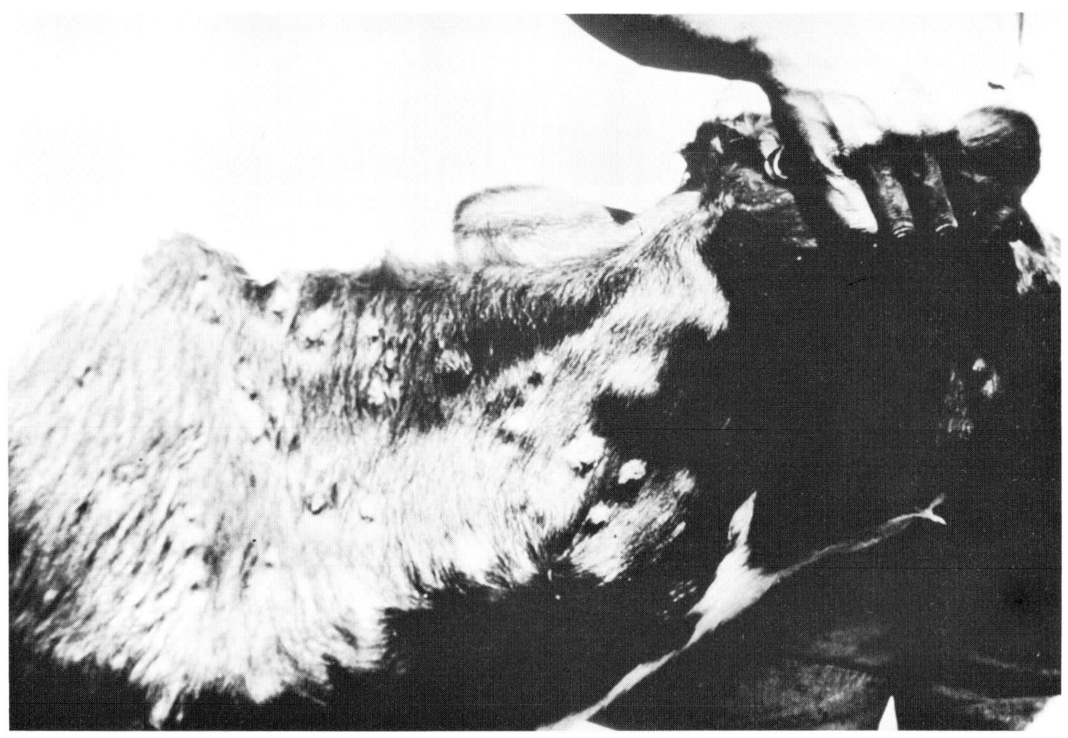

FIG. 30. Lumpy skin disease. Note lumps on neck of bovine. (Courtesy USDA.)

which may be the channel of entry of secondary bacterial and maggot invaders. Nodules may be found in the mucous membrane of the mouth, nostrils, pharynx, gastrointestinal tract, lungs, udder and genital organs. Involvement of the internal organs often gives rise to ulceration of the mucous membranes. Lesions of the respiratory tract may lead to death through suffocation. Mortality does not exceed 10 percent, but the economic losses from emaciation, damage to the skin, loss of milk, injury to reproductive organs, and pneumonia are heavy.

Pathology

The skin surface of the entire body may be involved in the nodule formation. The tissue is thickened locally, develops a creamy-gray color and sometimes encloses caseous necrotic material. The subcutis may be infiltrated with reddish-gray serous fluid. Edema of the lungs and occasional pneumonic lesions with adhesions of the pleura and peritoneum may also be observed.

Diagnosis

The mysterious way in which the disease spreads by jumping from place to place, possibly missing several farms and affecting only a certain number of cattle, the distinctive nodular eruptions on the skin and mucous membrane, and the swelling of limbs and lymphatic glands are characteristic of the disease. Where lesions are followed by necrosis and later by suppurative changes through secondary infection, the presence of the disease is more readily confirmed.

Most affected animals recover spontaneously. In mild cases animals may be ill but a few days. If large areas of the skin slough, secondary infections, such as those from clostridia, may prove fatal. In those cases where pronounced swellings develop around the head and neck, suffocation can cause death of the animal.

Subcutaneous injection of blood or suspension of nodular material from infected animals into susceptible cattle with reproduction of typical lesions is the only means of biological diagnosis.

Control

Quarantine regulations prohibiting animal movements have not been effective in preventing spread of the disease. Insecticides and repellents have proved useless. Despite strong suspicion that insects transmit lumpy skin disease, the possibility of direct contact between cattle and other related species which may be inapparent carriers cannot be excluded.

Lumpy skin disease spreads rapidly; therefore, the combination of slaughter and vaccination is initiated to control serious outbreaks. In Africa, a lyophilized attenuated virus vaccine is available. The vaccine is injected subcutaneously and immunity is established in about ten days, providing protection for one year.

PART 5

Poisonous Substances

48
Poisonous Plants

TOXICOLOGICAL problems are difficult to prevent, because there are many poisonous substances to consider. The poison may be a naturally occurring plant constituent, or a chemical introduced into and not normally found in the natural environment. It is helpful in diagnosing poisonings to examine the entire herd, observing the animals for any deviation from normal, while evaluating all known facts surrounding the problem. Pastures should be examined for poisonous plants, discarded paint buckets, fertilizer spills and other possible sources of poisoning. Overgrazing of pastures and ranges is probably the greatest single factor in losses from poisonous plants.

Livestock producers must consider their management procedures and shortcomings when multiple poisonings occur on a property, because most cases are the result of carelessness, poor management or ignorance.

On most properties the prevention of plant poisoning is, in general, a matter of livestock and pasture management. The main step is the eradication of poisonous plants from all parts of the property. If the farm is in a prairie region, this is relatively easy. If it includes woodland, natural meadows, or other areas where native plant life persists, the problem is more difficult. It is then necessary to know poisonous plants, to keep the number of them as small as possible, and to keep animals away from them at seasons when they may be eaten in quantity. Most poisonous plants are weeds and can be eradicated by the same general practices as those used for weeds. Where complete eradication is impossible, it is necessary to know more about poisonous plants—the stages at which they are poisonous, the seasons when they are dangerous, and the conditions under which they cause poisoning. Valuable animals can then be prevented from feeding on them.

Poisonous plants are a hazard to livestock in many native pastures when the right set of circumstances occur. Generally, most plant poisonings occur early in the spring before grass is adequate, or during periods of drought when green feed is scarce. The toxic substance of some plants is concentrated in the young growing leaves in the spring, while in others it is found in the seeds and stems later in the season.

Generally, there are only a few poisonous plants that are troublesome in an area, and producers should learn to recognize them. Bulletins or books are available from the state agricultural extension services.

Hydrocyanic Acid Poisoning

This can occur from several plants, such as arrow grass, Johnson grass, Sudan grass, common sorghum, wild black cherry, chokeberry, pin cherry and flax. All of these plants contain cyanogenetic glucosides which, when hydrolyzed by enzymes in the digestive tract, yield hydrocyanic acid (prussic acid).

Johnson grass and Sudan grass are considered good pasture grasses but, when normal growth has been interrupted by drought, frost, trampling or other causes, hydrocyanic acid may develop to a point where the plants become toxic to livestock. The cyanogenetic glucoside content is increased by heavy nitrate fertilization and excessive irrigation or heavy rainfall. Very young, rapidly growing plants are most hazardous. Neither freezing nor wilting increases the glucoside content, but both tend to increase the free hydrocyanic acid content, resulting in a temporary increase in toxicity.

Sheep and cattle may be poisoned by eating arrow grass, the leaves of which contain hydrocyanic or prussic acid. Species of arrow grass which poison livestock are widely distributed in marshy pastures and native grass-hay areas throughout the United States. As long as arrow grass has adequate moisture, it does not cause poisoning; when growth is stunted from lack of moisture or an early frost, however, plants quickly become toxic. Arrow grass grows best in soil covered with water and in such soil may spread over large areas. In moist soil or near springs, it sometimes grows in small patches.

About $\frac{1}{50}$ of an ounce of hydrocyanic acid ($\frac{1}{4}$ to 3 pounds of stunted arrow grass) will kill a 600-pound animal. The toxic dose must be eaten at one time to cause death, because the poison is not cumulative. Death results from respiratory failure.

Signs of poisoning are: nervousness, abnormal breathing (either very rapid or slow and deep), trembling or jerking muscles, blue coloration of the lining of the mouth, spasms or convulsions continuing at short intervals until respiratory failure causes death.

Bracken Fern Poisoning

This fern is widely distributed in North America. When ingested by cattle and sheep it causes cumulative poisoning, taking from 1 to 3 weeks to develop. Signs of poisoning may occur for two weeks or more after animals have been removed from fern foliage. Cases generally develop in late summer or fall following periods of drought.

Sheep and cattle show toxic signs after eating green ferns daily for a period of time. Cattle have hemorrhages in various parts of their bodies, develop a fever, and lose weight rapidly. They are affected by the so-called aplastic anemia factor which depresses bone-marrow function. Cases are irreversible. The onset of symptoms is sudden and of short duration, and death loss may approach 90 percent of those affected. Treatment should be under the direction of the local veterinarian, although few cattle recover after signs of acute poisoning appear.

Animals seldom eat bracken fern if sufficient forage is available. To eliminate livestock losses, do not overgraze ranges. Make sure sufficient forage is available at all times to animals in infested areas. If necessary, give supplement near the end of the grazing period. Without supplement, animals often eat toxic amounts of bracken to make up for the decreased nutrient value of mature plants.

Bracken fern can be eradicated. In areas where cultivation is practical, the plants can be destroyed by cultivating the soil for 2 to 3 years. Keeping the tops cut will starve the roots and prevent spread.

Crooked-Calf Disease

Toxic species of lupine weed eaten by cows during early pregnancy cause crooked-calf disease, a crippling disorder of calves present at birth.

Stricken calves have twisted and badly aligned leg bones, twisted backs or necks, or cleft palates. One or more of these defects can cause defects ranging from inability to move or eat to harmless bone alterations noticeable only on X-ray films.

Lupine, or beanweed, is a plant of the pea family with multiple leaflets radiating finger-like from a common point. A spike of white, pink, yellow or bluish florets projects from the top. Only a few of the more than 100 known species have thus far been found toxic. Lupine grows on foothills and mountain ranges in many areas of the west. The poisonous species are perennials, although some lupines are annuals. Poisonous species are dangerous from the time they start to grow in the spring until they dry up in the fall; most are especially dangerous during the seed stage in late summer. Pods and seeds retain their toxicity even when the plants are matured.

When cows graze on toxic lupines, they themselves may show moderate reactions. They exhibit a reluctance to move and a stiff-legged walk; coats are rough, noses are dry, and feces are hard. In many cases, these cows later produce deformed calves. There is no direct relation between severity of symptoms in the mother and severity of deformity in the offspring. Cattle are often poisoned by eating 1 to 2 pounds of lupine without other forage.

Comparison of cows fed lupine during various stages of early pregnancy showed that the worst time for grazing on contaminated ranges was between the 40th and 70th days of pregnancy. Slight to moderate bone malformation, however, has been shown to result during experimental feed trials when cows ate lupine after that time span.

Unfortunately, cows are likely to eat lupine just at the critical time, in August, when most of the herd is one or two months pregnant, range pastures tend to dry up, and good feed gets scarce. Cattle normally do not like lupine, but they eat it when there is no other choice. The best way for ranchers to avoid crooked-calf disease is to provide an alternative to lupine ranges, at least during the first 120 days of pregnancy.

Losses may be extremely heavy when hungry sheep are trailed through lupine ranges in the later summer. Supplemental feeding is helpful when animals are herded through lupine ranges.

Sweet-Clover Poisoning

Sweet clover, a valuable forage crop, may be used freely as pasture, but the feeding of damaged or spoiled sweet-clover hay or silage may cause death. Death losses from sweet-clover poisoning in a herd may vary from one or two animals to 15 or 20.

Prior to the isolation of dicumerol, the hemorrhagic agent in spoiled sweet-clover hay, an infectious agent was considered as a possible cause of the condition. The appearance of the symptoms does suggest a transmissible infectious disease because the condition occurs simultaneously in several animals on the same farm. Additionally, in feeding trials, the disease appears in cattle of the same age and after approximately the same length of time.

Dicumerol has been isolated from experimentally produced spoiled hays and from hays fatal to cattle in field cases. The substance is insoluble in acid media but forms salts in basic or alkaline solutions. The damaged hay is usually moldy, but not all moldy hay is poisonous. Dicumerol poisoning is usually seen in winter after cattle have been fed damaged sweet-clover hay for approximately two weeks.

In sweet-clover poisoning nothing in the appearance of cattle attracts attention until hemorrhages occur. Swellings representing subcutaneous hemorrhage are usually noticed first. The swelling is often great enough to cause lameness.

The mucosa are pale, and persistent bleeding occurs from superficial cuts and scratches. Progressive weakness follows anemia resulting from loss of blood. Affected cattle may remain bright and alert and continue to ruminate. Unless pressure from hemorrhage blocks the esophagus and stops eructation, bloating does not occur. With the hemorrhaging, the heart rate quickens and the increased force of the beat is obvious. Death results from anemia.

Animals dehorned or castrated while in the toxic state will bleed to death, as coagulation is inhibited. Bleeding is particularly severe during parturition if toxicity is present; both the dam and calf usually die.

Calves are more susceptible to the disease than are older cattle, but mature animals may show signs of the condition if the spoiled hay is fed to them over a long enough period. Because of their physiological deficiency of vitamin K, newborn animals and infants are particularly sensitive to the anticoagulant. Lactating animals, however, are usually resistant to the toxic substance. That the drug passes the placental barrier is shown by the fact that the prothrombin level is reduced in newborn animals from dams fed spoiled sweet-clover hay.

The characteristic lesion is hemorrhage into the tissue in all parts of the body. Blood in the tissues usually clots after death occurs, but that in the peritoneal cavity remains fluid. Most often the hemorrhages are found in the subcutaneous tissues and intermuscular fascia, but lesions have been seen in the brain and in the medullary cavities of the long bones.

There is much variation in the time required to produce sweet-clover toxicity, indicating that not all damaged clover hay is equally toxic. Coagulation of the blood is not usually retarded before 14 days of feeding moldy hay. The average time is about 15 days. If coagulation has not been adversely affected within three weeks, the hay is probably not highly toxic, in which case the onset of hemorrhaging occurs after about 30 days. Toxic hay does not lose its toxicity, and experiments have shown that it can still cause hemorrhage after four years in storage.

Herd history may immediately suggest a diagnosis of sweet-clover poisoning, or careful examination of affected animals and necropsies may be necessary to confirm the diagnosis. Sweet-clover disease should be suspected when sudden deaths occur in cattle fed on sweet-clover hay or when several animals die within a day or two after dehorning or castrating. Upon postmortem examination, excessive hemorrhages should substantiate the diagnosis of sweet-clover disease.

Properly cured sweet clover is not toxic and is a good feed, although it is unpalatable because of the woody fiber of its stems. Sweet clover is not toxic when grazed, and can economically be used in this manner.

Cattle alternately fed good hay and toxic sweet-clover hay may not be affected, depending on the toxicity of the hay and the ratio of substitution. With highly toxic hay, a 50:50 ratio may still produce the disease. If sweet clover is fed until a delay in clotting time becomes apparent, and a safe forage is then fed, trouble is not likely to be encountered.

Fescue Foot

Fescue foot in cattle is a peculiar disease in that the symptoms first appear in the left hind foot in a great number of cases. The condition is due to a toxic substance causing vasoconstriction in the animal's body and produced by tall fescue grass. Tall fescue is a valuable pasture grass, but cattle feeding on it occasionally develop lameness.

All breeds of cattle are susceptible to the condition, which resembles ergot poisoning but which has a predilection for the feet. The poisoning may appear as an outbreak, and many cattle on improperly managed pastures may be affected during droughts. When the grass has received little fertilizer or has not been previously grazed or mowed, it is of poor quality in late fall and winter. Cattle grazing on it are subject to extreme malnutrition if supplemental feed is not provided. Fescue foot is prevalent in animals suffering from malnutrition, and also occurs in cattle fed fescue hay or silage.

On the other hand, few cases of fescue foot have been reported in cattle rotated on well-managed pastures of fescue-legume mixture or vigorously growing stands of pure fescue.

The disease may appear 10 days to several weeks after cattle start to feed on fescue since they are most susceptible to fescue foot when first placed on fescue pasture.

Usually, the first clinical signs are general stiffness and soreness. Affected cattle are slow to move and refuse to graze. They become dull and listless as their rate of breathing increases. They lose weight rapidly. Cattle soon become lame in the hind feet. Hooves may split.

At this time fescue foot may be confused with foot rot. Cattle with foot rot usually develop distinct swelling and inflammation in the space between the claws. There is no such swelling in fescue foot.

As fescue foot progresses, dry gangrene develops in the foot tissues. Skin around the hoof breaks; a definite line marks the affected area. In severe cases, sloughing of foot tissue occurs at this time. Also, the switch, the end of the tail, and—in rare cases—the tip of the ears may slough off.

No medication is effective for cattle with fescue foot. In severe cases where sloughing has occurred, animals should be destroyed for humane reasons.

Cattle usually recover completely if they are removed from fescue pasture or fescue hay and given other feed as soon as the first signs of the disease appear. After they recover, cattle may be safely returned to fescue pasture if the grass is growing satisfactorily. These cattle should be checked daily for signs of recurrence.

Proper management of fescue pasture is the best way to prevent fescue foot. Pasture rotation will help prevent fescue foot during severe drought when forage is badly needed. To rotate pastures: Put cattle on other forage for 10 days; follow with fescue pasture for the next 10 days. Continue pasture rotation at 10-day intervals until the drought breaks.

Tall fescue is adapted to many soils and climates in the United States. Because it grows well on soils of low productivity, this pasture grass has made a major contribution to the agriculture of the south central and southeastern states. The grass may be maintained in legume-fescue mixtures or in pure stands. When fescue pasture is fertilized and well managed, cattle make satisfactory gains. On pure stands of fescue, young cattle gain 0.8 to 1.5 pounds a day. Cattle on legume-fescue mixtures make gains comparable to other cool-season legume-grass mixtures.

Cattle grazing fescue should have provided for free choice adequate amounts of salt, bone meal, and limestone and perhaps a mineral supplement containing minor elements.

Grass-Seed Nematode Poisoning

Grass-seed nematode poisoning of animals is a sporadic condition difficult to diagnose because the principal clinical sign is nervousness, followed shortly by death. The condition occurs in areas where grasses are subject to the grass-seed nematode disease caused by the larval stages of *Anguina agrostis.* In only two diseases, ergot and grass-seed nematode disease, are grass seeds replaced by sclerotia and galls toxic to livestock. The effects of ergot poisoning on livestock are well documented, but little is known about grass-seed nematode poisoning.

The clinical signs in cattle are neuromuscular, such as knuckling of the forefeet, lowering the head between the forelegs, sweating, staggering, falling, convulsions, and death. In dairy cattle the first sign is a drop in milk production, followed by the other symptoms if the toxic hay is not removed.

Farmers in central Oregon produce a variety of seed crops, and it has been their custom to feed the seed screenings to livestock in the winter months. The seed screenings resulting from the cleaning of Chewings fescue seed contain a large proportion of seed galls. The seed galls contain many larval nematodes which leave the galls after wet weather in the spring and migrate to the grass leaves. When the grass panicles develop, the microscopic nematodes penetrate the ovaries and stimulate the plant to produce galls. In any seed head, one or all of the seeds may be affected.

The infested seeds have been found to contain a heat-stable, alcohol-soluble substance that is toxic to livestock when added to their normal diet.

Many grasses may be infested sporadically by *A. agrostis.* Among these grasses are Chewings fescue, creeping red fescue, Kentucky bluegrass, annual bluegrass, velvet grass, sweet vernal grass, creeping timothy, red top, spike bent, highland bent grass, velvet bent grass, seaside bent grass, orchard grass and buffalo grass.

Wheat and rye are infested by another species of this genus, *Anguina tritici,* but it is not known if this nematode is toxic to animals. In wheat the nematode causes the formation of gall in place of the grain. The galls are shorter than the wheat grains and look like smut balls. However, the galls are hard, whereas the smut balls are soft and easily crushed with the fingers. In addition, other related nematode species infest seeds sporadically in species of *Calamagrostis, Dantonia, Elymus, Holcus, Sporobolus,* and *Stipa* throughout the country.

The disease in grass plants may be controlled only by drastic measures and by constant attention to prevent a recurrence. Effective measures include burning of fescue fields following the harvest of seeds to destroy galls in the stubble, rotation of crops for several years, and the use of costly chemicals. (The grass-seed nematode disease involves only the seed heads so that the grass may be utilized for lawn or turf.)

49
Poisonous Minerals and Mixtures

Urea Poisoning

MORE than half of all cattle in feedlots in the United States are probably fed some urea, according to findings of a survey recently reported by the United States Department of Agriculture covering more than 6,000 cattle feeders.

Urea is fed in commercial mixed feed, in a concentrate ration mixed by the cattle feeder or to his order, or in silage.

Until recently it was difficult to measure the urea used in livestock feed. Urea is widely used for fertilizer and industrial purposes as well as for feed, and technical problems formerly restricted feed use to "feed-grade" urea. However, these problems have largely been solved, and most commercial grades of urea have become multipurpose in use. Thus, commonly quoted estimates of feed-grade urea represent only part of the urea actually fed to livestock.

More than half of all feedlot operators who buy urea as a separate ingredient mix it on the farm with their own equipment. Local feed dealers mix for small feedlots.

Some guidelines for feeding urea to beef cattle:

1. Do not feed urea or supplements containing urea to newly arrived or shipped-in cattle for a period of 21 to 28 days, or to cattle that have been starved or off feed for 36 hours until they have had a chance to fill up with feed.
2. Feed a maximum of 0.15 pound of urea daily to growing or wintering cattle.
3. Feed no more than 0.22 pound of urea per head daily to fattening steers or heifers on grain and roughage.
4. Do not feed urea to young calves until after the rumen develops—at about 6 to 8 weeks of age.
5. Formulate complete cattle rations so that no more than 33 percent of the crude protein or nitrogen is derived from urea.
6. Do not feed urea over and above the protein requirements.
7. Mix urea in a properly balanced supplement or a complete ration; do not feed free-choice or self-feed urea supplements.

The recommendations for use of urea in dairy cattle are not so clear-cut as those for beef because there is a variation in the level of grain fed for different levels of milk production. Urea can be used to replace up to 35 percent of the protein of the concentrate ration of dairy cattle after rumen function has been established. A high-urea protein supplement up to 20 percent of urea or 90 percent of the protein from urea can be used, but it should be mixed in the ration so that the urea level does not exceed recommended allowances.

Urea is used by rumen microorganisms and supplies nitrogen for the synthesis of amino acids. Amino acids are eventually either incorporated into tissue protein or used to form ammonia. In the first process, the animal makes its own protein from a relatively inexpensive material. In the second, the nitrogen is not only largely wasted but the product is toxic and absorbed into the bloodstream.

The toxicity of urea largely depends on the energy content of the ration, the kinds of microorganism making up the rumen flora and the rate of consumption of urea. The rumen may be conditioned to convert urea to amino acids rather than to ammonia by starting at a low level and gradually increasing the amount fed. This presumably encourages multiplication of those bacteria which synthesize amino acids at the expense of those which do not. One hundred grams of urea in a single feeding will kill a 1,000-lb cow not previously fed urea. The same amount distributed over two or three feedings will not be lethal, since the ammonia concentration in the blood will remain below a critical level.

Under feedlot conditions, as much as 300 gm of urea per day per 1,000-lb animal may be fed to cows adapted to urea feeding. (It should be noted, however, that renal damage may result at this high level.) If animals are kept off feed for a short time, even 24 to 48 hours, they lose much of their adaptability to urea and may be killed by the same level they had earlier consumed safely.

The clinical signs of urea toxicity in cattle are severe groaning, shivering, staggering, labored rapid breathing, violent struggling, and death.

Nitrate-Nitrite Poisoning

Nitrate poisoning is often the consequence of a complex of mismanagement. It can result from careless handling of fertilizers or other nitrate-containing chemical mixtures or from the accidental ingestion of the chemicals. Secondly, animals may graze on pastures or ranges where nitrate-bearing plants are prevalent. Thirdly, the poisoning may result from drinking water, either from naturally nitrate-bearing spring water or from streams, ponds, or wells contaminated with nitrate-bearing run-off water.

Perhaps this problem is becoming more important through recent innovations and trends in modern agriculture. Natural waterways and surface drainage undoubtedly contain more nitrates leeched from surface applications of fertilizer products. Surface contamination from feedlot drainage, old manure piles and other sources is an important factor, especially in poorly placed farm wells.

Geological surveys and public-health surveys have shown that natural spring waters and wells less than 200 feet deep often contain levels of nitrate hazardous to animal and human health. Reports show that some Minnesota wells have a nitrate-nitrogen content of 190 ppm, which, under some circumstances, approaches the minimum lethal amount for swine. Some Missouri and Kansas wells show over 800 ppm. Such sources of water should not be used for any human or animal consumption.

Most water analyses are based on nitrate level. One must remember that swine can tolerate large amounts of nitrate, but are highly susceptible to nitrite. For the swine industry this introduces an additional hazard, since nitrate can be converted to nitrite by bacterial action, especially by organisms of the coliform group which abound at or near livestock sources of water. Zinc from storage tanks, coated water lines and waterers also act as conversion agents.

During the growing season, plants absorb nitrate from the soil; in the stems and leaves the nitrate is reduced to nitrite. Continuous nitrate absorption from the soil, coupled with retarded growth, may lead to nitrate or nitrite concentration because of incomplete reduction. (Examples of conditions leading to retarded growth include drought, shade, herbicide action, and plant disease or injury.) Accelerated nitrate absorption following rainfall—especially after a period of drought—may also cause such concentration, and heavy nitrate fertilization will add to the problem. Under such conditions, immature plants in particular tend to concentrate nitrate or nitrite.

Nitrate concentrations in silage are reduced, but not eliminated, by the fermentation process. Silage forages containing moderate amounts of nitrate can be fed safely, if offered in small amounts over a long period of time. In ruminant animals, carbohydrates hasten the conversion of nitrate into amino acids, hence reducing the toxic effects of excess nitrate in the feed. Feeding roughage containing nitrates should be supplemented with vitamin A. It should be remembered that small amounts of nitrate may affect feed utilization without causing clinical signs of toxicity.

In cattle, symptoms of nitrate toxicity are: a marked drop in milk flow within a week after chopped hay or silage is fed, increased urine production which is darker than normal, and apparent digestive failures. In a type of toxicity which appears slowly, milk flow declines and symptoms of vitamin A deficiency appear. When abortions are noted, they usually occur in the third to fifth month.

Abnormal births are common and calves carried to term are born dead or die immediately after birth. Nitrate-bearing oat hay and corn stalk poisoning appear to act similarly, in that sudden losses may occur when cattle or sheep ingest nitrates. Chemically, the nitrates are converted to nitrites in the paunch. The resulting nitrites compete with the oxygen, tying up the erythrocyte-oxygen mechanism in the blood. Blood from these animals will be chocolate brown. Feedstuffs incriminated in nitrate poisoning are corn silage or fodder, sorghum silage, oat hay or silage, Sudan pasture, hay or silage, and alfalfa hay.

Fluorosis

Fluorine is an active chemical element widely distributed in soil, water, rocks, and plants in many parts of the world, but most often encountered in water from deep wells in the more arid parts of this country. Fluorine combines with other elements to form fluorides. Toxic quantities of fluorides occur in a few products used in feeding animals, such as raw rock phosphates and phosphatic limestone.

Chronic fluorosis results from the ingestion of small amounts of fluoride over a long period of time. This occurs primarily where livestock consume water high in fluorine, and forage contaminated with wastes from nearby industrial plants. All types of livestock may be affected by excessive amounts of fluorides although cattle are the most susceptible, followed by sheep and swine. The severity of the lesions caused by fluorine poisoning depends upon the form of the fluoride ingested, the age and species of animal, the nutrient level, the level and period of consumption, and the state of reproduction and lactation.

The clinical symptoms associated with fluorosis include staining and mottling of the teeth with excessive wearing of the incisors. In severe cases, exostoses may appear at the joints, the shafts of the long bones may thicken, and the animal may exhibit intermittent lameness. Acute fluoride poisoning is characterized by diarrhea, sudden loss of appetite, loss of weight, and inflammation of the stomach and intestine.

Prevention of fluorosis depends upon

recognizing potential sources of consumption of the chemical and eliminating the possibility of excessive intake.

Wood-Preservative Poisoning

Pentachlorophenol (penta), a wood preservative, is toxic for swine. It does not stain wood, but a stain such as coal tar or creosote is almost always added. These compounds may be more dangerous than the penta. Arsenic or lead in boiled linseed oil, as an additive, may also constitute a hazard.

Readily absorbed through intact skin, pentachlorophenol causes increased metabolism, nervousness, rapid respiration, muscle tremors, and death. On contact it burns the skin and mucous membranes of pigs, and will irritate the skin of adult swine. Prolonged contact may slow growth in feeder pigs.

Typically afflicted newborn pigs nurse well but become ill with fever, muscle tremors, and labored breathing. Death occurs several hours later. Internal necropsy lesions are usually absent, but the skin may be red where it has come in contact with treated lumber. Survivors develop ulcers of the oral mucosa, knees, and soles of the feet. Reduced food intake and bacterial arthritis may follow.

Though adult swine are more resistant to the effects of penta, some sows become restless and, if not removed from the pen, may become hysterical. Prolonged contact of pregnant sows with penta reportedly causes weak or stillborn pigs. It has also been reported that, if sows are confined to treated farrowing crates for 7 to 10 days before farrowing, newborn pigs may bleed to death via the navel.

In one instance, a boardwalk treated with wood preserver 20 years previously but still in good condition was salvaged to build a slatted floor. Weaned pigs placed on this floor developed blood dyscrasias, and 10 percent died of hepatitis and anemia. The problem occurred in each group of pigs placed on the floor until the floor was removed. Arsenicals and coal tar may have been the poisons in this wood. Adding sufficient bedding to keep the pigs off the floor, washing with lye soap and allowing to weather for a year, in one instance, did not resolve the problem adequately.

Lead Poisoning

Lead poisoning is common in pastured animals. Old paint buckets are a common cause when dumped on trash piles, as are old batteries on which curious cattle may chew and lick. Signboards are another source, since cattle may make them a loafing place especially when the rest of the pasture is relatively shade-free.

Buildings that may not have been painted for years, and which may appear to be paint free, are often the source of lead poisoning—again because they are loafing areas. The licking of buildings by cattle is likely to occur in winter and early spring months before grass starts or in periods of drought when grass is in short supply.

The lead content on forage and other plants may reach levels toxic to livestock at the edges of heavily-traveled highways, especially if some of the common orchard sprays are used to control weeds.

Lead is a cumulative poison, and the toxic effects may not become evident until many small doses have equaled a toxic dose.

The clinical symptoms of acute lead poisoning appear in animals as two separate although related syndromes. First, there is a stage of inflammation due to the corrosive effect of the metal on the mucous membranes of the stomach and intestines. This leads to loss of appetite, salivation, intestinal pain, grinding of the teeth, and copious fetid diarrhea. The second syndrome involves the effects of the lead on the nervous system. Animals will appear deranged, walk in circles, stand with heads pressed against a wall or a tree, and bellow as if frenzied.

In the chronic stage, animals will be depressed, lose weight, and stagger when forced to move.

As with most other preventable diseases, the primary means of prevention is good management.

Arsenic Poisoning

Arsenic poisoning probably occurs less frequently now than in years past, but still must be mentioned. Sodium arsenite, lead and calcium arsenate have been used as herbicides and insecticides, and the improper disposal of dust or spray containers was a common cause of arsenic poisoning. Newer and safer pesticides have to a great extent, however, reduced this problem.

Arsenic is poisonous to animals both by absorption through the skin and by oral ingestion.

Clinical signs of arsenic poisoning include general weakness, muscle twitching, weak pulse and staggering gait. Diarrhea is an inevitable sign and results from the destruction of the mucosal lining of the gastrointestinal tract. Because of abdominal pain, animals get up and lie down, kick at the belly, and bite at the flanks. Feces may be copious, watery and flecked with blood.

50
Insecticide Poisoning

Organic Phosphate Poisoning

THE organophosphate compounds are sometimes spoken of as the "nerve gas insecticides" because of the origin of the compounds.

All breeds of livestock are susceptible to poisoning with organophosphate compounds. Neither age nor sex has any significant bearing on susceptibility, but young animals are more sensitive than adults.

Organophosphates may enter the body by inhalation of the vapor, by absorption of the liquid through the skin and eyes, and by ingestion with forage crops or other feedstuffs. However, poisoning usually results from the accidental consumption of an overdose of the insecticide. Inaccurate computation of the oral or dermal dose may cause poisoning. The products are dangerous if improperly used, not only because small doses may be lethal but because sublethal doses are cumulative. All animals exposed to excessive doses, even though symptomless, should be moved to noncontaminated areas.

The clinical symptoms may be local or systemic in origin and may appear a few minutes or several hours after exposure, the time lag depending to some degree upon the specific product, the amount absorbed, and the route of exposure.

Ocular and respiratory effects are caused by conjunctival exposure or inhalation of the insecticide and are evidenced by nasal discharge, prolonged wheezing, rapid respiration, constricted pupils, and, occasionally, protruding tongue.

Systemic symptoms resulting from absorption of higher concentrations are evidenced by sweating, loss of appetite, respiratory difficulties, muscle twitching, restlessness, depression, convulsions, paralysis and death.

To avoid poisoning, great care should be exercised in using insecticides or any other external medicament. Read the labels carefully and follow directions explicitly. Most insecticides are toxic, although none is likely to cause poisoning when used strictly according to label directions.

Other Insecticide Poisonings

The signs of poisoning of DDT, TDE, and methoxychlor are distinctive and easily recognized. The same can be said for other groups or related insecticides; therefore, they will be considered in outline form below.

General Symptoms	*Individual Symptoms*	*Chemical*
Muscular tremors very fine at first, progressing to coarse tremors, to steady shivering. Initiated by stimulant first but constant at later period. Loss of coordination, dyspnea, apprehension, and hypersensitivity.	Hyperirritability	DDT
	Hyperirritability	TDE
	Hyperirritability	Methoxychlor
	Hyperirritability	Perthane
	Hyperirritability	Dilan
Muscular spasms, twitches, jerks or convulsions, no steady tremors but may respond to sudden stimuli. Excessive salivation (mostly frothy). May be depressed but mainly apprehensive and hypersensitive. Onset may be abrupt but recovery sudden.	Odor of rosin or pine.	Toxaphene
	Musty or metallic odor.	BHC or Lindane
	Aromatic or pleasant odor.	Chlordane
	Odor absent or not well defined.	Heptachlor
	Odor absent or not well defined.	Dieldrin
	Odor absent or not well defined.	Aldrin
	Odor absent or not well defined.	Endrin
	Odor absent or not well defined.	Thiodan
	Odor absent or not well defined.	Telodrin
Excessive salivation, fluid or stringy, dyspnea, muscular stiffness or weakness, with or without tremors or trembling. Hypersensitivity and apprehension. Often demonstrate extreme nervous signs.	Excessive salivation.	Trichlorofon (Dipterex, Neguvon)
	Excessive salivation.	DDVP (Vapona)
	Excessive salivation.	Diazinon
	Excessive salivation.	Tepp
	Trembling or rage.	Sevin
	Abrupt onset, swift recovery.	Pyrolan
	Mild nervous signs.	Compound 4072
	Violent nervous signs.	Kuelene
	Progressive nervous signs.	Co-Ral
Great muscular weakness, inapparent until handled, dragging feet, limp tail. May develop dyspnea and excessive salivation.	Diarrhea	Ronnel

PART 6

Parasites

51
Parasitology

OBVIOUSLY the full scope of parasitology cannot be covered in this book; only the most dangerous parasitic diseases of livestock and those against which effective preventive measures have been developed will be considered.

The science dealing with the lives of parasites, their influence as biological irritants and the diseases they cause is called *parasitology*. Parasitic diseases are subdivided according to the zoological group to which their causative agents belong: ticks, lice, mites, roundworms, flatworms, tapeworms, protozoa, and insects. Parasitology as a discipline has as its task the freeing of man and animals from parasites.

Where agriculture is extensive, with intensive development of livestock and constantly rising productivity, the husbandman should be well versed in the general and theoretical problems of parasitology. He should know the causative agents of diseases, their biological and harmful effects on the body of the host, and the principal methods of combating these diseases.

Parasitic diseases are characterized by wide-scale distribution and extended duration. They are encountered in all countries of the world. On farms where parasitic diseases are not combated, considerable mortality occurs and productivity is drastically lowered. Parasitic diseases have a particularly deleterious effect on young animals, retarding growth and development. They make the animal prone to secondary infections, lowering resistance to and complicating the course of such infections.

Breeding healthy animals free of parasitic diseases is one of the primary goals of livestock producers. This can be done by regulating the conditions of the external environment. The surrounding environment determines on the one hand the possibility and degree of contact of the parasite with the host and, on the other, affects the health status of both host and parasite. During recent years, scientists have achieved considerable success in the study and control of parasitic diseases, and livestock specialists should assimilate these measures and apply them widely in animal husbandry.

Of great importance in combating livestock losses from parasitic diseases are properly organized prophylactic measures to prevent or curtail the infective stages of the harmful parasites. These measures are based on the interrelationships among various species of livestock, the life cycles of the parasites, and the factors of the external environment which influence the survival of the parasites; these include: conditions of feeding, maintenance, care, and use of animals, their age, the invasive ability of the larval stages of the parasites, the management of fields and sanitation of barns and feedlots.

Parasitism is defined as a complex relationship between two organisms during which one of them, the parasite, temporarily or permanently dwells in or on the other, the host, feeding on its fluids and tissues and causing the latter harm. Animals encounter great numbers of parasites of varying species—worms, ticks, lice, mites, protozoa—in all situations where livestock are maintained. Such parasites do not always penetrate the body of the host and develop there, however; in other words, an infestation does not always occur. For such an invasion to take place conditions of the external environment must be appropriate and certain conditions must exist in the body of the host (age, lack of resistance to stress, low state of nourishment) and in the parasite (virulence, ability to invade the host, number of invasive parasites).

Types of Hosts for Parasites

An animal in which a parasite lives either temporarily or permanently is called a *host.* The following types of hosts are recognized according to characteristics of development of the parasite and the adjustment to parasitism: (1) *final or definitive host*—the host in which a parasite reaches sexual maturity; (2) *intermediate host*—one in whose body the larval stage of a parasite develops; (3) *secondary host*—a host in whose body the successive stages of the larvae of certain types of parasites develop. Thus, for example, the liver fluke of cattle, *Fasciola hepatica,* requires three hosts for its development: the adult parasite is encountered in the body of ruminant animals (the definitive host); eggs of the *Fasciola* excreted in the feces of infected cattle or ruminants reach water and are swallowed by a water flea in the body of which the larvae develop (the intermediate host); and, finally, the snail eats the infected Cyclops and the second stage of the larva develops in its body (the secondary host). The definitive host becomes infected upon ingestion of the metacercariae encysted on pasture grasses after it leaves the snail. The metacercariae develop into the mature fluke in the definitive host.

Some parasites develop in two hosts, for instance a definitive and intermediate host, while others develop in one animal only and do not require the participation of an intermediate host.

Under the influence of external conditions during the process of evolution, some parasites gradually adjust themselves in a wide circle of hosts. The common liver fluke, *Fasciola hepatica,* is parasitic in a large number of definitive hosts, mainly domestic and wild ruminants. Other parasites develop in specific hosts.

Following sexual maturity, adult parasites produce embryos which either spread freely in nature or concentrate in particular types of animals where they do not undergo further development. These hosts are known as reservoir hosts.

The embryos of certain parasites may undergo the initial stage of development in the body of a nonspecific host, thereby causing temporary harm to the host animal. However, the larvae of such parasites do not find a suitable environment in this type of host and quickly die, sometimes causing local inflammation and itching. This occurrence is normally called transitory parasitism. It may happen with larvae of *Strongyloides,* which are able to penetrate through the intact skin of nonobligatory hosts, and migrate through the subcutaneous tissues without further development. It is also known that, from the eggs of ascarids swallowed by nonobligatory hosts, larvae immerge which migrate along the pulmonary vascular system and are expectorated with mucus into the external environment, providing a focus of infection for susceptible animals.

Localization of Parasites

Parasites localize in various places in the bodies of their hosts, primarily in the gastrointestinal tract and its associated digestive glands and, secondarily, in other internal organs and tissues, for example in the blood. On the whole, it may be assumed that there are no tissues and organs of animals that may not accommodate one or more types of parasites.

According to their mode of life, parasites are divided into temporary and permanent parasites. Temporary parasites undergo part of their life cycle on or in the body of the animal host. They attack their host in order to feed or multiply. Permanent parasites exist on the host for extended periods, frequently for the duration of the parasite's life. To this group belong most species of helminths, some protozoa and some external parasites.

The differentiation between external and internal parasites is by localization. The former, ectoparasites, dwell either temporarily or permanently on the skin of animals. The abode of internal parasites, endoparasites, is the internal tissues of the animal host. During the process of development, they migrate in the body of the host. Therefore, they may at first be internal parasites and then, during maturation, become external parasites, and in some instances the process may be reversed.

Parasitic animals themselves may occasionally harbor parasites in their bodies. Such occurrences are known as superparasitism. For example, worms may become infected with bacteria or viruses or protozoa which may be transmitted to the host animal as an additional infection.

Host—Parasite Relationship

Reciprocal relationships between parasites and their hosts are determined by phases in the development of the parasites and by the corresponding reactions of the body in which the parasites dwell. The effects of the parasite on the body of the host should be considered, while taking into account the conditions of the external environment. These effects are determined by the behavior of larvae on the body of the host while developing to sexual maturity, and also by the behavior of the adult parasite during the phase of multiplication, as in the asexual multiplication of protozoa. The parasite may attach itself to the body of the host by means of its attachment organs, frequently traumatizing the organs and the tissues of the host. When they accumulate in large numbers, parasites may block the lumen of intestines, bronchi or ducts, and cause the rupture or atrophy of organs through prolonged pressure. Embryos of many species of parasites are capable of penetrating into tissues and migrating within them. Of particular vital effect are products of the parasites' metabolism, that is, their endotoxins and exotoxins. Various metabolites are excreted by parasites at different stages in their development. In a number of cases, metabolites excreted by the larvae of the parasites are more toxic than those excreted by the adult form. Many species of parasitic worms, insects, and arachnids possess glands with hemolytic secretions. Toxins of parasites frequently cause severe reactions in the host.

When they attack an animal, arthropods may inoculate or introduce pathogenic microorganisms and viruses into the tissues of the host. Infection of the host may also be caused by the excretions and secretions of arthropods. Parasitic worms are also important as introducers of infection. In mass, the parasites affect surrounding tissues as biological irritants, and thereby bring about various changes in the body of the host. Severe diseases with fatal termination may appear in the host as a result of the parasite's effect. At other times, the action of the parasite inhibits the development of the host, that is, retards development in young animals and predisposes them to stressful conditions.

The condition of the host has, in turn, an important effect on development of parasites. When the host is resistant, it frequently fails to show harmful effects from the parasitic invasion. In such cases parasites may develop normally but, if they are few in number and acted upon by the protective mechanisms of the host, they have a limited effect. Animals harboring parasites with nonclinical manifestations of their presence may be termed *carriers* of parasites. Animal carriers, while not distressed themselves, are dangerous to surrounding animals since they serve as a source of spread. In some infections, carriers acquire immunity to reinfection.

A well-balanced, nutritious diet containing proper vitamins and minerals counteracts harmful effects of parasites to a considerable degree. Thus, well-fed animals may not develop adverse effects of an invasion by internal parasites, while underdeveloped animals—those with a poor dietary regimen—will have greater difficulty in resisting the invasion and may become severely stunted in growth. For example, poorly nourished young pigs heavily parasitized by ascarids die as a result of pneumonia. On the other hand, young pigs kept on a well-balanced diet are resistant to the sequelae of ascaridiasis. It has been established that most livestock infected with internal parasites free themselves from the parasites more rapidly when they are properly fed.

The age of livestock strongly affects the course of the invasion. In young animals the parasites develop rapidly, while in adult animals some parasites cannot develop at all. The resistance of the animal's body becomes considerably stronger with age, a phenomenon that strengthens its physiological state. At the same time, there are parasitic invasions into susceptible animals of any age.

In response to the irritation caused by parasites, the body of the host animal sets up defensive mechanisms, that is, immunity mechanisms. These are expressed as inhibitory effects on the parasites, decreasing their reproductive capacity and length of life, and creating conditions unsuitable for their further development in the body of the host. Immunity during parasitic diseases is most frequently of a nonsterile nature and, with the disappearance of the parasites, the immunity of the host to further invasions frequently disappears.

The external environment has a variable effect on parasites. Depending on external factors, the virulence of parasites rises and drops. The larvae of parasites discovered during periods of low temperature are less virulent than larvae discovered during the warmer periods of the year. The development of causative agents of various contagious diseases of cattle and sheep may occur unevenly in various species of intermediate hosts, such as ticks, that serve as the transmitters. The effects of parasites on the host change even within the same species, as seen in certain types of tapeworms which cause pernicious anemia in some hosts while in others they produce a carrier disease.

Spread of Parasitic Diseases

Natural conditions—climate, soil, vegetation linked with the pasture season, fauna, altitude, rainfall, humidity, and quantity and quality of water sources—have a great influence on the spread of parasitic diseases to livestock. For example, in rainy years there is considerably greater infection with flukes and lungworms in cattle and sheep. Thickets and marshy areas on the pasture allow the multiplication of snails, ticks and insects.

Wild animals play an important role in the spread of parasitic diseases, serving as reservoir and intermediate hosts for many parasites that are transmitted to livestock. Principal

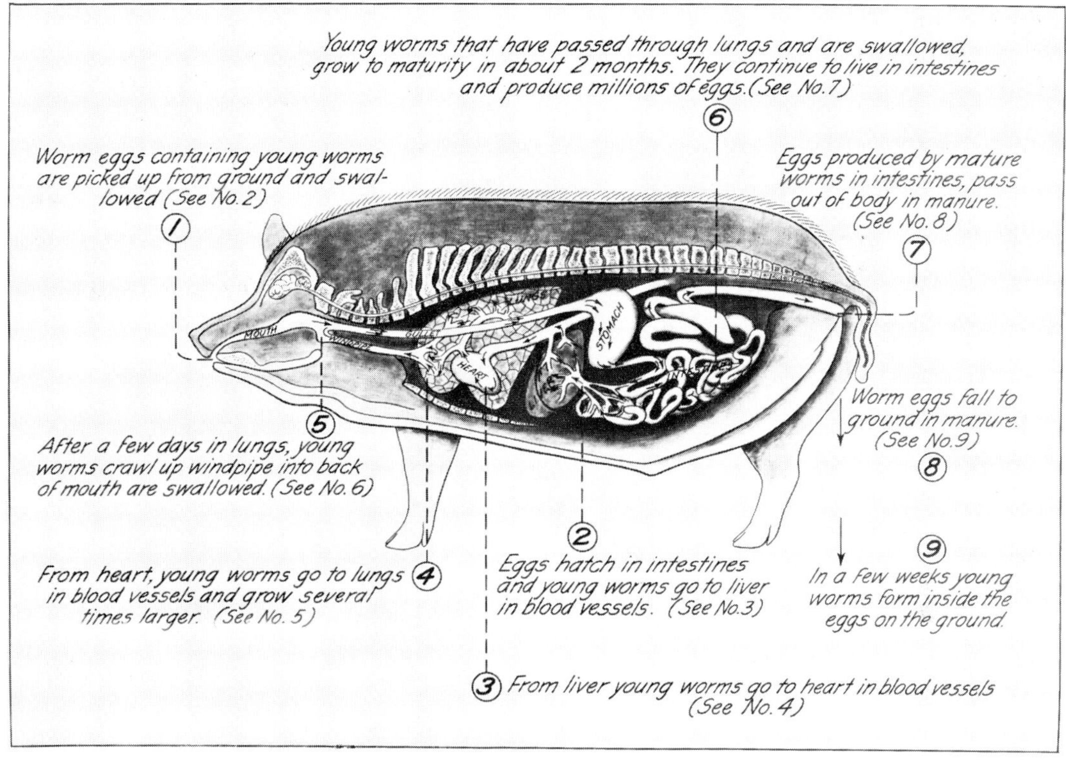

FIG. 31. Generalized life history of roundworm parasites in swine.

among these are the ticks. Factors in the external environment, that is, methods of maintenance and the state of health of the livestock, the presence of intermediate hosts and foci of infection, have varying effects on the parasites in different climatic regions of the United States. When studying invasive diseases for the purpose of deciding the most radical preventive measures against them, it is essential to know the stages of the developments of the parasites and their intermediate hosts, while taking into account the periods of appearance of parasites in any given locality, and optimum conditions for development. Most parasitic diseases are enzootic rather than epizootic. As distinct from infectious diseases, in which microorganisms multiply rapidly in the host, become distributed over a wide area, and run a severe course, the causative agents of parasitic diseases are essentially stationary, spread in a focal manner and have a long period of development, frequently with the participation of a vector or intermediate host. In the study of parasitic diseases, carriers are of very great importance.

Animal diseases caused by various parasites may be distinguished by frequency of occurrence and by pathogenicity. Many animal parasites are rarely encountered, but others are universal and afflict almost all animal species; examples of the latter are the ascarids and the fasciolae.

According to their pathogenic properties, the causative agents of parasitism may be arbitrarily divided into several groups. (1) Certain species of parasite are pathogenic and dangerous spreaders of diseases which take the form of mass enzootics with considerable mortality to animals. A number of highly infectious and widespread parasitic diseases are responsible for enormous economic losses since they are chronic in nature, cause mortality or great emaciation, and are responsible for a drop in the quality and quantity of the produce of livestock. (2) Less pathogenic parasites cause changes in the host which are neither noticeable nor considerable. (3) The host may be parasitized by species of rarely encountered parasites the pathogenic role of which is thus far undetermined.

Animals may become infected with parasites upon ingestion of contaminated food, water, or meat infected with larval stages of the parasite, and by contact with other animals harboring external parasites. A considerable number of parasites penetrate into the body of a host by the aid of vectors such as bloodsucking arthropods. Some species of parasites have the ability to penetrate into the body of the host through the intact skin; examples are hookworms, cattle grubs, and mites. Protozoan diseases such as coccidiosis become infectious when the immature organism is ingested with contaminated feed and water.

Geographic Distribution

The distribution of a number of parasitic diseases is related to the characteristics of a particular geographical environment, to the density of the population of livestock on a farm or ranch, and particularly to animal migrations; even birds may aid in spreading diseases among domestic animals. Diseases with causative agents spread by vectors are widespread. Their distribution is connected with the stage of development of the vector and the appropriate temperature thresholds at which the survival of the parasite and its transformation into the infective stage are possible. Some diseases are found only in subtropical zones where the parasite has become well adjusted to living conditions in the appropriate vector zone.

Individual invasive diseases are focal in nature and are found where parasites are abundant on farms and ranches. The geographical distribution of parasitic diseases in the United States has been investigated and found to be variable. Regional scientific parasitological laboratories and experiment stations give information concerning the presence of natural-focus parasitic diseases, and distribution of individual species of parasites that attack livestock and wild animals.

Preventive Measures

Experience has shown that eradication of parasitic diseases of livestock is possible only by (1) employing complex preventive measures aimed at the removal of parasitized animals, that is, carriers of the infection; (2) the destruction of the vectors and intermediate hosts of parasites; and (3) the removal of the infective stages of both external and internal parasites from pastures, livestock quarters, manure piles, and water sources. In this country, preventive measures against many invasive diseases caused by parasites are included in the federal and state eradication plans directed by the U.S. Department of Agriculture. Prophylactic measures to combat livestock scabies and tick infections are carried out on a similarly large scale.

Tactical measures to combat worm parasites include keeping pens and yards as clean as possible, and drenching all grazing animals three weeks following a good rain after a prolonged dry spell. Larvae of most species require about four weeks to develop to the adult stage; therefore, at three weeks they are at the susceptible stage and can be killed before they begin to lay eggs.

External parasites are especially vulnerable to strategic as well as tactical measures of control. With the advent of systemic insecticides the days of the cattle grub may be numbered. Depending upon the region, the activity of the heel fly may vary, but in general the application of organophosphate spray late in the fall will kill the minute larvae in situ, and will provide a measure of control against ticks and lice as well. Among the ectoparasites, lice and mites are most active in the winter months. It is advantageous routinely to dip or spray all stock, including very young animals, in the fall and again in the spring. The fall treatment will hold down an otherwise disastrous infestation and the spring treatment will catch those organisms that develop during the winter. Tactical sprayings and dippings may be done at any time when scabies or mange becomes a problem.

52
Helminthology

HELMINTHOLOGY is a science dealing with parasitic worms and diseases caused by them. Helminths comprise a large and varying group of invasive parasites which have been divided into several general groups, that is, flatworms, roundworms, tapeworms, and worm-like organisms. There are more than 800 species of roundworms and flatworms that can be encountered on farms and ranches, and any species of helminth when encountered in mass can cause diseases with specific manifestations. It is rare, however, that many different species of round- and flatworms are encountered in any particular area. To study the enormous number of helminths encountered in livestock would be a difficult and endless task. Therefore, this text will describe only widely distributed helminths of considerable harm to livestock.

The large losses to animal husbandry due to the presence of helminths on a large scale are indicated as follows. (1) Mortality is observed as a result of lungworms in sheep and calves, flukes in sheep and calves, tapeworms in sheep and calves, roundworms in swine, and thorny-headed worms in swine. The greatest losses from worms are reported in young animals and particularly those on a poor plane of nutrition. (2) Infection with helminths increases mortality from secondary infections through disruption of tissues and stress. (3) Many helminth infections are responsible for underdevelopment of young animals, which inhibits reproduction in the herd to a considerable degree, and decreases the yield of meat, wool and milk. (4) Animal flesh heavily infected with certain parasitic diseases is not fit for human consumption.

Immunity

Immunity during helminthiasis has not been sufficiently studied. It may, however, be stated with certainty that it exists and develops in accordance with general physiological regularities. It differs from immunity developed during many infectious and protozoal diseases mainly in that full resistance to infection with helminths is not acquired (does not occur). In animals infected intensively with helminths, and occasionally in animals that have undergone disease, a relative or incomplete immunity develops during certain infections, that is, a state of resistance is developed capable of protecting the host from reinvasion or superinvasion. Such immunity is characterized by being species specific.

The mechanism of immunity during helminthiasis is unclear. The metabolites in secretions released by helminths, and also the tissues proper of most species, constitute antigens under the influence of which antibodies are formed in the body of the host. Proof of this is the appearance of anaphylaxis in animals and sensitization to the antigen of helminths. It has been established that such antigens are also species specific.

The defensive organisms occurring in the invaded animal are incapable of completely destroying most species of helminths. Some survive for long periods of time in the body of the animal. The result of such antagonism between the host and the parasite is that the animal host develops defensive mechanisms while the parasite shows decreased virulence. By their metabolites and secretions, helminths act on the body of the host, the latter reacting by increasing its resistance to the parasite. This phenomenon is accompanied by the development of defensive mechanisms which result in resistance that limits the pathogenicity of the metabolic processes of the helminth.

The defensive mechanisms of the host limit the number of developing helminths, decrease their size and retard their growth, decrease the period of parasitization, slow down the migration of larvae in the body of the host, decrease the reproductivity capacity of the helminths and the metabolism of the eggs and larvae, and, finally, mitigate the clinical picture of the parasitism.

Under a well-balanced diet (particularly with a sufficient quantity of vitamins, mineral salts and protein in the feed) and appropriate conditions of maintenance, the defensive mechanisms of the host become considerably strengthened and have a deleterious effect on the embryos of helminths.

Diseases, improper maintenance, prolonged protein starvation, and shortages of vitamins and minerals in the diet are all factors that combine to disrupt the defensive mechanisms of an animal and lower its immunity potential against parasitism. Superinvasions are often encountered among such animals, parasites becoming long-lived and showing increased fertility and pathogenicity. Helminthiases are especially severe in young animals because their defensive mechanisms are not fully developed. Artificial immunization against helminths is not practical for a variety of reasons. However, recent research has indicated that a breakthrough may be imminent.

Basic Measures toward Eradication of Helminths

Successful eradication of helminthiasis in livestock is possible only through the use of preventive measures directed toward stopping the development of carrier animals and the spread of viable larvae. The form which such measures assume is determined by specific factors in the biology of the pathogenic agent, and, of course, by existing local conditions. Since there are many different helminthiases among animals, preventive measures should be designed along lines specific for each parasitic disease.

It is impossible to maintain grazing animals entirely free of worms under normal conditions. Indeed, this would be undesirable, as the young would not develop any immunity. Therefore, strategic measures include pasture rotation, spelling each field or area at least six weeks to eliminate large numbers of larvae, avoiding overstocking and overcrowding, plowing and discing pastures at frequent intervals to disperse fecal matter, sanitary handling of manure and waste products, maintaining a high level of nutrition, and routinely drenching all livestock twice each year, in the winter and in the summer, in addition to tactical drenching.

Drenching

Deworming of livestock is carried out with therapeutic as well as prophylactic goals in mind. Tactical drenching is carried out at any time during the year when helminth disease appears; it is done both to restrict the diseased animal from contact with other animals and to remove the worm burden. Strategic drenching is carried out according to plan during specific months of the year. Such a plan is devised well in advance and allows for no deviation. It is put into effect in spite of any recent tactical measures which may have been taken. The life cycles of the parasites and their particular characteristics are taken into account. The purposes of strategic drenchings are to free infected animals from a particular helminth when the parasite is most active on the pasture and to dilute the infective larvae within a given area.

Animals are usually prepared for drenching 12 to 18 hours prior to treatment with the therapeutic drug. They are denied food and are transferred to special quarters or special pastures where they are kept for 3 to 5 days, that is, from the time the drug is administered until they are free from helminths or their larvae.

53 Cestodes of Livestock

CESTODIASES are diseases the causative agents of which are ribbon-like helminths called cestodes or tapeworms.

ANATOMY AND LIFE CYCLE OF CESTODES

The body of a cestode is ribbon shaped (flattened and elongated), and consists of a head or scolex, a neck, and a chain of proglottids. Some cestodes have only a single proglottid; others have tens, hundreds, or even thousands. Cestodes may range from 0.5 cm to 10 m in length.

The scolex serves only as an organ for attaching the worm to the intestinal mucosa of the host. It is equipped with muscular organs (suckers or bothria) and chitinous structures by means of which it adheres, by hooking or suction, to the host's tissues. In several species of cestodes, the tip of the scolex, or rostellum, is armed with one or more rows of hooklets. The neck (the zone of growth) originates immediately behind the scolex. From its posterior portion there is continuous budding of new segments which form into a chain of proglottids (strobila).

The proglottids of different species of cestodes may assume various shapes (square, ovoidal, trapezoidal) and may also vary in length and width. Each proglottid contains a full complement of organs. There is no alimentary tract in cestodes, nutrition being obtained by osmosis through the entire surface of the body. Mature cestodes dwell mainly in the large and small intestines of animals, while the larvae are found in various organs and tissues.

The life cycle of a cestode involves one, two, or occasionally no intermediate hosts. The eggs are passed with the feces, enter the body of an intermediate host and transform into a larval stage. For some cestodes, the oncosphere within the intermediate host changes into a form called cysticercoid, while in other cestodes the embryos change into various larval forms—Cysticercus, Coenurus, and Echinococcus. Each species of cestode has its own particularly-shaped larva which may contain a single scolex or several scoleces

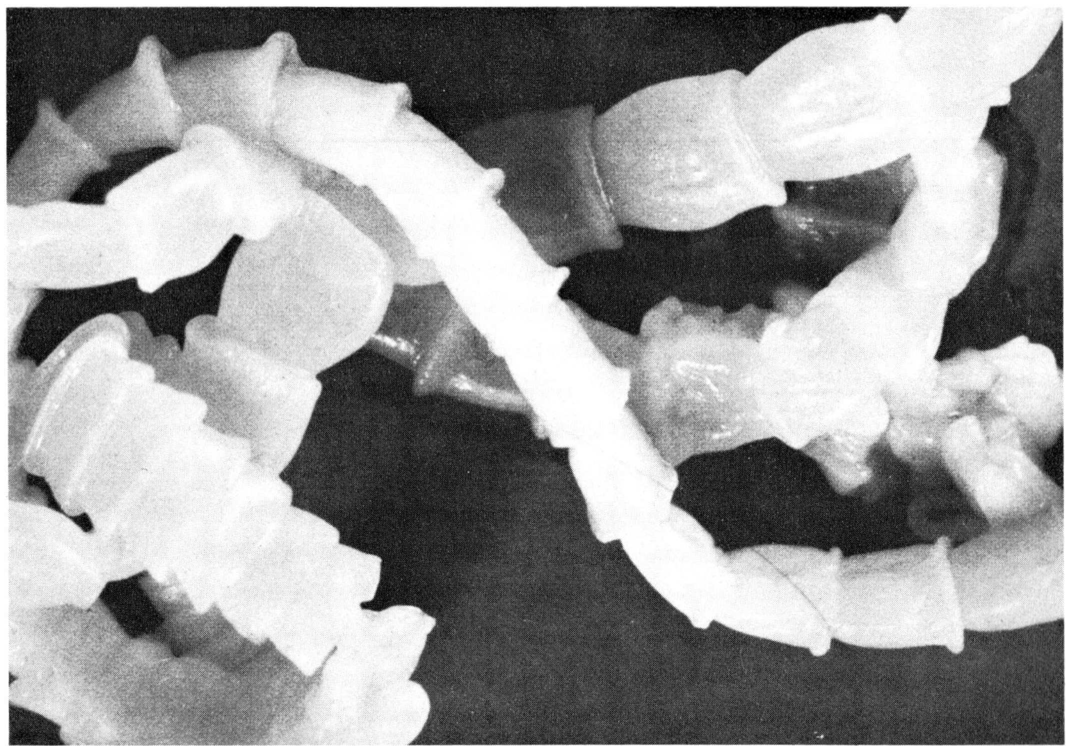

FIG. 32. Representative specimen of tapeworm infection of livestock.

equipped with sucking discs. Adult cestodes develop from the scoleces within the final host.

The larval stages of tapeworms take on several distinctive forms, which may vary in size within a specific form.

Cysticercoid is the most primitive type of larva. It has a broad anterior end and a tapering worm-like posterior end.

Cysticercus is a round bladder. Within the capsule of the bladder is a clear fluid within which a single, evaginated scolex may be seen attached to the wall of the bladder. The bladder may vary in size depending upon the tissue in which it is found—small in muscle tissue, and larger in organ tissue.

Coenurus resembles the cysticercus in shape and size, but the capsule is quite thick and the fluid contains many scoleces attached to the bladder wall.

Echinococcus is a complex form of tapeworm larva. It is a bladder-like cyst that varies in size from very small to very large. Sometimes it can be felt as a soft, movable cyst under the skin. The fluid within the cyst is clear. It contains many scoleces and daughter cysts capable of developing many secondary scoleces.

Cysticercosis of Cattle (Beef Measles)

The causative agent of cysticercosis of cattle is *Cysticercus bovis,* the larval stage of the cestode *Taenia saginata,* which dwells in the small intestine of man. In animals the chief tissues affected are muscles, mainly those of the tongue, jaws, neck, intercostals, heart, or, in massive infestations, all muscles.

Economic losses from cysticercosis are considerable. The flesh of moderately infected cattle decreases in value (it is sold as fit for consumption only under certain conditions), while that of severely infected cattle must be destroyed. Some cattle die while still in the early stages of disease.

Description of Parasite

Taenia saginata is quite long and consists of scolex, neck and many proglottids (up to 1,000). The proglottids become progressively broader the farther they are from the anterior extremity. An external feature of the cestode is the presence in the scolex of four powerful suckers and a rudimentary rostellum devoid of hooks. Because the cestode lacks hooks on the scolex it is called an unarmed cestode.

The eggs are rounded or oval, the outer shell is transparent and delicate, with 1 to 2 filaments. Since factors in the external environment such as mechanical action can rapidly destroy the egg of *T. saginata,* the latter is immediately infective upon leaving the host's body.

The larval stage of *T. saginata* is *Cysticercus bovis.* This is a liquid-filled vesicle the size of a pea or somewhat smaller (length 5 to 9 mm, width 3 to 6 mm). Within the vesicle is the head (scolex) of the future strobila, evaginated like the finger of a glove. When the cuticular coverings of the vesicle are torn away the four suckers on the scolex are easily visible microscopically. The cysticercus is immediately surrounded by a layer of connective tissue.

Development of Parasite

Man is the only definitive host of *Taenia saginata.* From raw or improperly cooked beef infected with the live cysticerci, the cestode develops in the intestine of man. The head of the cysticercus protrudes and attaches itself to the intestinal mucosa. Within 2½ to 3 months, the larva develops into a sexually mature cestode which liberates gravid proglottids. The gravid proglottids detach singly from the end of the strobila, then actively crawl over the body of man and on his bedding, scattering eggs in the process.

Cattle serve as intermediate hosts. They ingest the parasites with food or water. Within the gastrointestinal tract, the gravid proglottids are acted upon by gastric juices. The three shells of the eggs are dissolved and embryos escape. The oncosphere uses its six hooklets to penetrate the intestinal mucosa and enter blood vessels, eventually reaching the fibrillar tissue of striated muscles. The oncosphere becomes a cysticercus within six months. (The cysticercus may occasionally also be encountered in the lungs, liver, brain and adipose tissue.)

There are no exact data on the length of life of the cysticerci in muscles of cattle, although it is believed that the life span does not exceed 7 to 9 months. Following initial infection, animals become immune to reinfection for as long as two years. The disease is more frequently encountered in small farms than in large ones, as the infection is chiefly picked up around yards and houses of people lacking modern sanitation facilities, or using human excrement for fertilizer. Infected meat handlers, shepherds, and ranchers contribute to the spread of disease by passing the gravid proglottids. The infection may also be spread by unclean feet.

Pathogenesis

The toxins present in the proglottids of *T. saginata* in cattle produce symptoms of intoxication, fatigue, paresis of the feet, malfunctions of the gastrointestinal tract, and drop in body temperature.

Symptoms

Severe symptoms occur in the early stages of disease, but, because of the difficulty in diagnosing cysticercosis, these symptoms are usually mistakenly attributed to other sources.

If heifers and adult animals are infected for the first time, the body temperature rises a few days after infection and severe clinical manifestations, such as fatigue and occasionally profuse diarrhea that disappears upon the fourth or fifth day, occur. The animal lies down for long periods and has a capricious appetite. It ceases to ruminate by the fourth or fifth day, and there is atonia of the rumen and reticulum. The animal becomes restless and agitated when pressure is applied to the stomach or to the masticatory, foot, or lumbar muscles. Lymph nodes are enlarged. The mucocutaneous areas are dry and livid. Respiration and pulse rates are increased. After the sixth to seventh day the animal begins to recuperate, and by the eight to twelfth day most clinical symptoms disappear. Occasionally, the disease terminates in death. Animals that have overcome the acute course, however, show no clinical symptoms by the end of twelve days and to all appearances are completely healthy.

Pathology

Upon postmortem dissection, many small hemorrhagic spots are discovered in the connective tissue under the skin, in the region of the masticatory, thoracic and intercostal muscles. There are hemorrhages in the tissues of the udder, the heart, and most other organs. An excess amount of serous fluid is found in the peritoneal cavity. The small intestine and abomasum are in a state of hyperemia and inflammation. The lymph nodes are enlarged and spongy. The fairly large cysticerci are highly visible within the muscles.

To detect cysticerci in carcasses in abattoirs, sections from the heart and masticatory muscles are removed. If cysticerci are discovered, it is necessary to examine all musculature with particular attention to the intercostal muscles.

Cysticercosis of Swine (Pork Measles)

The causative agent of cysticercosis of swine is *Cysticercus cellulosae,* the larval stage of an armed cestode, *Taenia solium,* which dwells in the small intestine of man. In cysticercosis of swine (the intermediate host), muscle tissue is most frequently affected, abdominal organs and brain matter less frequently. *C. cellulosae* is encountered in dogs, cats and wild pigs as well as in swine. The larval stage of *Taenia solium* can also develop in man. Thus man may be both the definitive and intermediate host for *T. solium,* his intestine hosting the adult cestode while his muscles, brain and other organs contain the cysticerci.

Cysticercosis of swine causes heavy economic losses. Severely infested swine must be destroyed, while the flesh of those suffering mild infections can be used as meat only following special processing which diminishes its value.

Description of Parasite

Taenia solium is long. The scolex bears four suckers and is 1 mm in diameter. It differs from that of *T. saginata* in having 22 to 28 hooks arranged in two coronas. The strobila has close to 900 proglottids, and the gravid proglottids are filled with enormous numbers of eggs. They detach in groups of 5 to 7 segments and leave the body with the feces; they are incapable of independent movement and therefore cannot actively leave the host. The eggs of both armed and unarmed taenias are very similar.

The larval stage is a pea-sized vesicle. This cysticercus has a scolex bearing four suckers and two crowns of hooks.

Development of Parasite

Man is the only definitive host of *T. solium.* The infection is picked up by ingesting either raw or improperly cooked flesh of swine infected with cysticerci. In the human intestine, the cuticle of the cysticercus is dissolved, the scolex of the parasite protrudes and attaches itself to the mucosa with its hooks and suckers, starts to grow and reaches full development within $2\frac{1}{2}$ months.

Swine become infected by ingesting human

excreta containing proglottids and eggs of *Taenia solium*. The eggs come under the influence of gastric juices in the gastrointestinal tract.

Varying numbers of cysticerci may be in the flesh of infected swine. They are generally found in the same muscles as those occupied by bovine cysticerci. Man incurs cysticercosis in two ways: (1) the eggs reach his mouth with contaminated food or through contaminated hands; (2) in a man infected with *T. solium*, the oncospheres may get to his stomach directly from the small intestine through antiperistaltic movements (vomiting). In the acid gastric environment the proglottids are digested, the eggs within them are liberated, and their several shells are dissolved. The freed embryos use their hooks to penetrate through the intestinal wall into the vascular system.

In man, the cysticerci are usually located in the brain, eyes, and skin, and cause severe, frequently incurable disease.

Symptoms

The clinical picture of cysticercosis in swine is unknown. Usually, the disease passes without symptoms.

Pathology

The pathogenic effect of the cestode on swine becomes apparent at the onset of infection while the oncospheres are migrating through the body and traumatizing various tissues. The pathogenic action of the later-stage cysticerci becomes evident when embedded in the brains of swine, since they cause functional motor disturbances. The pathogenic effect is less pronounced when cysticerci are localized in muscles.

Prevention

Prophylaxis in cysticercosis of animals and taeniasis of man is a complex of veterinary and medical measures.

Among the veterinary measures, of principal importance are veterinary inspection of the flesh of slaughtered animals in meat-packing plants, abattoirs, slaughter centers, and meat-inspection stations, and the formulation of specific rules by local authorities forbidding the slaughter of animals and the sale of meat products that have not passed veterinary inspection.

Echinococcosis or Hydatid Cyst

Echinococcosis is a parasitic disease chiefly of sheep, cattle, pigs and, less frequently, other animals and man. Its causative agent is the bladder-shaped larva of the cestode *Echinococcus granulosus.*

The economic loss inflicted by echinococcosis is enormous. In severe infestations, animals die from the disease. In chronic cases, infected animals do not develop properly, resulting in lowered output of milk, meat, and wool. In addition, the liver, lungs and sometimes the entire body of animals infected with *Echinococcus* cysts must be condemned and destroyed.

Description of Parasite

The strobila is short and consists of a scolex and three or four proglottids. The scolex, 0.3 mm wide, is equipped with a rostellum and adorned by two crowns of hooklets, 28 to 50 in number. The scolex bears four suckers, each with a diameter of 0.13 mm. The terminal gravid proglottid is filled with 400 to 800 eggs. It reaches 1.5 to 2.5 mm in length and 0.5 to 0.6 mm in width. In the intestine of the final host, the strobila matures within $2\frac{1}{2}$ to 3 months, and the adult worm lives more than six months.

Development of Parasite

The adult worm parasitizes the small intestine of dogs, wolves and foxes. Dogs infected with the mature forms of *Echinococcus* (occasionally there are thousands of these in the small intestine) excrete an enormous number of proglottids and eggs in the feces. The eggs of the parasite may become dispersed on the grass of pastures, in barns, on the litter and feed of cattle, in cattle enclosures, and in the water of their drinking ponds.

Ripe proglottids of *Echinococcus,* excreted with fecal matter, are capable of creeping on the grass and may climb up the stems of plants. Individual specimens may remain in the anal folds, the perianal region and the perineum of infected dogs, causing irritation and itching. Gravid crawling proglottids liberate eggs which spread over the grass, soil, and hides of dogs. The eggs (oncospheres) of the parasite survive for long periods in the external environment (they survive in 0 C for 116 days). They are resistant to the action of chemicals, but high temperature (50 C for one hour) and direct sunlight kill them.

The parasite develops with the participation of an intermediate host where the larval forms develop from the oncospheres. The intermediate host may be sheep, cattle, northern deer, pigs and, less frequently, horses, donkeys, mules, rabbits, various wild animals, and man. Primarily young animals contract the infection.

Definitive hosts incur this cestode by ingesting the lungs and livers of animals infected with hydatid cysts and by feeding on the flesh of infected sheep.

The oncospheres reaching the stomachs of ruminants or other intermediate hosts are subjected to the influence of the hydrochloric acid therein which dissolves their membranes, allowing the larvae to emerge, to penetrate the gut wall using their six hooklets, and to migrate into the intestinal vascular system, arriving at the liver via the bloodstream. Some of the larvae remain in the liver, and form into cysts of *Echinococcus.* Other larvae pass with the portal circulation through the right side of the heart to the lungs and become lodged there. In some cases, the larvae may continue through the capillaries of the lung into the left side of the heart, and are then transported through the aorta into various organs and tissues where they transform into the cyst stage of *Echinococcus.*

The cyst of *Echinococcus* is either unilocular or multilocular, the structure varying with the age and condition of the organism. The unilocular cyst is frequently found. It consists of a "bladder" ranging in size from a pea to a man's head. Superficially, the cyst is surrounded by a white chitinous, striated membrane. Internally, a germinal layer surrounds the muscle fibers, calcareous bodies and excretory vessels. The cyst contains a transparent, colorless liquid.

Brood capsules are scattered through the germinal layer. Within the walls of these capsules scoleces develop which either fill the internal cavity of the capsule or form daughter cysts. Frequently, the scoleces break off from the brood capsules and swim freely in large numbers in the liquid of the cyst. This stage is frequently found in lambs and piglets, somewhat more rarely in cattle.

Some unilocular cysts are encountered only in adult animals (more frequently in cattle) and in man and are characterized by the fact that daughter cysts, developed from small projections in the germinal layer, are formed in the cyst. The daughter cysts may, in turn, form daughter cysts with scoleces on their walls. Thus, many daughter and granddaughter cysts may be formed within a single hydatid cyst, while on the outer surface of the cyst a connective tissue capsule may appear.

Multilocular cysts are frequently encountered in cattle, less often in man. They differ from unilocular cysts in that they do not form large cysts but consist of many small cysts devoid of any liquid. Granulation tissue develops in the intermediary spaces between the small bladders of the multilocular cyst and also around it, subsequently becoming fibrous connective tissue. In the small cysts of the multilocular cyst scoleces are not encountered.

Multilocular cysts should be regarded as pathological larvae that perish when the unity of the cuticular membrane is disrupted.

Pathology

By the pressure it exerts, the hydatid cyst, developing mainly in the parenchymatous organs (in the liver and lungs), causes atrophy of tissue and disruption of function. The presence of a large number of hydatid cysts (sometimes up to 50 and even 200) may cause total atrophy of the affected organ, and the animal dies. In addition to the mechanical action, the toxins present in hydatid cysts when they rupture are harmful to the body of the host, and frequently cause anoxia, elevated body temperature, diarrhea, and occasionally death.

Where the liver is heavily infected with hydatid cysts, digestion is disrupted as a result of interference with production and supply of bile. A greatly enlarged liver hinders the movement of the diaphragm; it may also cause obstruction of the esophagus and the portal vein.

When the number of cysts is low and they are within an organ, they may be detected by palpation. Occasionally the hydatid cysts become calcified or filled with pus.

Hydatid cysts are also frequently found in the kidneys.

Symptoms

During heavy infestations of the lungs in cows, chronic labored breathing is observed, and a protracted, dry, muffled cough—which may be artificially produced—causes the animal to walk with great effort. During the onset of disease, clinical symptoms are not readily noted. Respiratory disorders increase gradually and consecutively. Occasionally, particularly with rupture of the hydatid cyst, the general state of health deteriorates sharply, the animal weakens rapidly and dies of asphyxiation.

Infection of the liver is chiefly accompanied by disorders in the digestive processes. Marked changes in this organ exhaust the animal. In such cases, cows manifest sluggish rumination and frequently bloat.

In mild infections, disorders are not noticeable in cattle.

Sheep are more sensitive to the disease and die more frequently than cattle as a result of the infection. Heavily infested sheep are undernourished, their wool is stringy, and a characteristic cough is noted; when it occurs the sheep lie down on the ground.

Prevention

Control of echinococcosis is based on the control of stray dogs and wolves, compulsory registration of pet and watchdogs, and periodic deworming of these animals.

The feed and living quarters of animals should be protected from contamination with dog feces. Carcasses of infected sheep and other animals should be buried deeply in the ground or burned. It must be remembered that people who are in contact with dogs frequently become infected with *Echinococcus.*

Monieziasis of Ruminants

Two representatives of the genus *Moniezia, Moniezia expansa* and *Moniezia benedeni,* are parasites in the small intestine of sheep, cattle and goats and cause a disease called monieziasis, or tapeworm disease, which may occasionally appear in epidemic form and cause death in severely infected animals. However, for the most part *Moniezia* are nonpathogenic and cause trouble only in very young animals.

Description of Parasite

The strobila of *M. expansa* is composed of a scolex, neck, and proglottids, and may reach 1 to 5 m in length. The scolex is roughly ball-shaped, 0.7 to 1 mm wide and 0.4 to 0.9 mm long, and bears four oval suckers. The proglottids are wider than they are long.

The egg of *Moniezia* contains an oncosphere equipped with three pairs of hooklets. The latter are encased on a pyriform apparatus with two or more hook-like projections at one end. These projections may at times become fused at the tips and bear a number of fine, thin filaments which may similarly meet and fuse at the tips. The egg is 0.05 to 0.06 mm in diameter.

Development of Parasite

Moniezia, as are all cestodes, is a biohelminth; to complete its development it requires an intermediate host. Nonparasitic pasture mites serve as the intermediate host; in the United States, a species of oribatid mites qualifies as intermediate host.

The eggs or oncospheres of *Moniezia* are passed with the feces of an infected animal and are then eaten by the oribatid mite. Within the body of the mite, the embryo undergoes six larval stages of development before becoming a cysticercoid—the infective larval form.

Larval development to cysticercoid within the mite requires from 6 to 16 weeks. Lambs and heifers pick up the infection by swallowing mite-infested grass. Once the infected mite is swallowed, *M. benedeni* requires 50 days to reach sexual maturity within the final host; the equivalent period for *M. expansa* is 37 to 40 days. During a 24-hour period, the developing tapeworm may increase by as much as 8 cm in length. The length of life of the sexually mature worms within the final host is 2 to 6 months, following which the tapeworms actively leave the intestine and pass to the exterior.

Transmission

Monieziasis is a widespread disease, particularly prevalent among lambs 2 to 8 months of age. In lambs up to one year the infection rate with monieziasis may be quite high, but in adult animals the infection rate is low.

In the western regions, monieziasis makes its first appearance in heifers during June and July, and reaches a maximum infection in August.

The short time required for oribatid mites to reach sexual maturity (47 to 109 days at 20 C and 100 percent relative humidity) and their relatively long life as adults (14 to 19 months) assure perpetuation of infective material in nature.

Since optimum conditions are favorable both for the development of the mites and the preservation of *Monieza* eggs in the external environment, the chances of contact between eggs and mites are increased. Furthermore, most mites are found on the ground and, although omnivorous, subsist mainly on food of animal origin which may contain eggs of *Moniezia.*

The preservation of the eggs and the continuation of the life cycle of *Moniezia* is further assured by the fact that oribatid mites will climb up stems or down roots of plants to escape unfavorable environmental conditions.

Pathogenicity

Scores of the cestodes may be recovered from a single animal. Since they are localized within the intestine of a host animal, they may obstruct the passage of food, distend the walls of the gastrointestinal tract, and cause catarrh and tympanites. The tendency of the cestodes to form into closely packed balls may cause partial or complete blockage of the intestine, stasis of fecal matter, and invagination or even rupture of the intestine.

Metabolites of cestodes induce pathological changes in the body of an infected animal, primarily in the tissues of the intestine, mesenteric lymph glands and the kidneys. The general intoxication stunts the growth of sheep and lowers their resistance to various other pathogenic agents, thus increasing their susceptibility to secondary infections and reinfection by parasites.

Pathology

Upon dissection, an infected animal shows distension of the intestinal wall, invagination, inflammatory and degenerative processes in the intestinal mucosa and proliferative-degenerative processes in various glands, in the kidneys, spleen, and occasionally the liver. Frequently, there are hemorrhagic infiltrations in the brain, hemorrhages in the endocardium, and degenerative processes in heart muscle.. There are also subcutaneous infiltrations and transudates in the pleural and peritoneal cavities.

Symptoms

Clinical symptoms depend on the degree of infection. In moderate invasions, monieziasis may clinically pass almost unobserved. Massive invasions, on the other hand, exhibit marked symptoms and may terminate in death. Young animals exhibit diarrhea, anorexia and thirst. Proglottids or fragments of the cestodes are passed in the feces. Infested animals tend to lie down frequently and have trouble getting up again. The mucocutaneous regions are pale, the lymphatic nodules are enlarged, the hair loses its sheen and the animal loses weight.

Occasionally, symptoms suggesting damage to the nervous system are encountered, the animals suffering muscular cramps or moving around in circles. At the terminal stages of disease, the animals are totally apathetic, lie with heads turned up and back, and make masticatory movements of the jaw.

Diagnosis

Diagnosis is established by clinical symptoms and by the presence of proglottids and eggs of *Moniezia* in the feces of infected heifers and lambs.

The proglottids of *Moniezia* may be seen in feces with the unaided eye, since they are yellowish, fairly large and up to 1 cm in length. When present in small numbers, they may be detected by washing the fecal matter several times and placing the sediment in a dark pan.

Treatment

The veterinarian can prescribe the most up-to-date regimen for the effective elimination of tapeworms.

In the treatment of monieziasis, precautions should be taken to prevent eliminated cestodes from serving as new sources of infection. Infected animals are best treated in barns or special houses. All fecal matter should be buried, burned, or treated chemically to destroy all proglottids and eggs.

The elimination of cestodes following treatment continues for two days. Therefore, treated animals should be kept in barns or in isolation until all danger of transmission of the disease has passed.

54
Trematodes of Livestock

TREMATODIASES are diseases caused by helminths known as trematodes, or flukes.

Trematodes are flat, usually leaf-shaped worms. Some species measure only 0.1 mm in length, whereas others may reach 15 cm. The body is encased in a cutaneous muscular sheath within which all internal organs are enclosed. The anterior part of the body of the trematode bears an oral sucker with which the parasite attaches to the host's tissues. In many trematodes, an additional ventral sucker (acetabulum) serves to fix the worm firmly to the host.

Flukes feed upon the body fluids or mucosal secretions of the host, and some even live on the host's blood. Metabolites are eliminated from the fluke's body through an excretory pore in the posterior of the body.

Trematodes are generally hermaphroditic (bisexual) creatures. Eggs pass out of the host's body in feces and are deposited on the ground or in water where they undergo further maturation. The embryos forming within them emerge after a period of development.

Trematodes require a change of hosts for further development. Flukes that have reached sexual maturity can thrive only in the body of a final (definitive) host, whereas the larvae, once they have hatched from the eggs and reached the external environment, must undergo further development in the body of a different kind of animal host—an intermediate host. In the latter, asexual production of the various larval stages occurs.

The life history of flukes is, generally speaking, as follows. From the egg, a larva—miracidium—covered with cilia hatches in water. For a while it swims about before actively or passively penetrating into the body of an intermediate host. There, it transforms into sporocysts—larvae with a concentration of cells capable of multiplying asexually. Sporocysts produce rediae which, following further asexual reproduction, become cercariae.

Cercariae leave the body of the intermediate host, swim about for a while in water and are swallowed by the definitive host where they metamorphose into a stage capable of sexual reproduction. Some cercariae encyst on plants and while in that dormant state are called metacercariae.

Sexually mature trematodes are located mainly in the bile ducts, liver, gastrointestinal tract and, rarely, in the blood and other organs of the host animal.

The trematode diseases of greatest importance are fascioliasis, dicrocoeliasis, and paramphistomiasis.

Fascioliasis

Fascioliasis is an animal disease caused by trematodes, usually *Fasciola hepatica,* rarely *Fasciola gigantica.* Fascioliasis affects sheep, goats, and cattle.

The disease is usually characterized by a chronic, or occasionally acute, inflammation of the liver and bile ducts, accompanied by general intoxication and disturbances in feeding. Fascioliasis frequently assumes the proportions of an epidemic.

The disease is usually fatal to sheep, especially to younger animals. Severe forms of the disease are also encountered among cattle. The disease occurs most often in humid, swampy regions.

The economic loss caused by fascioliasis essentially is due to: (1) mortality during an outbreak; (2) loss of body weight in chronically diseased animals; (3) a drop in milk production in chronically infected cattle—10 percent in relatively mild cases and up to 20 percent in more severe forms of the disease; (4) destruction of liver tissue in animals slaughtered for their meat.

Description of Parasite

Fasciola hepatica, the common liver fluke, may reach 20 to 30 mm in length and 8 mm in body width. These measurements, however, are variable. The parasite is leaf shaped, the body encased in an integument within which are muscular layers. The integument bears many small spines. The oral sucker on the anterior end of the body measures 1 mm in diameter and connects the mouth to a pharynx leading into the esophagus which, in turn, opens into the intestine. The latter consists of two stems (branches), each terminating in a cul-de-sac. All waste food materials are excreted through the mouth, since the trematode has no posterior anal opening. The acetabulum serves only as an organ of attachment and lacks any connection with the intestine.

Flukes feed on capillary blood in the tissues of the host.

Fasciola gigantica differs from the common liver fluke in having a more elongated form and a larger size. The length of the body is about three times its width. The conical protuberance of the head is a direct continuation of the body and therefore the "shoulders" occurring in other trematodes are practically nonexistent in *F. gigantica.*

Development of Parasite

The common liver fluke dwells in the biliary ducts of the liver in animals (in cattle, however, it may also be encountered in the lungs). There it secretes an enormous quantity of eggs, estimated to run into hundreds of thousands. The eggs pass through the bile ducts with bile, enter the intestine, are mixed with fecal material, and excreted.

The eggs are oval, brownish-yellow, and covered with a four-layered cuticle. In the external environment, under optimal temperature, an embryo—the miracidium—develops. When other conditions such as oxygen, moisture, and light are satisfied, the miracidium develops and after 10 to 25 days emerges from the egg and moves about in liquid media (puddles, rivers, lakes). When subjected to darkness, the miracidum will not hatch but may survive for long periods of time within the egg.

The body of the miracidium is covered with cilia and measures up to 0.19 mm in length and 0.026 mm in width. The miracidium may live not more than 40 hours in water, and is sensitive to the action of various chemical substances. An intermediate host snail—*Lymnaea sp.*—is necessary for further development of the miracidium. The snails multiply in water and lay their eggs in large numbers upon stones, plants, and other objects within the water. After 8 to 10 days of development, young snails emerge from the eggs. They tolerate low temperatures and may even survive a whole winter under ice. They also withstand desiccation by submerging and burying themselves in the moist silt at the bottom or by fixing themselves to stems of grasses. However, they may survive up to 2 months in dry sand. Other snail species may also serve as intermediate hosts for *Fasciola.*

While swimming about, the miracidium encounters the snail and actively penetrates its body. Eventually, the miracidium reaches the hepatopancreas of the snail, sheds its ciliated epidermal covering and transforms into a saccular sporocyst (0.1 mm long). There are germinal cells within the sporocyst; after 15 to 30 days, these germinal cells grow and develop into rediae—elongated organisms bearing a mouth, esophagus and gut. As the sporocyst grows, the contained rediae reach 0.26 mm in length and may then rupture the walls of the sporocyst and emerge to settle in various organs of the snail.

By asexual reproduction, one sporocyst may give rise to 5 to 15 rediae. Each redia, in turn, is capable of producing a new generation of embryos, second generation or daughter rediae. The rediae continue to develop and increase in size, reaching up to 1 mm in length. After 35 to 40 days, they produce 15 to 20 cercariae. Each cercaria has two suckers, a long tail and a bifurcated intestine; it resembles a tadpole in shape. The length of time required for development from the miracidial to the cercarial stage is 50 to 80 days.

Briefly summarized, the complete development of an embryo of *Fasciola* is: (1) ovum, (2) miracidium within the snail, (3) sporocyst, (4) redial generations, and, from the latter, (5) cercariae. The complete life cycle from egg to cercaria takes about 70 to 100 days.

Cercariae measure 0.28 to 0.30 mm in length and 0.23 mm in maximum width. The number of cercariae in one infested snail may reach 600 to 800. Cercariae may continue to develop and emerge from snails over a period of several weeks.

After reaching a certain age, cercariae emerge from the snail and swim about, using their long tails. Several hours after emergence, they lose their tails, release a mucous material which hardens within minutes, and surround themselves with a hard, brown capsule. Some of the encysting cercariae become attached to leaves and stems of plants while others float on the surface of the water. They are spherical in shape and measure 0.2 to 0.25 mm in diameter. In this stage, the parasite is called a metacercaria.

The cyst of a metacercaria is thick and composed of two layers. Enclosed within is the motile *Fasciola* embryo with two well-defined suckers, a branched gut and an excretory bladder.

Animals on contaminated pastures swallow the metacercariae while drinking water from puddles, pools, or lakes, and by eating infested grass. The cyst walls of metacercariae dissolve within the intestine of the animal and the released embryos secrete a substance from their "penetration" glands that enables them to make their way to the liver, where they develop into the sexually mature *Fasciola.*

Fluke embryos penetrate into the bile ducts in two ways. Some of the embryos penetrate the mucosa of the intestine and enter the veins, then proceed by way of the portal vein into the liver. If they reach vessels of small diameter in the liver, young flukes are prevented from further progress. They therefore perforate the walls of the vessels and make their way through the liver tissue, reaching the bile ducts after several weeks of travel. In other cases, embryos may pass through the capsule of the liver into the bile ducts.

Three to four months are required in order for fluke embryos to develop in the liver of cattle; they then become sexually mature and deposit eggs. The mature flukes are capable of living 3 to 5 years within the host animal.

The life cycle of *Fasciola gigantica* resembles that of *F. hepatica.* The development of the miracidium to the stage of cercaria within the intermediate host lasts from 41 to 70 days. Other snails may serve as intermediate hosts for *F. gigantica.*

More than three months are required for the development of *F. gigantica* in the liver of sheep and cattle.

Animals are not believed to be susceptible to fascioliasis during early spring. Some larval stages of *Fasciola* may, however, survive the winter months in the body of *Lymnaea.* Such larvae may mature during June, after surviving for long periods at low temperatures. In water and moist hay mixtures, and under the normal temperature of the summer and autumn months, metacariae may be preserved for five months and more.

Infections of fascioliasis occur during summer and are most intensive during the last months of the grazing season. By then, the number of snails on the pasture has increased considerably. Cercariae and rediae that have managed to develop and multiply within the intermediate host during the summer now make their appearance in the water.

During rainy years, massive infections of animals with fascioliasis are encountered even in places where no swamps or pools exist. On the other hand, during drought years when all ponds dry up, the occurrence of fascioliasis is considerably reduced. Modern irrigated pastures, however, provide an ideal environment for snails and the perpetuation of this disease.

A large percentage of infection with flukes is encountered where sheep are kept over long periods on moist pastures, either marsh or irrigated. While on such pastures, infected sheep cause increased contamination of the pasture by passing eggs of *Fasciola* in the feces, and may, after a period of time, become reinfected. One should not forget that a single miracidium developing in the body of *Lymnaea* can produce 100 to 150 cercariae. Therefore, the presence of even a small number of infected animals on the pasture constitutes a serious danger.

Fascioliasis is not contagious during winter (in central and northern regions). During summer, however, infection in sheep kept in pens rather than put to pasture may be picked up when the animals are fed grass cut and gathered from pastures infected with metacercariae.

Pathology

The pathogenic effects of flukes on animals are manifested mainly by changes in digestive functions, poisoning by toxins or other toxic materials that are the result of the action of the parasite, hydremia, and transportation of bacteria from the intestinal tract to other host organs and tissues.

At the onset of infection, young flukes cause trauma to liver tissue and capillaries, bringing about loss of blood and sometimes damage to the spleen, lungs, lymph nodules, and pancreas. In their progress through liver tissue, the parasites destroy the tissue and create a liver inflammation which may progress into the connective tissue of the liver. When the liver of sheep contains a large number of parasites, as in massive invasions, symptoms of hepatitis and posthemorrhagic anemia develop, and mortality frequently occurs within a month from onset of the invasion.

Growing flukes pass from liver tissue to the bile ducts and cause obstructions. Jaundice consequently develops.

The parasites release toxins within the animal. Under their influence, changes occur in the walls of the bile ducts and in liver tissue. When these toxins enter the vascular system they cause a general intoxication of the host body.

Young flukes, during migration from the intestine to the liver and bile ducts, carry various bacteria with them. During multiplication in the bile ducts, the bacteria increase the intoxication and may contribute to the development of other infectious diseases.

By this transportation of pathogenic bacteria into the liver or other organs, fluke embryos are responsible for the development of inflammatory, purulent wounds in these organs.

The effect of toxins of *Fasciola* on the lobules of the liver is expressed through infiltration of fluid and cells into the lobules, followed by the appearance of new fibrotic tissue. Running the length of the walls of the lobules, the process also spreads to the biliary ducts, which become distended and thickened. In this manner, the normal functions of the liver are disrupted and additional metabolic disturbances occur. The flukes themselves, while present in the bile ducts, consume large quantities of blood. Observations have shown that cattle infected with fascioliasis undergo aggravated forms of other diseases, such as hemosporidiosis, tuberculosis, and other infectious diseases.

The pathological-anatomical changes in the liver depend on the degree of fluke infestation. If the invasion assumes massive proportions, the liver becomes acutely inflamed, increases in size and becomes hyperemic. Foci are seen on it, and in them are dark red knots up to 2 to 5 mm long, containing coagulated blood and minute flukes. Small hemorrhagic spots and, occasionally, fibrinous membranes may be discerned on the serosa of the liver. In cases of massive infestation, peritonitis occurs and occasionally profuse hemorrhages enter the peritoneum. The serosa becomes a dull gray.

A chronic liver inflammation occurs after 2 to 3 months. The liver becomes hardened and the bile ducts become dilated. A large quantity of serous, mucoid fluid and many flukes are found in the bile ducts. The serosa of the bile ducts becomes thickened due to hypertrophy of connective tissue. The walls become calcified and hardened and their inner surfaces assume a rough consistency. They protrude from the liver and become filled with a brown, murky fluid containing flukes and occasionally seropurulent material.

In mild invasions, changes in the bile ducts are practically invisible, superficially. By palpation of the liver, however, one can distinguish distended ducts within which flukes may be found. Fascioliasis is usually accompanied by a catarrhal, chronic inflammation of the entire liver. In cases of gross calcification of the biliary ducts, the flukes within the ducts die off or move to less affected areas of the liver. In a heavily infected liver, the worms are not encountered, and their previous presence can be attested to only by the state of calcification of the biliary ducts.

In cases involving cattle and sheep, there is loss of weight and general anemia. The flesh is gray in color and watery in consistency, the muscles being filled with a serous fluid. A clear transudate may be found in the peritoneal or pleural cavity, and in the pericardium.

Symptoms

Clinical manifestations of fascioliasis depend on the number of parasites in the liver. This number may range from a single fluke to 2,000 flukes per animal. Infestations with 250 worms are customarily considered to have an appreciable bearing on the state of health of cattle. The equivalent number for sheep is not less than 50 worms per animal. However, even a smaller number of parasites may affect the health of a young animal.

In sheep and goats, fascioliasis may assume either an acute or chronic form. The acute form occurs only during the fall. At the onset of the disease, a fever appears which frequently goes unnoticed. Diseased animals are depressed, tire quickly, stray from the rest of the flock and lose their appetite. There is increased sensitivity of the hepatic region. These manifestations are followed by rapid anemia, the number of erythrocytes decreasing sharply, and a pronounced drop in the percentage of hemoglobin.

The acute form of the disease is encountered among sheep only during massive infestation, and results in rapid mortality coupled with manifestations of hepatitis.

In the chronic form, infected animals do

not die rapidly. They develop anemia within 1 to 2 months, the wool becomes stringy, brittle and sheds easily, particularly over the chest and at the sides. Noninflammatory edema appears in the eyelids, in the intermaxillary space, on the chest, and in the lower abdominal region. The icteric index is not increased to any considerable extent. The sheep feed poorly, lose weight, and their milk becomes watery. Lambs do not suckle readily at the udders of a diseased mother. Individual cases may show symptoms of nervous disorders resembling gid, and there may be abortions during the terminal phases of pregnancy. Animals eventually succumb from exhaustion.

When the infection in sheep is of a less virulent nature, the disease process becomes prolonged. Diseased animals surviving the winter recuperate on the pasture during the spring, but when transferred back to the feedlot or barn lose weight once more. Such animals may contribute to the spread of fascioliasis. In cases of infection with a small number of flukes, clinical symptoms are nonexistent or extremely mild. Such parasite "carriers" also contribute to the spread of infection.

In cattle, the initial phase of the disease (during migration of the young parasites) is practically indistinguishable. Clinical manifestations appear only upon maturation of the flukes. Animals then lose weight even when kept on a well-balanced diet. The disease continues its chronic course and symptoms develop gradually. Afflicted cattle show anorexia and diarrhea. Nutritional changes or changes in feeding habits are usually observed. The appetite becomes poor or perverse, cattle lick objects which normally hold no attraction for them, and diarrhea, periodic gaseous swelling of the abdomen, and atonia of the rumen and reticulum occur. Body hair becomes harsh and loses its sheen. The mucosa becomes pale, with a peculiar luster. Dairy cattle show a drop of up to 50 percent in milk output, and abortions are frequent. In severe cases, fever, anemia, jaundice, and loss of weight are evident. When death occurs, it is usually the result of emaciation.

Moderate infection of fascioliasis in cattle may cause no overt symptoms of the disease, but even in such cases the productivity of the infected animals is lowered. Under poor maintenance conditions, especially with a meager diet, even a small number of parasites may produce the clinical picture of fascioliasis in weakened cattle. (A severe form of fascioliasis occurs in sheep with a diet poor in vitamins (vitamin A) and calcium salt.)

Prevention

Fascioliasis is prevalent among all livestock pastured where snails find a suitable habitat. Eradication of the disease requires stringent preventive measures. A preventive program includes: guarding pasture and water sources against contamination with *Fasciola*, preventing exposure of animals to the infection, culling infected animals, draining wet, marshy areas, fencing ponds and lakes, and treating snail-infested areas with approved molluscacides.

To check the spread of fascioliasis and prevent reinfection, animals are freed of parasites prior to being put to pasture. Therefore, on a farm infected with *Fasciola*, drenching of cattle, sheep and goats is undertaken during the winter and again in the fall when animals are brought back to their winter quarters. In the south, where animals are kept on pasture all year round, sheep undergo an initial drenching in January, a second five months later and a third $2\frac{1}{2}$ months later.

A fall drenching provides protection from adult *Fasciola* during the winter months when the plane of nutrition is lower. The preparations used, however, do not have any effect on immature parasites. Since, in an infection picked up during the fall, the flukes reach sexual maturity only by the end of January or February, a second, or winter, drenching is needed approximately 5 months after the first.

In regions where fascioliasis is endemic,

drenching should be performed thoroughly on all animals within any populated area.

Eradication of the parasite ova in manure is best accomplished by heat. This procedure is an extremely important prophylactic measure in combating *Fasciola* as well as other helminths. In all places where animals are housed, manure should be collected and stored at one place. Where there are no special facilities or structures for that purpose, the manure should be removed to high, dry sections of land where animals cannot come in contact with it. Manure is at first piled in stacks, to allow free access to air. As the temperature rises within the piles, they are gradually pressed, compacted and overlaid with fresh layers of manure. Continuing in this fashion for several months, the manure is eventually stacked in elongated rows until it is removed to the field. Under these conditions, larvae of *Fasciola* or other helminths which may have thrived in the original feces are quickly destroyed by the high temperature of the manure; the latter may, subsequently, be removed to the fields.

It is important to drain all moist, muddy pastures, and those frequently covered by water. Draining of the land alone, however, cannot bring about eradication of all snails, as these may survive and even thrive in some places between clods of soil. A chemical and biological attack on the snails should therefore be undertaken in conjunction with drying of the pasture.

A pasture which is partially swampy or frequently wet is not recommended. Where the use of such a pasture is inevitable, animals should be kept in it for not more than one or two months, then transferred to sections of pasture where no other animals had previously pastured during the particular season. Young animals (heifers and lambs), after weaning, should be kept in isolated pastures upon which, for the duration of the grazing season, no adult animals are allowed.

Hay processed from infected pastures may be offered to animals only following storage for at least six months.

To combat fascioliasis effectively, one must study the course of development of the disease in sheep and cattle under varying climatic conditions and determine the snail population in a given area, that is, determine the intermediate host, its ecology, and the invasive stage of *Fasciola* during the different seasons of the year. Furthermore, there is need to develop new, effective drugs against the disease, study the prophylaxis of pasture areas, and devise methods for making water sources safe for livestock.

Dicroceliasis of Ruminants

The disease called dicroceliasis is caused by the trematode *Dicrocoelium lanceatum,* which dwells in the bile passages of the liver and in the gallbladder. The disease is encountered among numerous wild and domestic animals. It has been reported in goats, cattle, buffalo, hogs, donkeys, horses, dogs, moose, rabbits, hares, small rodents, and bears. It may, on rare occasions, be encountered in man. The disease shows a severe clinical picture and appears in the form of epidemics, primarily among ruminants.

Description of Parasite

The flukes are lancet shaped, with a broad body slightly rounded at the tail but tapering to a sharp anterior tip. They are 5 to 15 mm long and 1.5 to 2.5 mm wide.

Development of Parasite

Dicrocoelium requires two intermediate hosts, a terrestrial snail and an ant.

The adult trematode deposits eggs in the bile ducts of the liver. These eggs enter the intestine with the bile and are then passed outside with the feces. They already contain fully formed miracidia which, unlike those of *Fasciola* and *Paramphistoma,* do not hatch but are swallowed by snails while still in the intact eggs. The eggs hatch only in the intestine of the snail, liberating miracidia which travel in the snail to the connective tissue of the liver where they shed their cilia and transform into mother sporocysts. Next, daughter sporocysts develop within the mother sporocysts, which disappear or shrivel up after liberating the daughter sporocysts. Cercariae developing within the daughter sporocysts undergo a period of maturation before leaving them. Following liberation, cercariae travel through the vena magna to the pulmonary system and then to the mantle cavity of the snail. Here, each cercariae encysts and then forms into aggregates of 100 to 300 individuals called mucous droplets. (Several investigators report the formation of the mucous droplets to occur outside rather than inside the snail.) When expelled through the pulmonary aperture, these mucous masses adhere to plants or other objects. They are next picked up by ants, carried to the anthill, and eaten. Once within the ant, the cercariae transform into metacercariae which become situated within the abdominal cavity. The final host picks up the disease by ingesting grass bearing infected ants.

The cycle of development within the snail lasts from 82 days to 5 months. The cycle of development within experimentally infected sheep ranges from 72 to 85 days. The length of time for development of *Dicrocoelium* within cattle has so far not been ascertained.

Transmission

Dicorceliasis, with a large number of intermediate and final hosts, exists practically everywhere. It is, however, encountered more frequently in the northern regions.

Animals are usually infected while on pasture; the initial infection of young animals is usually caused by larval stages of the parasite that have passed the winter within ants. Eggs of the parasites may be encountered in the feces of animals two months after they are put to pasture.

The eggs of *Dicrocoelium*, with their semi-permeable inner walls, are more resistant to the external environment than those of *Fasciola*.

Pathology

At the onset of disease, the only detectable changes are those in the system of the bile ducts. In these, catarrhal and inflammatory processes develop, with proliferation of the epithelium and connective tissue. The basal layer of the connective tissue within both small and large bile ducts becomes appreciably thickened. Changes in other organs with the exception of the pancreas, however, are not observed.

Macroscopically, the changes appear essentially as a diffuse affliction of the minor ducts of the hepatic lobes. Major ducts appear as uniformly thickened tubes.

Prevention

No full program of therapeutic and preventive measures is available, since there is no effective treatment for the disease.

Strategic measures include drainage and improvement of pasture and eradication of snails through destruction of vegetation and small growth which tend to harbor both snails and ants.

Paramphistomiasis of Ruminants

The disease caused by the trematode *Paramphistomum cervi* is called paramphistomiasis.

The parasite is found in the rumen of sheep, goats, cattle, reindeer, buffalo, and several other mammals.

The disease has a wide distribution and occasionally, especially during the migration of the young paramphistomes in the body of the animal, is fatal to the host.

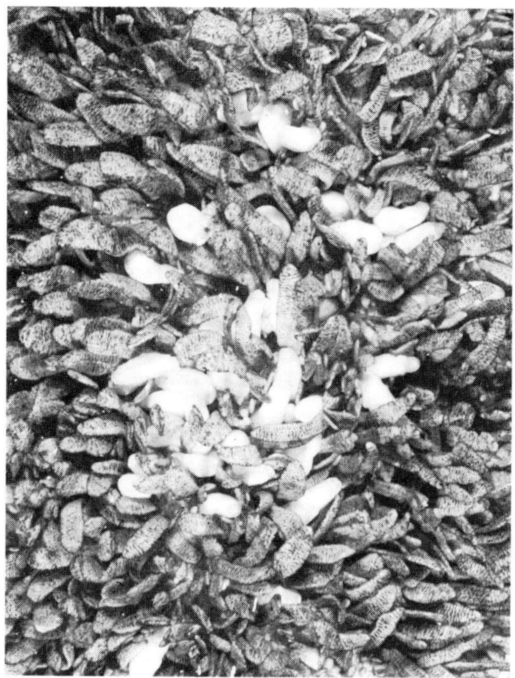

FIG. 33. Rumen flukes (adult) in papillae of anterior dorsal sac. (From Jensen, R., and Mackey, D. R.: *Diseases of Feedlot Cattle.* Ed. 2, Philadelphia, Lea & Febiger, 1971.)

Description of Parasite

P. cervi is a fairly large, reddish, cone-shaped trematode measuring 5 to 12 mm in length. The immature stage of the fluke is 1 to 3 mm in length and does considerable damage to the small intestine of infected cattle before moving forward to the rumen.

Development of Parasite

Paramphistomes require intermediate hosts which are fresh-water molluscs. To date nine species of snails in various countries have been found to serve as intermediate hosts.

The eggs, which are probably laid in the rumen, enter the intestines and are passed out with the feces. Given the proper temperature and humidity, miracidia develop and hatch to enter the intermediate-host snail. Within the latter, miracidia transform to sporocysts. Each sporocyst gives rise to 9 rediae and each redia, in turn, gives birth to 20 cercariae. One miracidium may thus give rise to 180 cercariae.

The young paramphistomes undergo migration in the body of the definitive host prior to settling in the rumen. They have been found in various parts of the intestine, in the abdomen, the bile ducts, gallbladder, large intestine, and in a transudate of intraperitoneal fluid. Single specimens have been recovered from the kidney.

Pathology

Paramphistomes inflict damage upon the rumen when attaching to it by means of their powerful acetabula. Especially severe traumatic effects are inflicted upon the mucosa of the intestine and other organs by the young migrating paramphistomes. The latter cause further complications by introducing pathogenic microflora into the organs. The metabolites of paramphistomes are also responsible for marked changes in organs and tissues—swellings, wounds, hemorrhoidal clots, infiltrations, and the formation of bile clots as a result of stagnation.

Postmortem findings reveal pathological and anatomical changes brought about by exhaustion of the animal prior to death. The mucosa is white, and there are superficial sores on the lips, nose, and various parts of the mouth. In the intraperitoneal cavity large quantities of a reddish fluid on occasion may contain floating young paramphistomes. Mucous and young paramphistomes are found in small hemorrhagic areas. The duodenal mucosa is catarrhal-hemorrhagic or hemorrhagic and young paramphistomes are found either floating in the exudate or embedded under the mucosa. The bile is pale yellow, becomes watery and often contains paramphistomes. The liver is somewhat swollen and hard; the spleen becomes hard and dry, and hardly palpable. The heart is enlarged, its muscles generally lacking consistency, with occasional hemorrhages in the endocardium and the pericardium.

Symptoms

At the onset of disease, the animal exhibits apathy or depression. Several days later, diarrhea and weight loss occur, and in many heifers the hindlegs and tail become smeared with liquid fecal matter. The mucocutaneous regions of the nose, eyes and mouth are pale. In the nasal cavity there are superficial ulcerations of variable size. Body temperature usually remains normal. Occasionally, however, during the seventh to tenth day of disease, the temperature may rise to 104 to 106 F. In some diseased animals, hemorrhages may occur on the conjunctiva or in the mucous membranes lining the mouth and nose. In severe cases, profuse diarrhea occurs and occasionally bloody feces are passed. The diseased animal is in poor condition, the hair turns lusterless, and the eyes become deep-set and dull. Atonia of the rumen is manifested in many infected animals and there are signs of abdominal pains. Animals groan, gnash their teeth, try to lie down but rise immediately. There is progressive loss of weight with emaciation. Heifers showing severe paramphistomiasis, as a rule caused by young paramphistomes, die within 5 to 30 days. Some heifers may recover and show no clinical symptoms of the disease, but never return to a normal, sound state of health.

In paramphistomiasis caused by adult parasites, or in chronic cases of the disease, progressive emaciation, anorexia and continuous diarrhea are manifested. In addition, in many animals, edema appears in various parts of the body and the visible mucous membranes become pale, although the body temperature remains normal.

A postmortem diagnosis is based on pathological and anatomical changes, recovery of the adult trematodes from the rumen, and recovery of young forms from various other organs.

Prevention

Since the intermediate host is a fresh-water snail, it is obvious that any combat measures effective against fascioliasis are equally effective against paramphistomiasis. Thus, the basic methods are: (1) drying of the ground; (2) biological warfare on the snails (raising ducks and geese on the pasture helps with this); (3) keeping young cattle off swampy pasture; (4) chemical warfare on the snails; and (5) prophylactic drenchings of animals while in their winter quarters.

55
Nematodes

NEMATODIASIS is a disease caused by one or more of the many species of roundworms parasitizing various parts of the digestive tract of domestic animals.

The body of a nematode is elongated, thread-like, or spindle shaped; it varies in length from 1 mm to 1 m. Externally, nematodes are covered with solid cuticle. The surface of the cuticle is frequently covered with longitudinal and transverse striations, and in some species the cuticle may bear spines, combs, and tuberous processes by which the parasite attaches to host tissues. Under the cuticle are single layers of epithelial cells and muscle fibers.

Females, following fertilization, may discharge either ova or larvae, and for this reason nematodes are divided into oviparous and viviparous types. Oviparous nematodes discharge ova in various stages of development with the feces and urine of the host. These may be in segmented form or contain a formed larva. Viviparous nematodes discharge living larvae which may be passed to the external environment with the feces or may enter the bloodstream, depending on the location of the mature nematode in the body of the host. The larvae picked up from the bloodstream by bloodsucking insects are transmitted to other hosts.

Trichinella differs from all other nematodes in that it gives birth to living larvae in the intestine. The larvae do not leave the host but penetrate into the intestinal mucosa and from there into the lymphatic or blood vessels; they arc carried with the bloodstream to various muscles where they remain permanently. Thus, the same animal may serve initially as a final, and then an intermediate, host for the parasite.

Roundworms may develop with or without the participation of an intermediate host. The life cycle of oviparous nematodes varies. The ova of many nematodes, when passed outside, require time for maturation. In the external environment, under favorable conditions, larvae develop in these ova. When this happens, the eggs become infective to animals. Ova bearing larvae are swallowed with feed and are subjected to the action of gastric

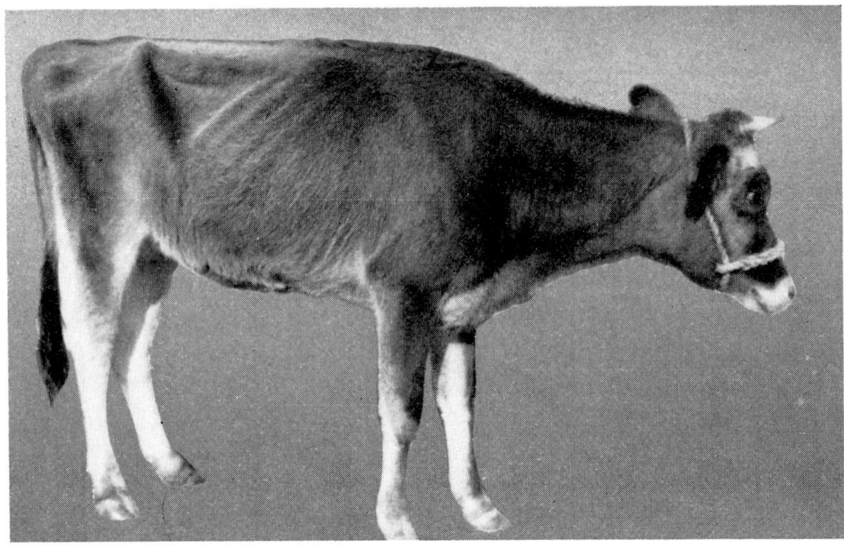

FIG. 34. Poor condition resulting from parasitism. (From Gibbons, W. J.: *Clinical Diagnosis of Diseases of Large Animals.* Philadelphia, Lea & Febiger, 1966.)

juices within the host. The wall of the ovum dissolves and larvae are liberated in the stomach. The liberated larvae of the various nematodes behave differently in the body of the host. For example, the larvae of oxyurids immediately attach themselves to the intestinal mucosa and become sexually mature. The larvae of ascarids and other nematodes migrate from the intestine into the blood vessels and, passing through the liver and heart, into the lungs. They penetrate through the walls of the lung capillaries to the bronchi, from which they are expectorated with bronchial mucus and then reswallowed. Only after having reached the intestine for the second time do they begin to grow and develop into sexually mature ascarids.

The larvae of many nematodes emerge from the ova in the external environment, grow, undergo several molts, and finally become capable of invading the final host.

Nematodes developing without the aid of an intermediate host, especially when the embryos are liberated from the final host onto the ground, in water, or in manure, are called geonematodes; the diseases they produce are called geonematodiases. Many nematodes require intermediate hosts for their development, and are called bionematodes; the diseases they cause are bionematodiases.

Swine Ascariasis

Ascariasis is an invasive disease widespread among swine, particularly among piglets 2 to 6 months old. The causative agent is the helminth *Ascaris suum* or *Ascaris lumbricoides.*

The economic damage inflicted by ascariasis involves (1) loss due to disease and mortality of piglets; (2) drop in pig-breeding productivity. Stricken piglets are undernourished and die when heavily infested. Ascarids from cattle and horses are superficially like those of swine, but the swine ascarids found in sheep are much smaller.

Description of Parasite

Ascaris suum is a large worm. The male reaches 12 to 25 cm in length and 3 mm in width; the female is 30 to 35 cm long and 5 to 6 mm wide. They are robust, cream colored and vigorous. On careful observation, both sexes have three lips at the anterior end.

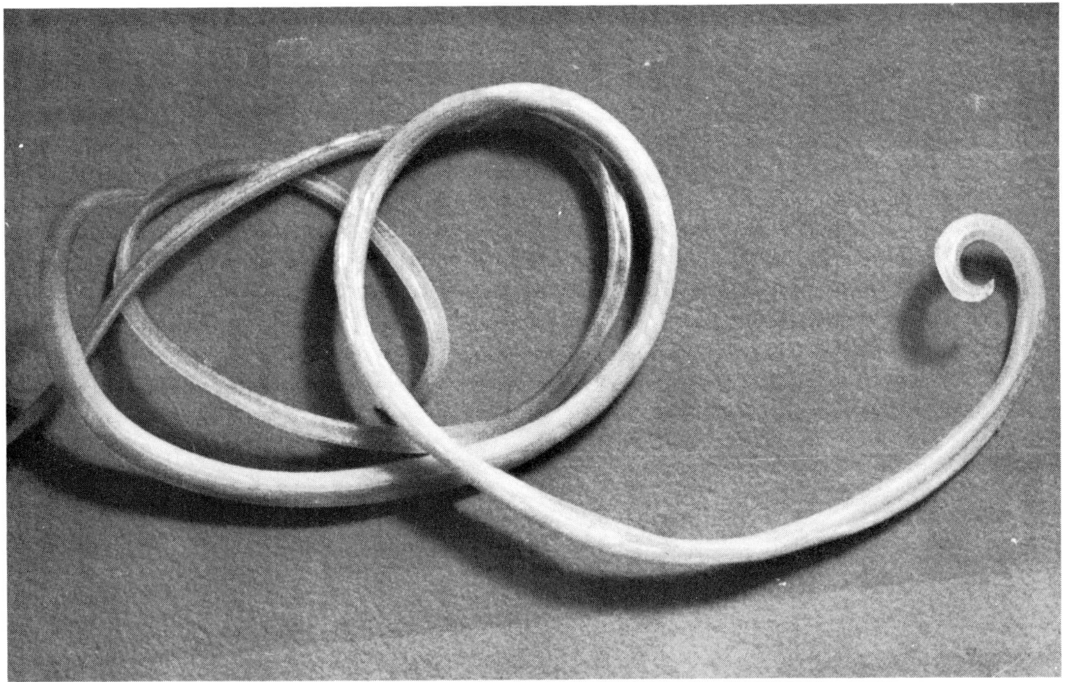

FIG. 35. General appearance of roundworm of livestock.

DEVELOPMENT OF PARASITE

Ascarids parasitize the small intestine. Following fertilization, the females discharge an enormous quantity of eggs (100,000 to 200,000 eggs in 24 hours) which are mixed with the intestinal contents and excreted with the feces. In the external environment, with an adequate supply of oxygen, moisture, and the appropriate temperature, the ova complete their development within 15 to 30 days; during this time the larvae in the ova become infective. At low temperatures, the period of ovum development is greatly prolonged.

Infection occurs chiefly in the pigsty when swine swallow the infective ova with contaminated feed and water. The infection may also be picked up on the pasture and in the vicinity of the pigsty, the soil around which may be heavily infected with the ova of the parasite.

Maintenance of pigs in unsanitary and congested quarters, poor feeding, and especially an insufficiency of vitamins, fosters large-scale infection, which may occur any time during the year and may spread to piglets of the very youngest age group.

The larvae emerge from the infective ova within the intestine of the host. They penetrate through the mucosa into the intestinal venules and pass with the bloodstream, via the portal circulation, into the liver. Subsequently, the larvae get into the vena cava and are transported to the right side of the heart, from which they are carried through the pulmonary artery to the lungs. After migrating through the capillary network of the lungs, they molt and increase in size. From the lung capillaries larvae penetrate into the alveoli, migrate to the bronchioles and trachea, and are passed with mucus into the buccal cavity. Larvae are next swallowed with saliva and are carried to the small intestine. There they gradually increase in size, and, 2 to $2\frac{1}{2}$ months from initial infection, become sexually mature males and females.

Ascarids can live only in the small intestine; they do not attach to the mucosa, but

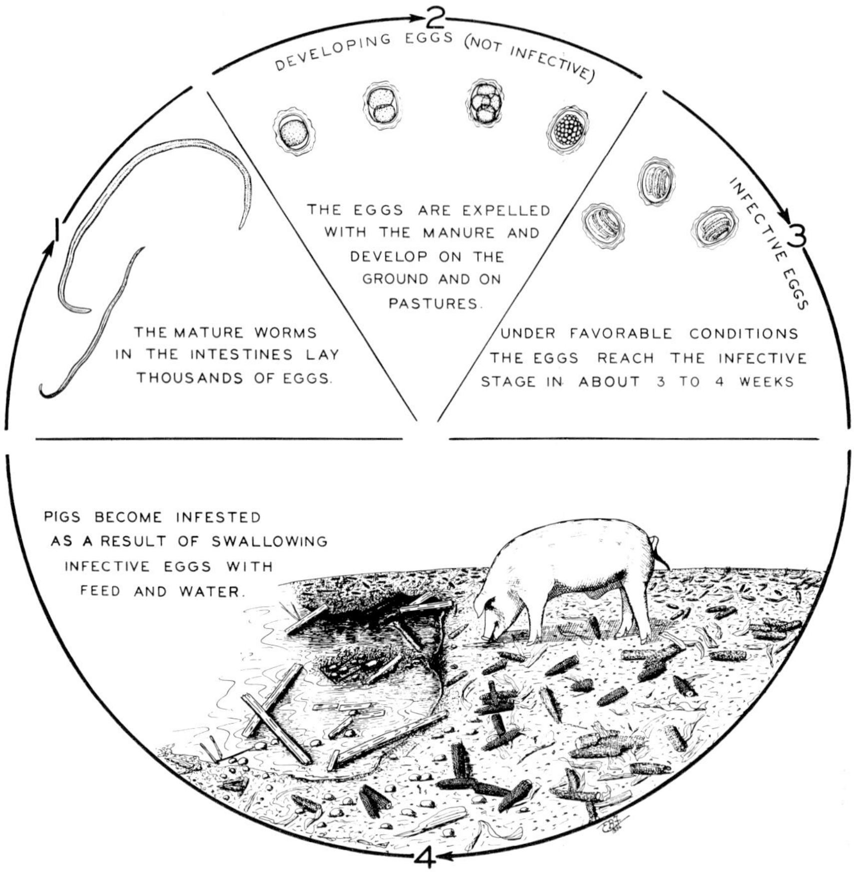

FIG. 36. Life cycle of ascarids of swine.

can, nevertheless, withstand peristaltic movements by bending their bodies into an arch and pressing their extremities against the gut walls. Ascarids feed on the surface of the mucosa and on the contents of the intestine. After 7 to 10 months, the parasites leave the intestine voluntarily and are expelled with the feces. When conditions are unfavorable (infectious diseases in piglets, elevated body temperatures), the ascarids leave the body of the host shortly after maturing. The quantity of parasites in the intestine of infected piglets may vary from a few to thousands under optimum conditions.

The ova of ascarids are resistant to adverse external factors because of their thick four-membrane cover. This development is possible only in an environment in which the temperature is higher than 45 F; at low temperatures the embryos survive but do not develop. The ova of ascarids do not endure prolonged desiccation, however, and high temperatures, above 100 F, rapidly destroy their infectivity. The sizes of *Ascaris* ova vary considerably; they are thick walled and brownish. The surface is bumpy and irregular and is covered by sticky albuminous material.

Pathogenesis

Ascarids have a pathogenic effect on the body of the pig in both the larval and sexually mature stages.

Sexually mature helminths localize in the small intestine and mechanically irritate the mucosa, causing severe pain. When they accumulate in considerable numbers, they fre-

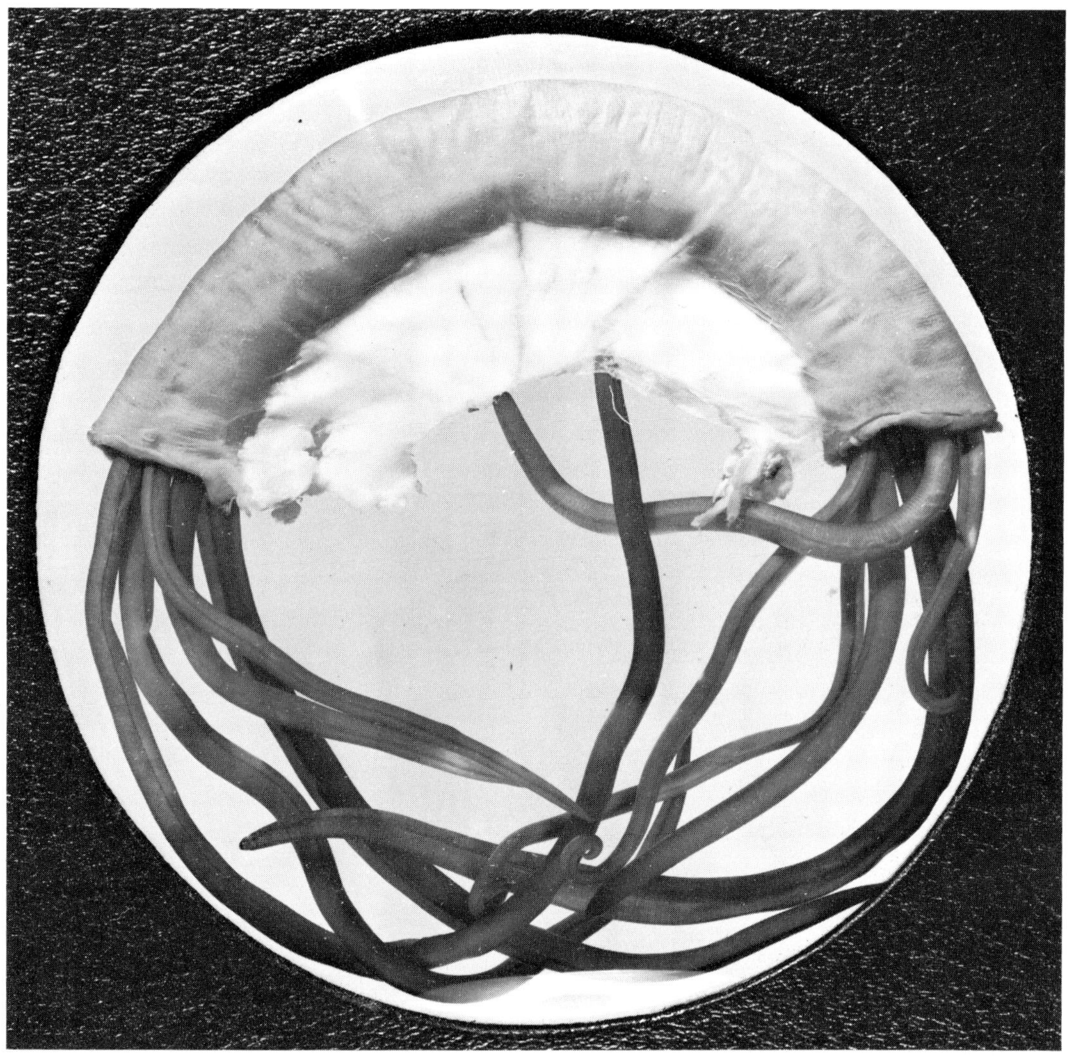

FIG. 37. *Ascaris suum* in the intestine of swine.

quently intertwine into a ball and block the lumen of the intestine; as a result, rupture of the intestinal wall may occur. Intestinal ascarids frequently invade the bile duct, causing various pathological changes.

Pathology

In the initial stages of ascariasis, symptoms of pneumonia are observed. The congested lungs show a spotty exterior and occasionally are dark in color. Many *Ascaris* larvae may be found in the alveoli. Mature ascarids, when accumulated in large numbers, cause mucosal catarrh. When single parasites are present, no vital changes are manifest. If the intestine ruptures, peritonitis and hemorrhage may be detected in the abdominal cavity.

Symptoms

Clinical symptoms of the disease appear chiefly in piglets 2 to 6 months of age, which endure the invasion with difficulty. *Ascaris* pneumonia is characterized by persistent coughing, elevated body temperature, rapid breathing, and poor appetite. These manifestations last 6 to 15 days. In heavy infestations, pneumonia, digestive disorders, and vomiting occur, chiefly in unweaned animals. The piglets begin to cough five days following infection, their appetite is sharply reduced, and they lie down and bury themselves in litter. During this period, heavy breathing, vomiting, and general depression and pneumonia occur.

Ascariasis takes a different course once the adult parasites become settled in the intestine. In most infected piglets (those 4 to 6 months old) which do not manifest clearly expressed symptoms, improper development, insufficient growth, decrease in weight, and gastrointestinal disturbances are observed; in a few days, symptoms of rickets appear. In heavy infestations, obstruction and rupture of the intestine may occur. In some piglets, anaphylactic manifestations such as convulsions, nervous seizures, rash and eruption on the skin and cough may appear but rarely last up to one hour. Adult pigs do not suffer from the acute symptoms but are carriers of the infection.

Prevention

On farms afflicted by ascariasis, planned prophylactic drenching of pigs is carried out during the spring and fall. At first, all breeding females, all adults, and piglets after weaning are subjected to a fecal examination. Those found infected undergo drenching, with sows treated at least three months before farrowing.

The pigsty is thoroughly mechanically cleaned and washed. The troughs, brooms, spades, and scoops are rinsed daily in hot water and periodically scalded with boiling water. The stalls in the pigsty are sterilized with a hot alkaline solution every ten days.

Manure from the pigsty is heaped in a manure yard which is removed from the pigs and subjected to biothermic sterilization. The area of the pigsty, after a thorough spring cleaning of the feces, is deeply plowed and abundantly overlaid with lime.

Before being taken to pasture and again before return to winter quarters, the pigs undergo fecal examination. Infected animals undergo prophylactic deworming. To prevent *Ascaris* infection on the pasture, pasture plots are rotated every 10 to 15 days during June to August, and animals are not returned to the same plot during the same grazing season.

When ascariasis is recognized clinically in pigs, the required deworming is carried out immediately upon diagnosis of the disease. Prophylactic treatment is carried out in the animal quarters, and the treated animals are not allowed to leave their quarters until five days after administration of the anthelmintic. The expelled parasites, with the feces, are collected and destroyed. A week after treatment, the living quarters and adjoining pens and yards are again sterilized to destroy the ova that have emerged during this period.

Haemonchosis of Sheep and Goats

The causative agent of this disease is *Haemonchus contortus,* often called the barber-pole worm. The parasite is usually localized in the abomasum, although it is also frequently encountered in the small intestine. In addition to sheep and goats, the helminth may parasitize cattle, northern deer, and other wild animals.

In sheep, haemonchosis frequently occurs as an enzootic disease. As such, outbreaks result in high mortality, especially in lambs, and are accompanied by a sharp drop in productivity in diseased animals. The disease is, therefore, regarded as one of the most dangerous helminthiases of sheep in all sheep-producing areas.

Description of Parasite

Haemonchus contortus is a thread-like nematode of reddish color. The cephalic end is equipped with a rudimentary oral capsule containing a chitinous lancet. Two large cervical papillae are situated at a distance of 0.4 to 0.5 mm from the cephalic end.

The male is 10 to 20 mm long, while the female, 18 to 33 mm long, has an elongated tail.

Development of Parasite

Females lay eggs in the abomasum; these are subsequently passed with the intestinal contents and excreted with the feces. At optimal temperature and sufficient moisture, larvae are formed within the ova and free themselves from the eggshells after 14 to 17 hours. Not leaving the feces, they undergo two molts and become infective. The period of metamorphosis, from the deposition of the

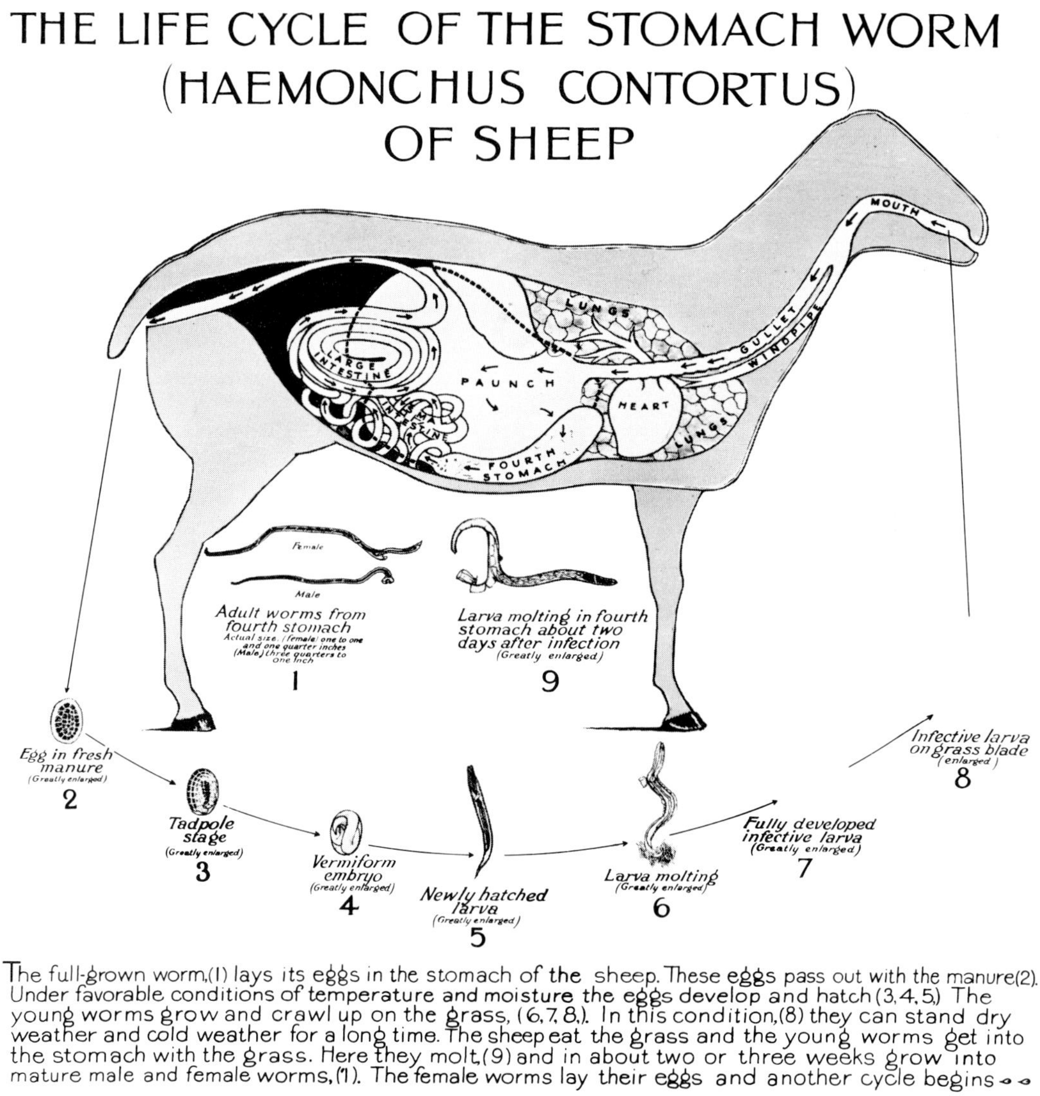

FIG. 38. Life history of the stomach worm of sheep.

ova to formation of infective larvae, takes $3\frac{1}{2}$ to 4 days. Under the influence of raised or lowered temperature, development is accelerated or retarded, respectively. At very high temperature, the embryos perish without becoming infective.

Following a rain, the infective larvae leave the feces. Crawling along the ground, they may climb plants and thus become more accessible to animals. They may also be washed away from the feces and scattered on the pasture by the rain.

Sheep become infected by swallowing infective larvae with food or water. Following two molts in the body of the final host, the larvae become sexually mature males or females within 2 to 3 weeks. The length of life of the parasite in the body of sheep or goats is not known; they are assumed to live not longer than one year.

Transmission

The infection of sheep and goats with haemonchosis may occur (1) as a result of ingesting grass contaminated with larvae, or (2) through drinking from small, nonflowing reservoirs, i.e. chiefly on the pasture, in the spring, summer and fall. Infection, as a rule, does not occur in barns or feedlots.

The resistance of infective larvae to external factors promotes a mass infection of sheep. (In the desiccated state, the infective larvae may remain viable for more than $1\frac{1}{2}$ years; in moist surroundings infective larvae die at a temperature of 122 F, while in a dry environment they succumb at 140 F.) The intensity of infection may be so high that the parasites overlie the mucosa of the abomasum like thick felt and it becomes difficult to determine their exact number.

Young animals are most heavily infected and endure the disease with the greatest difficulty. In lambs allowed on the pasture for the first time, the disease is clinically detected at the end of summer and fall.

Pathogenesis

The adults of *Haemonchus* are bloodsuckers. They traumatize the mucosa of the abomasum with their teeth, which are located within the oral capsule. As a result of their toxic effects, functions of the animal's nervous system are disturbed, making way for atrophic-degenerative changes in the abomasum and progressive anemia. Secretory and motor functions of the gastrointestinal tract are disrupted, and the reaction of gastric contents becomes neutral or even alkaline.

The clinical signs of disease are more sharply expressed in undernourished animals. Severity also depends on intensity of infection and conditions of maintenance.

Pathology

Haemonchosis is characterized by emaciation, anemia, and changes in the nervous system, the mucosa of the digestive tract, the hematopoietic and parenchymatous organs, and the endocrine glands. Edema is observed in the meninges of the brain and spinal cord.

The abomasal mucosa is atrophied and attenuated. The mucosa of the small intestine and cecum shows catarrhal inflammation. The muscle fibers of the heart are degenerated.

Symptoms

The disease is characterized by depression, anorexia, and diarrhea alternating with constipation. The temperature is usually normal but may sometimes reach 104 to 105 F. Anemia is accompanied by a decrease in the number of erythrocytes and quantity of hemoglobin, and by disruption in the formation of hemoglobin.

Control

Of great importance in combating haemonchosis are prophylactic drenchings carried out in the spring before leading the sheep to pasture, and in the fall after returning them to winter quarters. Other measures that may be applied successfully are chemical prophylaxis with therapeutic doses of anthelmintics, the changing of pasture plots every 5 to 6 days (in certain months, every 10 days) and general sanitary precautions.

Infections are a constant threat to livestock. Even if all worms could be eliminated by the use of chemicals, from all animals at the same time, a speck of manure harboring infective ova could reestablish a serious worm problem. Helminth infections with even a few worms can cause considerable economic loss through slower gains, wasted feed, and lowered resistance to other diseases.

Bunostomiasis

This disease is caused by the nematodes *Bunostomum trigonocephalum* and *Bunostomum phlebotomum.* Both are active bloodsuckers with well-developed buccal capsules by which the parasites attach to the mucosa of the small intestine.

Description of Parasite

Bunostomum trigonocephalum is a large nematode equipped with a funnel-like oral capsule bearing two semilunar ventral cutting plates situated at the margin of the oral opening.

The males are about 12 to 17 mm long with a funnel-like sexual bursa on the caudal end, with well-developed lateral rays but asymmetrical and poorly developed dorsal rays. The spicules are equal in length, 0.6 to 0.64 mm, and brown. The gubernaculum is absent.

The females (20 to 25 mm long) have a short, rounded, caudal end, 0.25 to 0.27 mm long. The vulva is situated in the anterior third of the body.

Bunostomum phlebotomum males are 10 to 12 mm long, the females 16 to 19 mm long. The spicules are 3.5 to 4.0 mm long. The length of the caudal end in the female is 0.4 to 0.5 mm.

Development of Parasite

The females of these parasites deposit ova into the intestine of the final host which are passed to the exterior with the feces. Larvae formed subsequently emerge from the eggshells. They must molt twice to become infective, within periods which depend on local meteorological conditions. In a moist environment at 80 to 90 F the larvae become infective on the fourth day; at 55 to 75 F, also in a moist environment, they become infective on the ninth to eleventh days; at 75 to 85 F, on the seventh day. Larvae of *Bunostomum* are able to migrate over wet grass.

Animals pick up the infection on pastures (1) when swallowing infective larvae with water or food, and (2) when the larvae penetrate through the intact skin of the host.

In oral infections, development of the parasites to sexual maturity and oviposition requires 24 days whereas, in cutaneous infections, the first ova of the parasite are detected in the feces of the host within 17 days. These data were obtained by infecting sheep with larvae of *Bunostomum trigonocephalum.*

Bunostomiasis is widely distributed throughout the United States; however, the disease is epizootic only in limited foci and infrequently. Young animals are most susceptible to infection, although on stricken farms adult sheep and cattle may be seriously affected. Under temperate conditions, symptoms of the infection appear initially about the beginning of August, and by the end of the month and the beginning of September a severe clinical picture is already observed in infected animals. The intensity of infection may reach 5,000 to 6,000 parasites per animal.

Hookworm infestation of young calves is generally associated with crowding in small,

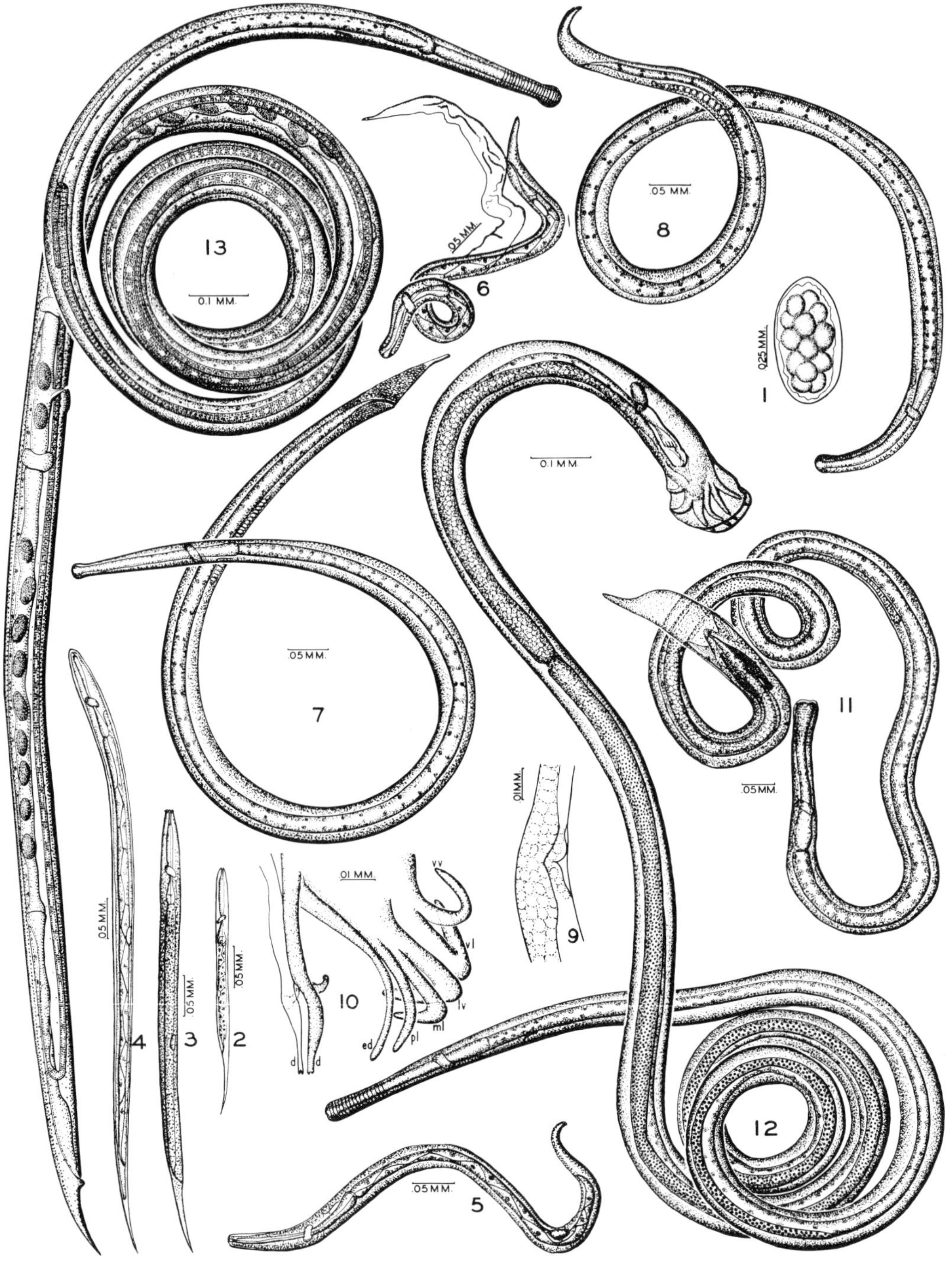

FIG. 39. Life history stages of *Cooperia curticei.* 1. Egg. 2. First-stage larva. 3. Second-stage larva. 4. Third-stage larva. 5. Third-stage parasitic larva. 6. Third-stage larva undergoing third molt. 7. Fourth-stage larval male. 8. Fourth-stage larval female. 9. Formation of vagina from cells in the body wall. 10. Bursa of fourth-stage larva. 11. Fourth-stage larval male undergoing fourth molt. 12. Adult male. 13. Adult female.

muddy calf pens and barnyards, in close association with adult cattle. The mixture of mud and feces makes a good medium for the development of the infective larvae and the adhering quality of the mixture allows easy entry of larvae through the skin. Low-lying swampy areas have the same effect as muddy yards and lead to heavy hookworm infestation in dairy cows, beef herds, and sheep flocks.

Pathogenesis

The parasites attach to the mucosa of the intestine by their powerful buccal capsule, traumatize the latter with their chitinous plates, and cause great blood loss.

The parasite is considered an active bloodsucker. It has been experimentally established that an extract made of *Bunostomum sp.* has hemolytic action on the erythrocytes of various animals. Penetration of pathogenic bacteria into the body of the host with the infective larvae may cause infection of the mucosa. Upon postmortem examination, anemia and emaciation are frequently found.

The subcutaneous tissue shows serous infiltration and the mucosa is swollen, with numerous hemorrhagic spots. The contents of the intestine are streaked with blood.

Symptoms

Adult animals suffering from the disease lose weight, while in young animals development is retarded. The disease is characterized by profuse diarrhea, symptoms of anemia, edema, and the development of a bottle jaw. Other symptoms include paleness of the mucous membranes of the eyelids and mouth, pale skin, and swellings in the dependent parts of the body. Occasionally, mass mortality of lambs and calves occurs but, generally, infections severe enough to cause death are rare in this country.

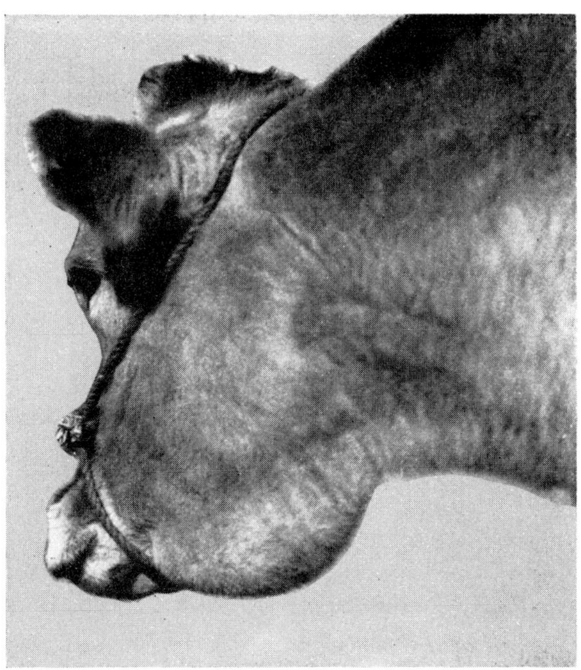

FIG. 40. "Bottle jaw" in the bovine resulting from parasitism. (From Gibbons, W. J.: *Clinical Diagnosis of Diseases of Large Animals.* Philadelphia, Lea & Febiger, 1966.)

Diagnosis

Diagnosis on a living animal is difficult, since the clinical symptoms of the disease are not specific. The exact nature of the disease may be established by finding large numbers of parasites in the intestines of dead or slaughtered animals.

Control

Control of hookworm infection must be based on preventive measures—strategic drenching, pasture rotation, adequate diet, and general sanitation. Calf pens, lambing yards, and pastures should be on high ground away from damp, swampy, or muddy areas. Particular attention must be given to young animals. They should graze on clean pastures, restricted from swampy areas, and should be rotated from area to area regularly. Avoid overstocking. Introduce new stock only after thorough treatment and sufficient quarantine period, and separate all obviously sick animals. A regimen of good food and therapeutic drenching is necessary whenever hookworm infection is diagnosed.

Oesophagostomiasis of Ruminants

Nodular worm disease is caused by three species of nematodes—*Oesophagostomum radiatum, Oesophagostomum venulosum* and *Oesophagostomum columbianum.* All three species are encountered in cattle, but *O. radiatum* is the most frequently observed; in sheep and goats *O. venulosum* and *O. columbianum* are more frequently encountered. The parasites are localized in the large intestine, the small intestine, and the cecum and colon, causing conspicuous nodules.

The disease is found in the north central states and in coastal areas. It causes a drop in the productivity of sheep, goats, and cattle, and is occasionally lethal to the animals. In nonfatal cases the infected intestine is not suitable for the preparation of sausages.

Description of Parasite

Oesophagostomum columbianum is a large, whitish nematode. The cephalic end bears a ring-like capsule wider than it is long. Two leaf crowns and a cuticular vesicle are present. The latter is marked off from the rest of the body by a ventral constriction. The vesicle bears an excretory pore on its surface. There is no esophageal funnel. The mouth is situated at the apex, while the cervical papillae are located anterior to the end of the esophagus. The forward part of the body is hooked. The female grows to a length of about 1.5 cm, and the male is a little shorter.

Development of Parasite

All three species develop directly. The female deposits ova in the intestine of the host; these are subsequently passed with the feces to the outside where, at a temperature of 75 to 80 F, larvae hatch within 10 to 17 hours. After undergoing two molts, the larvae become infective on the seventh to eighth day. (Eggs do not develop in the exterior at a temperature of 45 F and perish at a temperature of 95 F.)

Animals become infected chiefly on pasture, especially during spring and summer, by swallowing infective larvae with food and water. On reaching the large intestine, the larvae penetrate the mucosa within 24 hours and become encysted. After undergoing a third molt, by the sixth to eighth day (occasionally later), larvae leave the mucosa and enter the lumen of the intestine. Here, they continue to grow and undergo a fourth molt; on approximately the 32nd day, they transform into sexually mature males and females. In sheep infected repeatedly, some larvae remain encysted for several months.

In some permanently infected areas, 100 percent infection with oesophagostomiasis is encountered in sheep and cattle. *Oesophagostomum radiatum* must be present in large numbers, however, to produce clinical nodular worm disease in cattle. Although widely

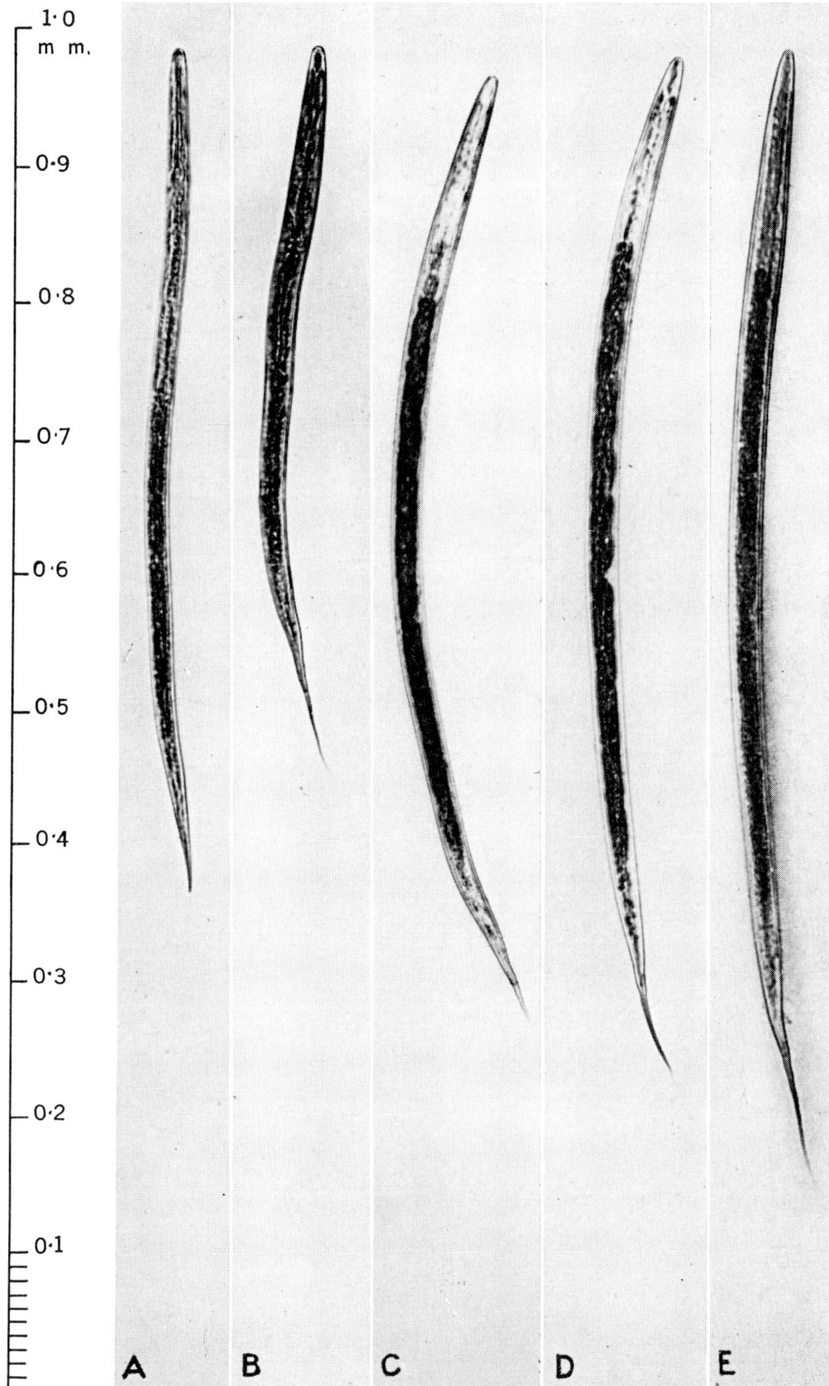

FIG. 41. Infective larvae of nematode parasites of cattle. *A: Strongyloides papillosus; B: Bunostomum phlebotomum; C: Trichostrongylus axei; D: Haemonchus contortus; E: Haemonchus placei.* (From Whitlock, J. H.: *Diagnosis of Veterinary Parasitisms.* Philadelphia, Lea & Febiger, 1960.)

distributed in the United States, the disease is more common in the southern states where humidity and temperatures are high. While all breeds and sexes are susceptible, animals under two years of age are more commonly affected. Lambs and calves younger than three months, however, do not suffer from this disease unless they have grazed upon heavily infected pasture.

Pathogenesis

The parasites are most pathogenic while in the larval form, because of deep penetration of the mucosa and formation of numerous nodular cysts. Because of this, the disease is often referred to as nodular worm disease. These nodules frequently necrose, apparently because of introduction of pyogenic bacteria by the larvae. Thus, in cases of disease, there are three ways in which the causative agent manifests pathogenicity on the body of the animal: through mechanical and toxic action, and by introduction of pathogenic microflora.

Pathology

The intestinal mucosa is hyperemic and edematous. On the fifth day of infection, the nodules are visible to the unaided eye, with small hemorrhages which have a yellow spot at the center. These hemorrhages are surrounded by a slightly hyperemic mucosa and constitute nodules containing larvae of the parasite. Occasionally, necrotic changes may occur in the nodule, and ulcers and pus may appear. On the seventh or eighth day it is possible to detect an ulcerous and inflamed colitis, the ulcers reaching 1 to 3 mm in diameter. From the serosal surface traces of necrotic changes may be seen in the intestinal wall.

Thousands of nodules may be encountered. They may range from the size of a pinhead to that of a pea, and consist of thick, connective tissue fibers with caseous contents. The nodules occasionally become calcified. Larvae are detected only in early nodules.

Symptoms

Two stages are recognized in the clinical picture of the disease: an acute phase connected with the penetration of the larvae into the mucosa, and a chronic phase determined by parasitization of the sexually mature helminths.

The acute stage is characterized by diarrhea, colic, anemia, frequent spasmodic urination, and a marked rise in body temperature when the larvae penetrate the intestinal mucosa. The animals refuse food, lose weight, and respond painfully to palpation of the abdominal wall. The mucous membranes are pale, although the anemia develops gradually. Acute diarrhea results in emaciation and death. Although the usual course is for diarrhea to develop slowly, in 1 to 3 weeks, it may persist for up to 6 months.

The chronic phase is accompanied by intermittent diarrhea, but is frequently symptomless.

Diagnosis

Diagnosis is difficult on a living animal, since the clinical symptoms of the disease are not specific. Diagnosis is more precisely carried out during necropsy of infected animals, with detection of the pathological and anatomical changes specific to oesophagostomiasis, and the presence of the parasites themselves in the lumen of the intestine or within the nodules.

Control

On farms permanently infected with nodular worm, feeding and maintenance of the animals should be improved; it has been shown that when animals are properly fed and maintained the disease in livestock is nearly symptomless. All manure should be removed from cattle yards and sheep pens daily, since this is the main reservoir of infection on the farm. The manure should be subjected to biothermic sterilization in manure dumps, collected in sewage lagoons or manure pits under slotted floors.

Animals should be subjected to several drenchings prior to being taken out to pasture, so that only ruminants free of *Oesophagostomum* are on the pasture. This measure alone is sufficient to eradiate the disease from farms in many districts where winters are severe and summers are hot and dry. Larvae perish on the pasture during periods of extreme heat and cold. Little infection is carried over from one season to another except in adult breeding stock. Where sheep and cattle are housed indoors during the winter, or where dairy cattle are confined close to coolers during hot weather, the use of slotted floors effectively lowers the incidence of infection because the animals do not come into contact with infective larvae.

An effective means of combating oesophagostomiasis is rotation of grazing plots, taking into consideration the periods of development of the larvae in the external environment. If 10 days are necessary for maturation of the larvae, then a plot should be grazed for not longer than 9 days. Return to a used plot should take place only after the death of the discharged ova and larvae. The length of life of larvae on pastures differs with degree of moisture and temperature of the air. In the south the parasites are relatively short lived, but in more temperate regions they may live for several months. (In northern regions some protection is afforded by the fact that long, hard winters virtually eliminate pasture contamination. At the end of a moderately severe winter, no infective larvae survive on unused pasture.)

On farms where it is impossible to change the grazing plots, or where it is necessary to utilize lowland pastures, chemical prophylaxis is carried out by use of anthelmintics, as follows. Approximately one week before the start of the pasture season, and then throughout the summer until the onset of the winter weather, sheep and goats are given periodic doses of anthelmintic in the amount recommended by the veterinarian. The drug may be mixed with sodium chloride or with initially concentrated feeds such as oats and bran. Anthelmintics effectively remove adult worms from the intestines. The removal of adult nodular worms immediately benefits diseased animals to some extent and helps to prevent the disease in susceptible animals by reducing the risk of infection.

Such treatment is essential to the control of nodular worm disease. Nothing can cure it once animals are infected. Young worms in nodules in the intestines are not affected by the drugs and no known treatment will remove the nodules.

Cattle, sheep, and goats on pasture should not be permitted to drink from puddles and ditches nor from small ponds and standing-water reservoirs in which the water has become brackish. Clean water must be provided during the pasture period.

Dictyocauliasis of Cattle

The causative agent of this disease is the nematode *Dictyocaulus viviparus,* commonly called the lungworm because it parasitizes the bronchi and trachea of cattle and sheep.

Dictyocauliasis, or husk, is chiefly a disease of young animals 4 to 18 months of age, although it may sometimes be encountered in adult animals. Frequently, the disease assumes the form of an outbreak and terminates in the death of numerous calves and lambs.

Description of Parasite

The male is 17 to 53 mm long and 0.4 to 0.7 mm in maximum width; the caudal end is supplied with a cuticular bursa with characteristic, evenly distributed rays. Two spicules, 0.22 to 0.27 mm long and 0.048 wide, of a brown-yellow color and spongy structure, are present. A gubernaculum is also present, 0.06 to 0.08 mm long, and is cellular in nature.

The female is 23 to 75 mm long and 0.4 to 0.6 mm in maximum width, with a vulva situated close to the middle of the body. The eggs are ellipsoidal, and may reach 0.085 mm in length and 0.051 mm in width.

Development of Parasite

Fertilized females deposit their eggs in the bronchi and trachea, where some ova develop larvae that emerge and are coughed up into the mouth and swallowed with the saliva. During passage through the digestive tract, chiefly while in the small intestine, the remaining larvae emerge from the ova and are passed with the feces to the outside.

Under proper conditions, the larvae undergo two molts, a fact easily confirmed by the loose skins present at both the anterior and posterior extremities of the larval body. Only after molting do the larvae reach the third or infective stage, when they are capable of infecting the final host. The period required for development is entirely dependent on the temperature of the air and the moist medium surrounding the larvae, but under optimum conditions is about five days.

Infective larvae are swallowed by calves and lambs with food and water. Upon reaching the small intestine they penetrate through the mucosa and enter the lymphatics and circulatory system in which they are carried to the lungs, the site of parasitization of the sexually mature organism.

In the lungs, the larvae leave the capillaries by rupturing the walls and pass into the alveolar system and the bronchioles. The period required for reaching sexual maturity, from the moment of ingestion of infective larvae by young animals to the production of ova by female lungworms, is 21 to 25 days.

The length of time the parasites remain in the body of the animal varies in different species from 2 to 4 months, and depends primarily on conditions of maintenance and nutrition and, secondly, on the physiological state of the host. In well-fed animals this period is short, but in emaciated animals the infection may persist. It is possible to shorten the period of parasitization by improving maintenance and feeding.

Dictyocauliasis of cattle and particularly of calves is widely prevalent. The sources for cattle of all ages are carrier animals and larvae of the parasite. To infect the host, larvae must free themselves from the expelled feces; this is accomplished by rainfall, which washes and scatters the larvae over the pasture, and also by fog and dew, which create minute rivulets in which larvae are carried away. Some investigators maintain that larvae are actively capable of covering distances up to 0.5 m. Other authors, however, believe that the larvae may be spread over the pasture by various insects. The likelihood of these last two modes of distribution requires experimental confirmation.

Dictyocauliasis is a seasonal disease, found mainly during the summer in high rainfall areas. Calves born in the current year, and adult groups of cattle which become infected during May and June in ever-increasing numbers, reach the maximum infection rate toward August and September. During that time, the clinical picture of disease is sharply manifested. Subsequently the disease declines naturally, and toward the winter months few infected cattle are observed. High temperatures will kill larvae in a few days on pasture, but it has been demonstrated that the larvae can survive through the winter. They live longer on wet than on dry pastures; therefore, it is obvious that irrigation can result in an increase in incidence and severity of lungworm disease unless proper preventive procedures are implemented. The same conditions apply for sheep as for cattle.

Pathogenesis

The larvae of the parasite, migrating through the body to the point where they will become sexually mature, traumatize the mucosa of the small intestine, the lymph nodes, the lymphatic and circulatory vessels, and the walls of the aveoli, bronchioles, and bronchi.

Furthermore, developing or already sexually mature parasites may cause irritation of the bronchi which results in congestion, mainly of the posterior portions of the lungs.

Irritation from large numbers of helminths causes excessive exudate in the bronchi and larynx which occasionally results in death due to asphyxiation.

As a result of irritation of the mucous membranes, hyperemia, swelling, progressive loss of weight, febrile reactions, depression, and various other abnormal signs are observed.

By disrupting the unity of the intestinal wall, circulatory and lymphatic vessels, and the tissues of the lung, the migrating larvae prepare the way for the invasion of pathogenic microflora, via the digestive and respiratory systems, into the vascular system and other organs and tissues, thus fostering the development of secondary infections. The atelectasis caused by the parasites is suitable for the development of microorganisms and corresponding inflammatory, purulent and necrotic processes.

Symptoms

The first and more or less constant symptom of dictyocauliasis is coughing. At the beginning it is infrequent and dry, but later becomes frequent and moist, often accompanied by a mucous nasal discharge. The appetite decreases or disappears completely. Animals lose weight, become sluggish, lag behind the herd, and are prone to lie down. Occasionally, the body temperature rises to 103 to 104 F. Rapid respiration is manifested, with an increase in heart rate.

When the disease is complicated by purulent pneumonia, symptoms become more pronounced. The disease frequently terminates in death.

Diagnosis

Usually, even clearly expressed clinical symptoms of dictyocauliasis are insufficient to diagnose the disease, since the same symptoms may occur in pulmonary diseases from other causes. The finding of relatively large worms in the bronchi upon postmortem is significant when associated with other symptoms. Pneumonia caused by unsatisfactory maintenance is characterized by localization of the pathological process in the anterior portions of the lung, whereas in dictyocauliasis congestion is, as a rule, in the posterior portions. Diagnosis by isolation of ova or larvae from feces and nasal secretions of infected animals is positive, but this is not always easy to accomplish.

Control

Control consists of general and specific organizational, therapeutic, and prophylactic measures to prevent the spread of infective larvae. War against the disease starts with the diagnosis of carrier animals and their treatment, control of pasturage, sanitation, and adequate feeding and watering of calves and lambs. At times these measures alone will not only eradicate but also prevent the reappearance of the disease on farms.

Dictyocauliasis is chiefly a disease of young animals; consequently, prophylactic measures should be aimed at the protection of this age group. This is accomplished by isolated maintenance and pasturing of young stock born in the current year, apart from adult cattle and especially apart from young animals born in the previous year which have already been to pasture. Young animals may also be maintained in stalls (with slotted floors) without pasturing.

Prevention may be accomplished by drenching all infected carriers during winter maintenance; carriers should be detected before allowing the animals to return to pasture in periods of low temperature not conducive to the development of larvae. Drenching is repeated when necessary 2 to 3 times, at intervals of 10 to 15 days, until all infected animals are free of parasites.

A vaccine developed against lungworm infection may prove to be successful in combating the disease where livestock are concentrated in numbers which preclude periodic drenching and pasture rotation. The vaccine is made by partially inactivating *Dictyocaulus* larvae by exposure to X-irradiation. The irradiated larvae are unable to develop to sexual maturity, but can migrate to the lungs and stimulate an immune response. The vaccine is both safe and effective, and when used properly can aid appreciably in the control of lungworm disease.

Best and most rapid results may be obtained by simultaneous application of the first three measures, namely, improved feeding and maintenance, strict isolation of animals born in the current year, and drenching of all infected carriers during the winter period.

Once the disease is controlled on the farm, in one way or another, measures should be adopted to prevent recurrence due to the introduction of infected replacements. All incoming livestock should be examined for the presence of dictyocauliasis during the quarantine period and infected animals subjected to treatment until completely free of parasites.

Trichinosis

Trichinosis is a parasitic disease of animals and man which affects the striated musculature. It is caused by a small nematode, *Trichinella spiralis,* and is important as a public-health problem.

The disease is encountered in pigs and rats, and occasionally in dogs, bears, foxes, mice and cats. Trichinosis is found in man in districts where pigs are infected with the disease, and people frequently die from this parasite.

Description of Parasite

Trichinella is a minute roundworm. The male is 1.4 to 1.6 mm long by 0.04 mm wide, while the female is 3 to 4 mm long and 0.06 mm wide. The esophagus is made up of a layer of closely juxtaposed cells. The females of *Trichinella* are viviparous. The males lack spicules, and have two papillae on the posterior part of the body just behind the cloaca.

Adult *Trichinella sp.* are found in the small intestine and are called intestinal trichinae, while their larvae parasitize the striated musculature and are called muscular trichinae.

Larvae of the parasite reach 0.08 to 0.12 mm in length and 0.006 mm in width following birth. The cephalic end is equipped with a stylet to aid in penetrating striated muscle. In the muscles, the larvae elongate to 0.1 to 1.15 mm, form into a spiral and become encapsulated.

Development of Parasite

Swine, dogs, cats, rats, mice, and man, when ingesting meat containing encapsulated larvae of *Trichinella,* become infected with trichinosis. The capsules of the parasites are digested in the stomach, liberating larvae 1 mm long which settle in the duodenal and jejunal portions of the small intestine. They grow rapidly and within two days the muscular trichinae transform into sexually mature parasites. Copulation occurs in the lumen of the intestine, the males die, and the fertilized females attach to the mucosa with their cephalic ends. They enter the lumina of the glands of Lieberkuhn or the intestinal villi, and on the fifth or sixth day begin to produce an enormous quantity (1,500 to 10,000) of living larvae. Occasionally, some of the female *Trichinella* may wander into the mesenteric lymph glands, the lymphatic vessels, and the submucosa of the intestine.

Newly hatched larvae are small. They travel initially into the lymphatic system, then into the circulatory system. Via the bloodstream they scatter over the entire body of the host, settling in enormous quantities in the striated muscles where they penetrate under the sarcolemma of the muscle fibers. At first they grow, then form into a spiral and become encapsulated. Larvae of *Trichinella* remain enclosed in the capsules until the flesh of the host is eaten by animal or man. In the intestine of mammals, the muscular trichinae develop into sexually mature forms. The larvae of *Trichinella* are unable to develop in cardiac muscle because the fibers of the latter have no sarcolemma. Trichinae are encountered in adipose tissue, the large thoracic peripheral muscles, and the esophageal muscles of swine. However, those reaching other than muscle tissue are destroyed by local inflammatory reaction.

Once it stops depositing larvae, between the 25th to 45th day of its life, the female leaves the intestine and dies. Following death, the adult worms are digested and are found only rarely in the feces. However, larvae encysted in muscles are able to survive for long periods (up to 25 years) without losing their viability. Trichinae also remain viable for a long time in the muscles of butchered swine. However, thorough cooking destroys them rapidly.

It is apparent from the above that an animal infected with trichinosis may simultaneously serve as a final and intermediate host.

Medical and Sanitary Significance

Man becomes infected with trichinosis only by eating uncooked, infected meat. The disease is focally distributed; however, in man it is encountered frequently in almost all countries where large numbers of swine are raised for meat.

Trichinosis is encountered in a large number of species of carnivores and rodents. The most important vectors among domestic animals are rats. The sources of swine infection are the bodies of dead rats, mice, and sometimes abattoir wastes.

Larvae of *Trichinella* are resistant to the influence of external factors. They remain infective for a period of 120 days in decaying meat exposed to air, but die quickly when the meat decays in water. A temperature of 160 F kills them, but at freezing temperatures they are effectively preserved. Curing of meat with dilute salt solution does not destroy the parasites.

Pathogenesis

Adult parasites and their larvae have a pathogenic effect. The larvae, as biological irritants, traumatize tissues during the period of migration and development, and thereby cause many hemorrhagic spots. The number of parasites which, when swallowed, causes a lethal course of the disease is 10 per kg live weight per pig, 30 for the rat, and 5 for man.

Larvae of the parasite are capable of transporting pathogenic bacteria into deeper tissues when they migrate from the intestine.

Pathology

Muscle fibers penetrated by trichinae larvae swell into spindle shapes. The transverse striations of such affected muscle fibers gradually disappear. The nuclei become enlarged, while the muscle substance transforms into a granular mass. The larvae of the parasite grow and increase, and an envelope forms around them as a result of thickening of the sarcolemma and proliferation of connective tissue. After 20 to 30 days the larvae complete their growth in muscles, begin to form into a spiral, and become enclosed in a capsule. After 5 to 6 months such capsules become calcified.

Trichinella larvae are detected mainly in the diaphragm, and in lingual, laryngeal, intercostal, and thoracic muscles. Occasionally, they may be found in parenchymatous organs and adipose tissue of swine.

Symptoms

The symptoms of the disease usually become manifested on the third to fifth day following infection, but only when the invasion is very heavy. The symptoms express themselves in elevated body temperature, diarrhea, and occasionally vomiting. Pigs show rapid emaciation, and frequently die after 12 to 15 days. In most cases the disease becomes chronic in nature. Pains in the muscles occur. Emaciated animals lie for long periods without movement, with extended extremities. Shallow respiration and occasionally edema of the eyelids and extremities are observed in diseased animals. The disease lasts for 1 to $1\frac{1}{2}$ months until the larvae are encapsu-

TABLE 4. Common Worm Parasites

Worms in swine	Watch for	Effect	Treatment
Large roundworm	Nonspecific. Soft, moist cough, lack of appetite, slow gains, runts. Found in intestines. Yellow to pink. Up to foot long.	Damage intestines, white-spotted liver, bleeding internally, pneumonia. Worm eggs are eaten and worm inhabits liver, lung and intestine.	Strict sanitation. Treatment with any of a number of drugs on schedule recommended by local vet or extension service. Antibiotics useful.
Nodular worm	Loss in feed efficiency, diarrhea, watery feces, loss of appetite. Less than 1 in long, thread-like in appearance.	Damage to intestines, loss of flesh, death.	Same as for roundworm.
Lungworm	Coughing, difficult breathing, loss of appetite. Inhabit trachea, bronchi, air passes of lung. White to pink, up to 2 in long.	Parasitic pneumonia. Swine influenza, general weakening of condition.	Strict sanitation, keep animals off infested land. No effective medicinal treatment.
Thorny-headed	Usually found in small intestine. Very long, thick, with flat back and underside.	Ulcers on intestine. General weakening of condition.	Same as for lungworm.
Threadworm	Short, whitish, thread-like. Causes anemia, diarrhea.	Migrating larvae damage heart, lung, intestine; can cause death.	Strict sanitation. Some antibiotics in feed effective.
Whipworm	Slender front end portion; short thick posterior. Found in cecum and colon. One to two in long.	None noted in light infestation. Heavy infestation can cause loss of weight, etc.	Strict sanitation, sound diet. Medicinals effective.
Kidney worm	Found in kidney, liver, lung, spleen, pleural cavity, spinal canal and loin muscle. Thick, shows sign of internal organs through skin.	Loss of flesh, hindlegs may be paralyzed, may make internal organs unfit for consumption. Pigs die.	Strict sanitation. Keep sows and pigs off infested soil to permit eggs to die from exposure. Feed sows and pigs in separate areas.

Worms in cattle and sheep	Watch for	Effect	Treatment
Tapeworm	Found in liver, lungs, intestines in adult and larval stages. Often cause diarrhea. Tapeworm cysts also found in muscles. Most serious in calves.	Unthriftiness, loss of vigor, tissue subject to attack by other disease agents. Condemnation of meat products.	Most effective measure is to keep pastures free of eggs. Study life cycle of pest and keep calves off infested land.
Lungworm	White, thread-like, infest bronchial tubes of lung. Taken in grazing. Difficult breathing, coughing spells.	Serious infestation causes death. Loss of appetite, weakness.	Strict sanitation, program to rotate grazing to keep cattle off infested areas if possible. Use vaccine for calves and lambs.
Stomach worm	Parasite of the fourth stomach. Up to 1.25 in long, size of a pin. Taken in grazing. Other species smaller in size.	Loss of flesh, weakness, anemia, diarrhea, irritation of stomach, gastritis.	Strict sanitation. Keep animals off infested pasture if possible.
Hookworm	Found in upper small intestine, sometimes in fourth stomach. Bloodsucker. Taken in grazing.	Similar to stomach worm.	Similar to stomach worm.

lated. Following this, no symptoms are noticeable except the sequelae of previous damage—muscle stiffness, nervous disorders, and respiratory distress.

In man, the disease is accompanied by fever, gastrointestinal disorders, facial edema, particularly in the eyelids, and muscular pains. Trichinosis is frequently mistaken for abdominal typhus because of the similarity in symptoms of these two diseases. The disease lasts for 3 to 6 weeks and may terminate in death.

Prevention

To safeguard people against trichinosis, and to prevent its spread, pigs should not be allowed to eat dead rats, and all garbage containing raw meat scraps should be thoroughly cooked before being fed to swine. Home economists, teachers, and public-health officials should stress the fact that viable trichinae may be found in any pork products that have been smoked or subjected to only "partial" heat treatment, and that inspection of meat at time of slaughter has not proved to be an effective means of discovering the infection. As there is no treatment, prevention is the only prophylactic measure.

Summary

Table 4 is an attempt to summarize the animal diseases caused by worm parasites, their symptoms and effects, and suggested treatments.

56 General Characteristics of Arthropoda

ARTHROPODS are invertebrates with jointed appendages. They are widely distributed throughout the world, and have attracted human attention for a long time. Though some arthropods are useful, others are harmful to animals and man.

A great many arthropods cause enormous economic losses to agriculture and animal husbandry. These are harmful organisms that infest forests and various forms of cultivated land, such as vegetable plots and gardens. They parasitize man and animals, causing severe diseases, and may also serve as vectors of infectious diseases.

Arthropods are characterized by movable, jointed appendages and metameric body segmentation. The body segments may be fused into a single whole (as in many ticks), divided into three sections—head, thorax, and abdomen (as in insects), or formed into a cephalothorax and abdomen (as in arachnids). The arthropod body is encased in a hard, chitinous cuticle which represents the exoskeleton. Striated muscles are attached to the internal surface of the exoskeleton, while 3 or 4 pairs of appendages are connected to its outside. The body cavity is regarded as a degenerated or vestigial coelom, rather than a true coelom. The bodies of several representative arthropod species are equipped with some additional structures—antennae on the head or cephalothorax, 1 or 2 pairs of wings originating from the thorax. The mouth is an opening at the anterior extremity of the body, while the anus is at the posterior end. The vascular system is not closed. The blood is usually colorless, but may be variously colored. The nervous system consists of paired supra-esophageal dorsal ganglia and a double chain of ventral ganglia which cross-connect in each body segment.

Arthropoda are divided into many classes, the most important of which are Insecta and Arachnida.

Insects have jointed legs, a body divided into a head, thorax, and abdomen, a single pair of antennae, and three pairs of legs; most of them are equipped with one or two pairs of wings. They breathe through tracheae. Insects may be either terrestrial or aquatic.

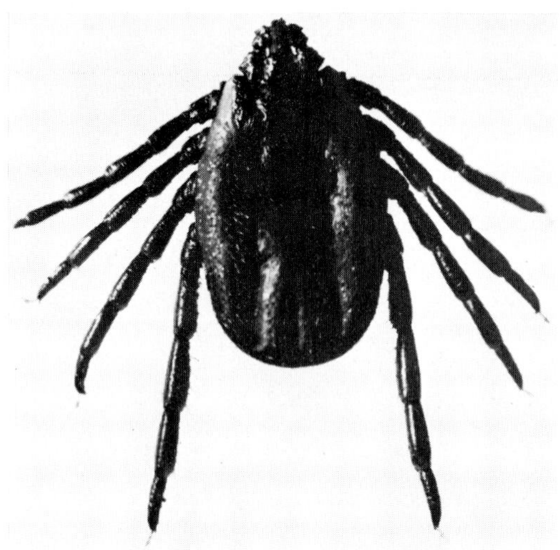

FIG. 42. Adult tick *Boophilus annulatus.*

There are approximately one million species of insects; those of importance to domestic animals include flies, fleas, lice, and mosquitoes.

Arachnida have jointed legs and a body either fused into an unsegmented whole (ticks and mites) or divided into a cephalothorax and abdomen (spiders). They lack antennae, breathe through tracheae and have four pairs of legs in the adult stage. They are usually terrestrial organisms and number about 28,000 species.

The study of parasitic arthropods has shown that some of them are permanent parasites of animals (lice and mites) and others are temporary (fleas, flies, ticks, and others). Parasitic arthropods feed on the host's blood, damage its wool, feathers, or skin, impair its growth and productivity, and hinder its development.

During infestation, the mouth parts of many parasitic arthropods wound the skin of the host and inject saliva and other secretions into the wound, resulting in inflammatory manifestations at the site of the bite and producing toxic effects on the animal.

Certain parasitic arthropods may produce specific diseases in animals (mange, gadfly disease, myiases), causing severe damage to the individual animal and considerable economic loss to the livestock producer. Losses to economy and industry are at times reckoned in millions of dollars and are the result of insufficient production of wool, skins, meat, fat, butter, milk, and the loss of valuable breeding stock.

Many species of arthropods serve as intermediate hosts for causative agents of a number of parasitic (invasive) diseases of man and animals. Fleas, flies, and dragonflies may harbor larval stages of helminths in their bodies; trypanosomal stages may be found in fleas and the sheep ked (*Melophagus ovinus*). Plasmodia of avian malaria are found in mosquitoes, while bloodsucking ticks may harbor the causative agents of hemosporidioses, spirochetosis, and various other diseases. Some nonparasitic armored ticks may harbor larval stages of cestodes.

In some cases, the causative agents of infectious diseases are picked up with the blood meal by the intermediate host while feeding on a specifically diseased animal (insects ingest helminths, trypanosomes, and avian plasmodia while ticks pick up hemosporidia and spirochetes). In other cases, arthropods pick up the infection from the external environment (armored ticks ingest eggs of cestodes with food material).

Of extraordinary importance is the role of arachnids and insects as transmitters of parasitic and viral diseases of animals and man. Two categories of transmitters are distinguished, mechanical and biological. In the former, the pathogenic microorganisms undergo no development or reproduction but are simply transferred from diseased to healthy animals. In biological transmitters, however, there is development and even multiplication of the microorganisms, after which the latter are introduced into healthy animals. These vectors may often serve simultaneously both as pathogens and intermediate hosts of pathogens.

Although an infection may at times persist for several generations as a latent, passive infection in carriers, it is passed on from one generation to the other. The presence of such a reservoir of infection is conducive to the circulation of the causative agent in nature and the maintenance of unfavorable, permanent, natural foci for future outbreaks. When infected alien cattle wander into an infested, unhealthy focus of infection, there is, on the one hand, a renewed infection of vectors, and, on the other, the acquisition by local cattle of specific immunity or resistance to further reinfection. The explanation for this immunity lies in the fact that young animals infested by ticks in the natural focus undergo a mild form of the disease which, in turn, creates mechanisms of immunity to further reinfection that might occur in heavily tick-infested pastures.

Postembryonal development of arthropods includes four stages: (1) larval, (2) and (3) nymphal, and (4) adult. In parasitic tick species the number of nymphal stages may be reduced (one stage only in Ixodidae) or increased (three or more stages in Argasidae).

Ticks

During various stages of development, ticks may attach in the hundreds and thousands to domestic and wild animals for feeding purposes. They are then for several days temporary ectoparasites. Once gorged, the ticks drop onto the ground where they reproduce and hibernate through the winter months. Most ticks, in various developmental stages, infest pastures, but some may, on rare occasions, infest dwellings. Most ticks are active during warm periods of the year and go into hibernation or become dormant during the cold periods; they hide within fissures in the ground, under rocks or in cracks in buildings.

The adult and nymphal stages of the tick have four pairs of legs while the larval stage has only three pairs. These legs are composed of six movable segments: trochanter, prefemur, femur, tibia, protarsus, and tarsus. The legs are joined to the ventral surface of the body by means of immovable coxae. The coxae of the anterior pair of legs may be bifurcated into two minute roots or teeth. The tarsi terminate into two hooks and a suction pad; these structures are particularly well developed on the tarsi of the first pair of legs. The aforementioned suction pads enable the tick to move vertically and upside down, while the long legs of some ticks enable them to move rapidly for considerable distances. The articulations of the legs are frequently white in color, giving the legs a striped appearance. Haller's organ, a special olfactory organ, is situated on the dorsal surface of the tarsi of the first pair of legs.

Life Cycle

Ticks are oviparous; the female may lay 10,000 to 15,000 eggs. The eggs are small, primarily oval, and yellowish-brown. They are deposited on the ground following engorgement of the female on animal blood. Oviposition is continuous and uninterrupted, and the female dies shortly thereafter. Minute, six-legged larvae hatch from the eggs.

After obtaining a blood meal from animals, the larvae molt into eight-legged nymphs which superficially resemble adult females. Larvae and nymphs have undeveloped genital systems and are incapable of reproduction. Larvae further lack respiratory organs, respiration taking place through the body surface. Nymphs, on the other hand, have a tracheal system opening on both sides of the body through spiracles. Following a blood meal and engorgement, the nymphs molt into adult males or females. Thus, Ixodidae undergo two molts and exhibit three active stages: larval, nymphal, and adult.

Larvae and nymphs feed on the blood of small wild animals and birds. Adults feed on bigger, usually domestic, animals. In some species of ticks, the different stages feed on the same host, usually a domestic animal. Ticks in all stages of development invariably feed on animals a few days after molting. During the blood meal they remain attached to the host, allowing their chitinous body coverings to harden. Unengorged larvae, nymphs, and adults crawl through the grass or bushes, using the hind legs for locomotion while the anterior pair of legs is held high and is constantly vibrating. Ticks, apparently, sense out the proper host animal with the aid of Haller's organ, attach securely to the host with the hooks on the free legs, pierce the skin of the animal with the hypostome, and proceed to feed.

Ticks at any phase of development, but particularly adult females, suck up a considerable amount of host blood. The female, while engorging, may increase 200 times in body weight, at the same time increasing considerably in size. The period of engorgement and length of time on the host averages 3 to 7 days for larvae, 3 to 10 days for nymphs, and 8 to 10 days for adults. Larvae may take a month or more to develop. The periods when larvae molt into nymphs and nymphs into adults may range from several days to a month.

Ticks in various stages of development may hibernate when natural conditions are unfavorable; even the eggs may frequently undergo a period of hibernation. Thus, eggs deposited during the fall may hatch only the following spring.

Some adult ticks either hibernate on domestic animals or remain active while on the body of a host animal.

The males suck up only small quantities of blood and are usually not firmly fixed to any one spot on the body; they wander from place to place in search of females. They also pass from one host to another. Thus, when they harbor pathogens such as *Haemosporidia,* male ticks are capable of transmitting the disease from animal to animal. The females of some species, especially *Amblyomma sp.*, may also serve as vectors of disease.

By their mode of development and manner of feeding, *Ixodidae* ticks may be divided into three groups: one-host, two-host, and three-host ticks.

One-host ticks (*Boophilus microplus*) undergo full development on a single host without leaving its body.

The larval stage of two-host ticks must find a host animal (first host). Following engorgement, larvae molt into nymphs while on the host's body. The nymphs obtain a blood meal and drop off the host, molting on the ground into adults. Adult ticks then attach to another animal (the second host), usually of the same species as the first but occasionally a different species altogether. Following engorgement, adults drop to the ground, lay eggs, and thus complete their life cycle. Among the two-host ticks is *Rhipicephalus bursa.*

Three-host ticks successively use three host animals. The larvae parasitize one animal (first host), then drop off and molt into nymphs. The nymphs, after gaining in strength, hook onto another animal (second host), gorge on its blood, and drop off to molt into adults. The adults, in turn, hook onto a third animal (third host) to obtain a blood meal, then drop off and deposit eggs on the ground. This mode of development is characteristic for all ticks of the genera *Ixodes, Haemaphysalis,* and *Dermacentor,* for several species of the genus *Rhipicephalus,* and others.

As hosts, the larvae and nymphs of two- and three-host ticks usually employ small wild mammals (mainly rodents), birds, and rarely lizards and snakes, while the adults may either feed on large domestic animals or, at times, on wild mammals (elk, deer, wild boars, wolves, foxes, and hares).

Ticks show fairly good adaptation to particular terrains. Some species will adapt to bush-forest areas, others to plains, semiarid or desert regions, and mountainous terrain. Some species have adapted to life within burrows of wild animals, while others will infest not only pastures but even living quarters of domestic animals, where they reproduce and multiply in cracks and crevices. We may therefore conclude that ticks are adaptable to widely different environmental conditions.

Prevention

Knowledge concerning the life cycle, host chain, and length of time on the host of the various ticks is essential for planning appropriate measures to combat adult and younger stages. It should be borne in mind that the salivary glands of unengorged ticks are at first (1 to 3 days) nonfunctional, becoming functional only during engorgement of the tick. In a tick infected with protozoa, large numbers of the pathogens accumulate in the salivary glands following a blood meal. Consequently, the infective tick is capable of injecting the parasites into the bloodstream of a host animal with its saliva.

To prevent possible infection, domestic animals should be subjected to daily inspections during which they are either freed manually of adhering ticks or treated with chemicals.

Extermination of Ticks in Nature

Ticks may be exterminated in nature by changing and isolating the grazing places, creating conditions unfavorable for the development of the parasites in the latter, treating tick-infested areas with chemical acaricides, and employing the natural enemies of the tick. Maximum success may be reached by combining the measures mentioned widely into animal husbandry.

Isolation means not allowing cattle to graze on land infested with ticks. Parasites which are not given the possibility of feeding on animals will die of starvation.

To free grazing land from one-host ticks which are vectors of diseases of livestock, the following procedure is adopted. If the only pastures on the farm are tick-infested, these are divided into two sections: one is allowed to stand fallow until the following year, while all animals are grazed for the entire season on the remaining land. During the following year, livestock are grazed on the first section and the second is isolated. All tick larvae will perish on the isolated first section in the first year, because they cannot live more than 6 to 7 months without food. Livestock are thoroughly dipped before being moved to the plot for grazing the following year. The second section, isolated in the second year, is then freed of ticks by the next grazing period. Thus, the whole grazing area is rendered tick-free in two years.

If some grazing lands are infested with ticks and others are free of them, the free areas are divided in the spring into four regions. Livestock are pastured 25 days in succession on each of these, calculating that, from the moment that larvae attach themselves to the animals until their transformation into gorged females, 21 to 24 days are needed. Infested lands remain unused for the entire period, and, by the time the four designated sections have been grazed, the infested lands have remained isolated for more than 7 months (from the fall of the preceding year). Livestock are then grazed over those fallow pastures, now free of ticks, after the passage of 100 days of the grazing season. The first four sections are then isolated until the following year. In this way, the entire area of grazing land is freed from ticks in one year.

Lice

The life history of all species of lice is similar in many respects. They are all obligate parasites and are normally found to be species specific. Biting lice reproduce parthenogenetically while the bloodsucking species must be fertilized before reproduction. The eggs are glued to the hair of the host, where they hatch in one to two weeks. Nymphs are similar in appearance to adults except for smaller size, light color, absence of sexual characters and certain other minor differences. In all species there are three nymphal stages, and adults are produced 2 to 3 weeks after hatching. Lice removed from the host will die in less than a week under normal barn or pasture conditions. The eggs attached to tufts of hair rubbed from the animals against posts and other objects around barns or corrals may take as long as three weeks to hatch.

The bloodsucking lice pierce skin and suck blood almost continuously; the biting lice feed around the base of the hair, causing blood to seep from injuries produced by the sharp mandibles and claws. These lice feed on the dried blood, scurf and skin of the animal.

The feeding of the parasites and the injuries produced by their claws cause severe irritation, and the host animals rub and scratch to the extent that frequently large areas of skin are denuded of hair and other areas are bruised and raw from rubbing against posts and other objects.

During the fall, with cooler weather, lice populations increase as the animal's hair coat becomes thicker and longer and the skin relatively dry. At this season, all sizes of lice and their eggs may be found on an infested animal.

Mites

There are four stages in the development of mites: the egg, the larva, the nymph, and the adult. Eggs are usually laid upon or under the skin (stratum corneum) of the host. After varying periods of incubation the larva hatches in the form of a six-legged creature, often quite unlike the parent. After a single meal the larva rests, sheds its skin, and appears with an additional pair of legs and a body form more closely resembling that of the parent, but without developed sexual organs. The nymph thus produced feeds and molts once or several times and finally, after another period of rest during which the body is once more remodeled, molts again as an adult male or female. The feeding and burrowing activities of the various species cause considerable irritation to the skin and underlying tissues of livestock, resulting in itching and thickening or wrinkling of the skin.

57
Ticks, Lice, Mites

Ticks

Ticks are external parasites of domestic and wild animals, widely distributed and usually seasonal in their activities. They are responsible for serious economic loss and are vectors of several viral and protozoan diseases. Tick infestation causes local irritation and discomfort leading to loss of production of meat, milk, wool and fiber. The injury to livestock, in most cases, varies with the total number of parasites; animals heavily infested with ticks which feed exclusively on blood rapidly become weakened and anemic. In attempting to rid themselves of the worrisome parasites, they may rub themselves vigorously against stationary objects, causing bleeding wounds and sores, which in turn may become infected with screwworms.

There are two families of ticks: the hard-shelled ticks, or *Ixodidae,* and the soft-shelled ticks, or *Argasidae.*

The *Ixodidae* of importance in the United States are: the Lone Star tick, the Gulf coast tick, the Rocky Mountain wood tick, and the cattle fever tick. Of the *Argasidae,* only one, the spinose ear tick, is of significance to domesticated animals.

The Lone Star tick, *Amblyomma americanum,* is found in the southern part of the country, and attacks all farm animals as well as wild species. It is a three-host tick and prefers to attach to parts of the body sparsely covered with hair. It is active from spring until late fall and is capable of transmitting Rocky Mountain spotted fever to humans.

The Gulf coast tick, *Amblyomma maculatum,* attacks horses, deer, sheep and hogs, but is most important as a parasite of cattle. It is prevalent in the southern states from the Atlantic to Texas. This tick is a three-host tick and infests livestock during the summer and fall; it attaches mainly to the ears and face. Ticks feed in clusters, causing intense irritation to the ears accompanied by painful swelling.

The Rocky Mountain wood tick, *Dermacentor andersoni,* is a serious parasite of cattle, horses, and sheep and less seriously of swine. The tick is primarily found in the northwestern part of the country and is of public-health importance as a vector of Rocky Mountain spotted fever in humans. This tick is a three-host tick with a long life cycle. The immature stages may overwinter and then become very active in the spring and early summer, when they attach to the head and ears of their host. Ticks invading the ear canal cause great distress, leading to head shaking, crying and inappetence in affected animals.

The cattle fever tick, *Boophilus annulatus,* once occurred in the southern states but was eradicated many years ago because of its ability to transmit babesiosis, or Texas fever. A related species, *Boophilus microplus,* is found in southern Texas, and attacks the softer parts of the animal body. This parasite is the main vector of Texas fever in Australia.

The spinose ear tick, *Otobius megnini,* affects cattle, sheep, and swine in the arid and semiarid regions of the southwest. These soft ticks are more common in cattle kept in small enclosures and feedlots than in range cattle. The larvae invade the ear canal in large numbers; they require several months to develop to the nymph stage, at which time they emerge from the ears and drop to the ground. On the ground, they molt into adults, mate, lay eggs, and start the cycle over again. In cold weather, ticks move from the outer part of the ear deep into the ear canal and often cause middle-ear infection by penetrating the ear drum.

Life History

The life history of the different varieties of hard ticks is quite similar except for the number of hosts required for development, even though the number of blood meals may be the same. Therefore, the cattle fever tick will be used as an example.

Cattle fever ticks spend the early part of their lives on the ground. They then infest cattle, or occasionally horses, swine, sheep, goats and deer. Ticks must have blood from an animal host to complete each stage of their life cycles.

Moisture and temperature affect the tick's development. In spring, summer, and early fall, a tick may complete its life cycle in 6 to 10 weeks. If growth is delayed by cold, a tick may take a year to complete its life cycle. Ticks are ordinarily killed by temperatures of 12 F, and eggs are destroyed at 2 F.

The newly hatched seed ticks, or larvae, are barely visible to the unaided eye. These waxy-brown, six-legged ticks crawl up grass or plants, where they wait for an animal to pass by. If they do not find a host they eventually die of starvation. In summer, seed ticks may starve in 3 to 4 months; in colder periods, they may survive for six months.

Seed ticks attach to soft skin inside the animal's thighs, flanks, and forelegs, or along the belly or brisket. Here, they gorge on blood, molt twice, and then become tiny white, eight-legged nymphs. After gorging about a week, nymphs become adults. Many adult ticks are olive green; others are mottled yellow or olive brown.

Mature ticks mate without leaving the host animal. At this time, the adult female is about $^1/_{10}$ in long; the male is slightly smaller.

After mating, the adult female pierces the host animal's skin and sucks blood until she is about $^1/_4$ to $^1/_2$ inch long. Then she drops to the ground where she deposits her eggs. Ticks remain on cattle 3 or 4 weeks; under favorable conditions, however, the period on the host may be shortened to 15 days.

The female tick dies after producing a cluster of several thousand amber-colored eggs on the ground. In warm weather, eggs usually hatch in 13 to 42 days. They may incubate in unfavorable weather for as long as seven months.

Infested cattle develop a rough coat, lose weight, and have a worried appearance. They become weak, stunted, and anemic from continuous loss of blood. When ticks locate in the ears, animals shake their heads, rub ears against fence posts or other objects, and try to scratch the ears with a hind hoof.

Diagnosis

Tick infestations can be diagnosed by finding the ticks on the host. Ticks may be found on all parts of the body but most often around the head, neck, flanks, and in the ears. They may vary appreciably in size as several stages of the developmental cycle of the ticks may be on an animal at the same time.

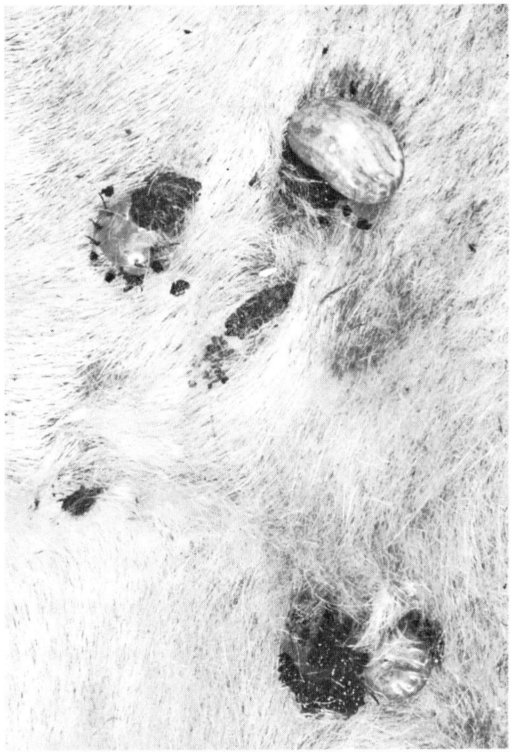

FIG. 43. *Dermacentor andersoni* attached to bovine skin. (From Jensen, R., and Mackey, D. R.: *Diseases of Feedlot Cattle.* Ed. 2, Philadelphia, Lea & Febiger, 1971.)

Control

Control of ticks in cattle herds is of prime importance to a good manager because of the losses caused both directly and indirectly by these parasites.

Control is usually directed toward treatment of an entire herd or flock with appropriate chemicals, either by dipping or spraying, although the same treatment may be applied to individual animals.

Although many chemicals are useful in combating ticks, some of them leave undesirable residues in meat or milk. Because no residues or pesticides are tolerated in milk under the regulations of the U.S. Food and Drug Administration, and only minimal amounts are permitted in the fat of meat-producing animals, the use of many effective materials has been suspended. The U.S. Department of Agriculture provides a list of acceptable dips and sprays.

Tick control may also be accomplished by the application of acaricides to small areas such as hedgerows, lanes, grassy plots, and small pastures. The application of acaricides to large pastures or wooded areas is not practical, and the methods of tick eradication mentioned in the previous chapter should be undertaken.

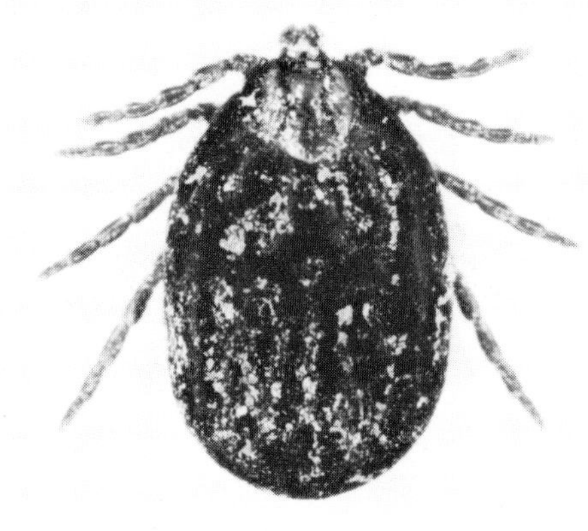

FIG. 44. *Dermacentor andersoni.* (From Jensen, R., and Mackey, D. R.: *Diseases of Feedlot Cattle.* Ed. 2, Philadelphia, Lea & Febiger, 1971.)

Lice

Pediculosis is a general term to designate an infestation with one or more species of lice. Depending upon the habits of the species concerned, the symptoms and lesions are variable. In most instances, lice are host-specific and may even be area-specific upon a given host. There are two types of lice: biting lice and sucking lice.

Lice are small, flattened, wingless insects which cause skin irritation from their piercing or biting feeding habits. Lice are dependent upon the host for their nutrition, and will die within a few days if removed. They are insidious and seasonal parasites, although they spend their life span upon the skin of the hosts. Infestations usually appear in the fall, increase slowly during the winter months, and then wane in the spring; the lice population gradually declines as the weather becomes warmer and the animal's skin temperature increases. Lice do not completely disappear from a herd or flock, however, until effective insecticide treatment and preventive control measures are exercised.

Adult lice lay their eggs by attaching them to the hair of the animal. The eggs of sucking lice hatch in 17 to 21 days, but eggs of biting lice require only 10 to 14 days. The nymphs reach sexual maturity in about two weeks and start a new generation. Thus, several generations occur during the winter.

The eggs will not usually hatch if they become detached and fall to the ground unless the weather is unusually warm. Even so, they must find a host in 2 or 3 days or they will die. The life cycles vary from 20 to 30 days, although the eggs may exist for 35 days. When removed from their natural hosts, some species will feed upon human blood, if hungry.

Each year, lice cost livestock producers millions of dollars in profits through morbidity and lowered production. These losses are incurred in all parts of the country, and any herd or flock may be affected. Primarily, the losses result from anemia, unthriftiness, reduced rates of gain, inefficient feed utilization, occasional loss of life, a predisposition to other disease—because of the numerous bites upon the skin—and expensive control measures.

Lice are transmitted primarily by direct contact, although occasionally indirect transmission through infested bedding, blankets, or brushes may occur. Although lice are generally host-specific, and several species of lice may commonly attack the same host either simultaneously or sequentially, only a few will infest more than one type of animal.

Cattle Lice

Four species of bloodsucking lice and one species of biting lice are pests of cattle in the United States. The bloodsucking lice feed by piercing the animal's skin and drawing blood. Biting lice feed on particles of hair, scabs, and excretions from the skin. The bloodsucking lice attacking cattle are *Linognathus vituli, Solenopotes capillatus, Haematopinus eurysternus,* and *Haematopinus quadripertusus.* The biting louse is *Bovicola bovis.*

The bloodsucking louse *H. quadripertusus,* commonly called the tail louse, was discovered in Florida; by 1956, it was found only in the southern states in areas along the coast. All other species of lice occur throughout the United States.

The other three bloodsucking lice are commonly called the short-nosed louse, the little blue louse, and the long-nosed louse. The short-nosed louse is the largest of these and is gray, while the others are blue. The biting louse, sometimes called the little red cattle louse, is distinguished from the sucking species by its reddish-brown color, broad head, and chewing mouth parts.

Although nearly all untreated cattle harbor lice to some extent, the heaviest infestations are generally found on a few especially susceptible individuals; the reason for this susceptibility is not known. The damage lice cause to cattle depends on the degree of infestation.

Lice-infested cattle can usually be detected because they rub against fences and other objects. Infested animals are usually in poor

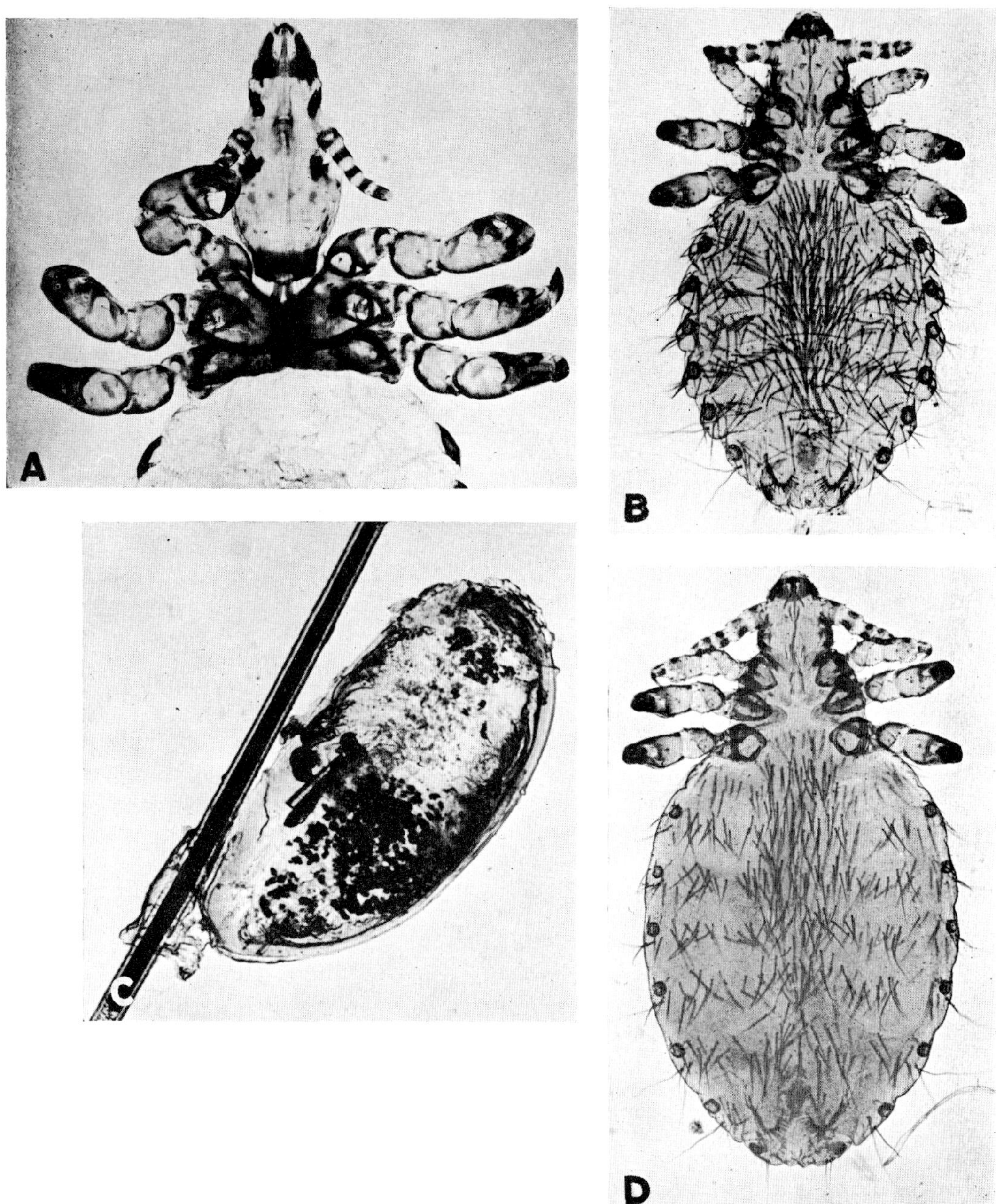

FIG. 45. *A, Hematopinus.* Note the tarsal claws on first two pairs of legs. *B, Linognathus* (male). Note small tarsal claw on first leg. *C,* Nit. *D, Linognathus* (female). (From Whitlock, J. H.: *Diagnosis of Veterinary Parasitisms.* Philadelphia, Lea & Febiger, 1960.)

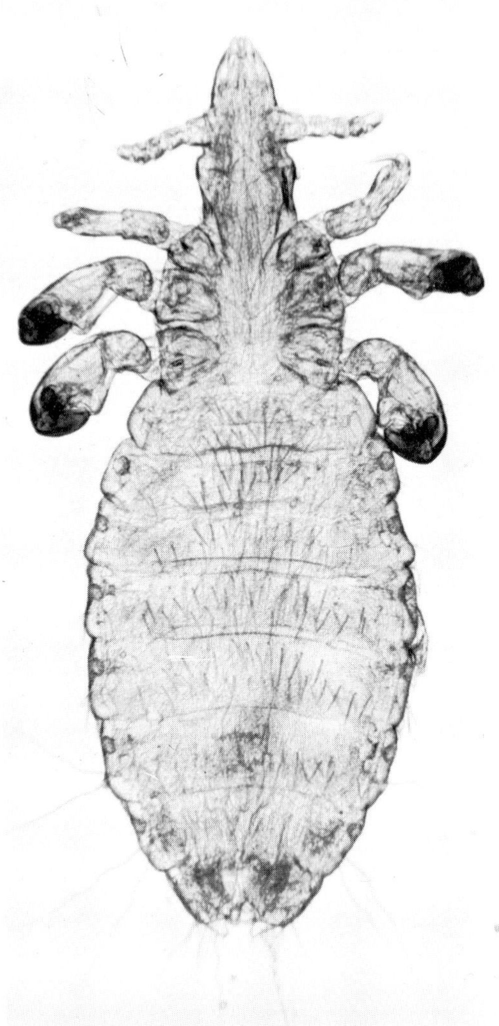

FIG. 46. The biting louse of cattle, *Bovicola bovis.* (From Jensen, R., and Mackey, D. R.: *Diseases of Feedlot Cattle.* Ed. 2, Philadelphia, Lea & Febiger, 1971.)

condition. Calves, yearlings, and old undernourished cattle suffer most. Weight gains are decreased or stopped, milk production decreases, and death may even occur, particularly in thin range cows of low vitality that have been exposed to bad weather. Lice infestation is usually heaviest and noticeable along the brisket, neck, and around the ears, eyes and tail head. Biting lice will cut off patches of hair and leave many bare spots.

Swine Lice

Swine are attacked by only one species of louse, *Haematopinus suis.* This is the largest of the lice found on domestic animals. It is grayish-brown with prominent brown and black markings. The female is 4 to 6 mm in length and the male is slightly smaller.

Pearly white ova are laid singly and attached to the bristles. Within a few days the ova change to an amber color, and hatch in 12 to 20 days. During her lifetime the female may deposit up to 90 ova, laid over a period of a month. Thus, all stages of the life cycle may appear on the host at the same time.

Since lice feed frequently, the continual puncturing of the skin to suck blood and lymph gives rise to considerable irritation. In severe infestations the constant irritation and itching induce hogs to seek relief by scratching and rubbing vigorously against any available object. This leads to skin laceration, bleeding, and a concentration of lice around the traumatized areas. As the louse population increases, the hogs become restless, do not feed properly, become unthrifty, and fail to make normal growth and weight gains. A general lowering of vitality and resistance makes them susceptible to attack by other parasites and contagious diseases. It is generally considered that the hog louse is the transmitting agent of swine pox virus.

Sheep Lice

Sheep are infested by both sucking and biting lice. The biting louse *Bovicola ovis,* and the sheep foot louse *Linognathus pedalis,* a sucking louse, are the two species most commonly found in the United States. Two other species of sucking lice—*Linognathus ovillus,* the face louse, and *Linognathus africanus,* the body louse—are also incriminated in pediculosis of sheep.

Females attach their ova to the fleece about one inch from the body. The ova are pale, translucent, and vary in color from yellow to brown. They hatch in 1 to 3 weeks, liberating nymphs which must molt three times before they become mature adults, mate, and produce ova.

The biting lice move about the body, from hair to hair, chewing at the epidermis and causing irritation and restlessness. The sucking lice are usually less mobile, although equally irritating, but are seen with their piercing mouth parts embedded in the skin.

The principal damage caused by sheep lice is to the wool. The fleece is often broken from rubbing and scratching and presents an unthrifty, ragged appearance. As the sheep continue to rub or chew at the infected areas their coats become progressively ragged, filthy, and matted, and sometimes shed in large patches.

CONTROL

Control of lice requires direct and persistent application of approved insecticides to the skin of infested animals. As lice are permanent parasites and spread by direct contact, control methods must be directed toward eradication of the parasite on the host. For strategic control, treatment is best initiated in the late fall before the onset of cold weather, although tactical measures should be started whenever lice are discovered. Treatment in the fall and again in the spring prevents a buildup of the louse population during the winter and catches those that escaped the first treatment.

Dipping of livestock is the most effective method of treatment, but in many areas dipping vats are no longer maintained. In northern latitudes, dusts are popular. Power sprayers provide a convenient means of applying both liquid and dust insecticides. Spraying equipment may be moved easily from place to place, which is more efficient than moving livestock to a central dipping vat. One disadvantage of the spraying method is the possibility of incomplete coverage with insecticide; in dipping, complete coverage is assured.

Because of current regulations concerning the use of pesticides and ecological concerns, great care must be exercised in their use.

Mites

Acariasis is a chronic, contagious skin disease of livestock and man caused by parasitic mites. It is characterized by severe inflammation of the skin and intense itching. Five species of mites infest livestock, each causing slightly different skin reactions known generally as scabies, scab, or mange.

The morphological differences of mites of similar appearance are so slight that they are considered to be varieties of the species form. There is a considerable degree of host specificity within each genus of mites, and biological races probably exist. However, most varieties can be transmitted from one host to another and established on the new host. Usually, they live for only a limited time on the unusual host, but during that time they cause annoying and serious skin reactions.

Of the five species commonly parasitic to livestock, three mites—*Sarcoptes, Demodex,* and *Psorergates*—burrow under the surface of the skin and produce what is commonly called mange, while two others—*Chorioptes* and *Psoroptes*—live upon the skin and cause the condition commonly called scabies.

Infection occurs primarily by direct contact of infested animals with healthy ones; the fully developed mites or their larvae or ova develop on the healthy skin, protected by hairy coverings or hidden between the folds of skin. Mites may be transmitted indirectly by infested blankets, harness, grooming tools, or clothing coming in contact with affected skin or touching the encrusted parts. Infection by immediate contact happens primarily when many animals live close to or in contact with one another, in feedlots, holding yards, or barns.

Although the infested animal is the most important factor in spreading mites, infested premises should not be overlooked. Owing to the varying conditions affecting the ability of the mite and its ova to remain alive when separated from a host, it is impossible to determine the length of time premises may remain infectious after the removal of infested

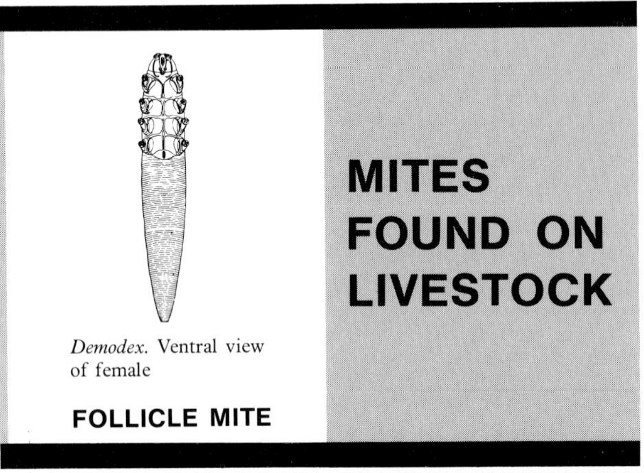

Demodex. Ventral view of female

FOLLICLE MITE

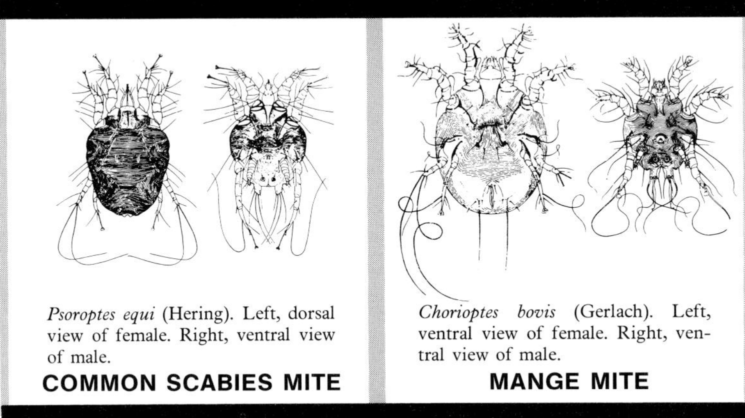

Psoroptes equi (Hering). Left, dorsal view of female. Right, ventral view of male.

COMMON SCABIES MITE

Chorioptes bovis (Gerlach). Left, ventral view of female. Right, ventral view of male.

MANGE MITE

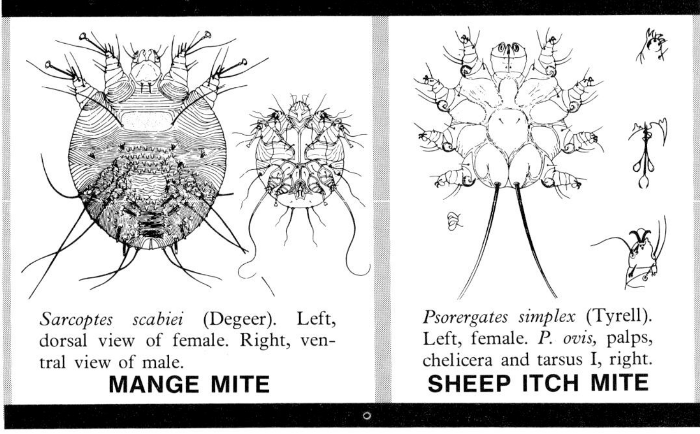

Sarcoptes scabiei (Degeer). Left, dorsal view of female. Right, ventral view of male.

MANGE MITE

Psorergates simplex (Tyrell). Left, female. *P. ovis*, palps, chelicera and tarsus I, right.

SHEEP ITCH MITE

FIG. 47. Mites found on livestock.

animals. Therefore, it is advisable to clean and disinfect all infested sheds, barns, yards, or small enclosures thoroughly before reintroducing clean animals.

Cattle, sheep, goats, and hogs are the hosts with which livestock owners are primarily concerned. All classes, ages, and conditions are susceptible to acariasis in one form or another, but usually the disease is less severe and spreads less rapidly in well-fed, vigorous animals than in weak animals. Ordinarily, the disease spreads fastest in winter when the animals may be closely confined or crowded together.

The seasonal occurrence of mange mites follows a set pattern. The mites multiply rapidly in winter and cause severe skin lesions. The lesions appear to clear up in the spring and disappear with hot weather. When cattle shed their winter coats, and sheep are shorn in the spring, most of the mites are destroyed by sunlight and drying. However, a few manage to localize and reproduce in protected sites where they will survive until the next cold season, when conditions will again be favorable for their rapid multiplication.

Sarcoptic Mange Mites

Mange mites spend their entire lives on the host animal. Sarcoptic mange mites are burrowing forms, living in galleries or tunnels in the horny layers of the skin. They are minute in size, roughly circular, whitish-gray, and scarcely visible to the naked eye. They are about 0.5 mm in length. The cuticle of the upper surface of the body is sculptured with fine wavy transverse folds or lines. In the female numerous, short, backward projecting spines may be seen on the dorsal surface.

The mature mite has four pairs of short, stumpy, thick legs provided with sucker-like organs at the tips of long unjointed pedicles on the first two pairs of legs in the female and the first, second, and fourth pairs in the male. Other legs terminate in long bristles.

A new host is infested by a mature female which penetrates the skin and works toward the inner layer of the skin. Egg-laying proceeds as the female burrows. The ova are oval, 0.15 by 0.1 mm, and 2 or 3 are laid daily over a period of about a month.

After laying 40 to 50 ova the female dies; she may usually be found at the end of a tortuous tunnel 0.5 to 3.0 cm in length. The eggs hatch in about five days and the larvae either remain in the parent tunnels, escape and wander back to the skin surface, or make new burrows. The larvae transform into the nymph stage, molt, and, finally, pubescent males and females are produced. Mating occurs either in the molting pockets or near the skin surface, whereupon the fertilized females start out to make new burrows. The life cycle from ovum to mature female may be completed in 10 days, though the average period is probably from 14 to 15 days.

Although the mites do not reproduce except when on the host itself, they can live for 2 to 3 weeks when removed from the host. Ova or mites that become dislodged and drop in moist, protected places may remain viable for 2 to 4 weeks in mild weather. They are, however, very susceptible to dessication and, if in dry surroundings and exposed to direct sunlight, are not likely to survive more than a day or two.

Sarcoptes scabiei var. *suis* causes mange and is the only mite of any significance to occur on swine.

Swine usually become infested with *Sarcoptes* by direct contact with infested animals. However, infestation may occur when clean hogs are placed in pens and yards where infested swine have recently been kept. The possibility that hogs may pick up the mite from contaminated premises should be kept in mind at all times.

All types, breeds, and ages of swine are susceptible to sarcoptic mange, though well-fed, healthy, and well-cared-for animals appear to have considerably more resistance to the devastating effects of the parasite than do unthrifty animals.

The first lesions of sarcoptic mange are usually seen around the snout, eyes, ears, or any place where the skin is tender and the hair is thin. In older pigs, lesions are frequently seen around the ears, tail, and on the inside of the hindlegs, in the region of the groin and shoulder pits. From these areas the mites spread and multiply until large areas of the skin become involved. Lesions may be observed six weeks after original exposure, or a much longer period may elapse before they appear.

As a result of sensitization of the infested

animal, considerable irritation, itching, inflammation, and swelling of the tissues occur. The intense itching causes the animal to scratch and rub vigorously. Scratching liberates the tissue fluids from the small vesicles around the burrow of the mite. This serum coagulates, dries, and forms crusts on the surface of the skin. Excessive keratinization and proliferation of connective tissue occur, so that the skin becomes thickened and wrinkled. In advanced cases, the heavily scabbed areas may crack, blood and serum may ooze out, and an offensive odor may be noted from the moist lesions.

Sarcoptes scabiei var. *bovis,* the mites causing sarcoptic mange in cattle, are found more often in dairy cattle and purebred bulls than in range cattle, although the incidence of the disease is low and it is not found at all in some states.

Sarcoptic mites, in establishing themselves on cattle, prefer areas where the hair is thin and the skin is tender. These first lesions are frequently found on the escutcheon or the inner surface of the thighs. From these regions the mites spread to the inside of the flanks and, as the disease progresses, along the abdomen to the brisket, posteriorly over the outer surface of the legs, upward on the root of the tail and downward on the legs. If the disease is not checked, the mites may cover the entire surface of the body. The affected areas show loss of hair and the skin becomes covered with heavy crust or scabs. In extensive and chronic cases, the involved skin becomes thickened and wrinkled, and takes on a typical elephant-skin appearance. The animals lose flesh, become emaciated and greatly weakened, and unless properly treated many of them die, especially under unfavorable weather conditions.

The parasites burrow into the skin, each mite making a separate gallery over which the skin becomes inflamed and swollen. The swollen areas are somewhat larger than pinheads and often a yellowish granule of dried serum adheres to them. As the mites multiply, the diseased area increases and the granular or raised areas come closer together. The hair over the affected part stands erect and some

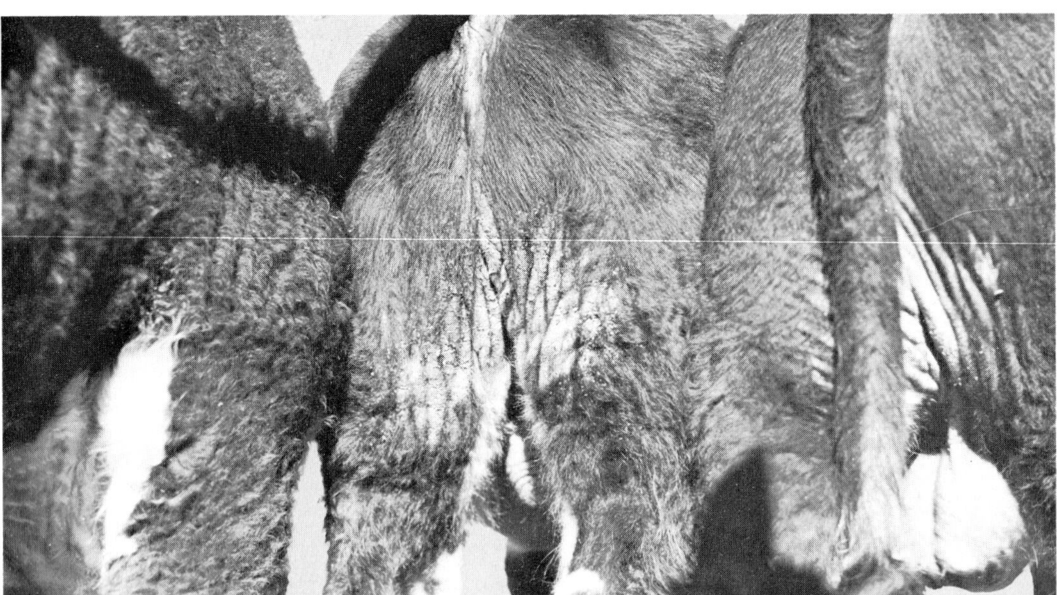

FIG. 48. Feedlot cattle with sarcoptic scabies. (From Jensen, R., and Mackey, D. R.: *Diseases of Feedlot Cattle.* Ed. 2, Philadelphia, Lea & Febiger, 1971.)

of it drops out or is rubbed off, although usually a few scattered hairs remain even in advanced cases. When the mites are inactive, the skin takes on a dry, scurfy, or leather-like appearance.

To relieve the intense itching, the animals lick, scratch, and rub the affected parts until the skin becomes raw. The mechanical injury results in a running together of the small lesions, and large scabs are formed. When the disease reaches this stage it resembles psoroptic mange and can be differentiated only by identifying the mite. Most of the lesions disappear during the summer, but on careful examination small lesions may still be found around the base of the tail or on the underside of the abdomen.

Sarcoptic mange in sheep, caused by *Sarcoptes scabiei* var. *ovis,* commonly called head scab, is not very important, but when it does occur the mites frequent only the nonwooly areas of the skin.

Psoroptic Mange Mites

Psoroptes bovis, the mite causing common cattle scab, may attack any part of the body covered thickly with hair, the first lesions usually occurring on the withers, over the back, or around the root of the tail. It spreads to other areas, and unless checked may involve practically the entire body. These mites are unable to burrow, and therefore complete their life span on the skin of the host.

The psoroptic mites prick the skin to obtain nourishment and in so doing cause a slight inflammation, but this early stage of the disease is rarely detected. As the mites multiply, large numbers of small wounds are made in the skin and are followed by intense itching, formation of papules, inflammation, and exudation of serum. The serum oozing to the surface becomes infected with microorganisms. This mass soon hardens into yellowish or gray-colored crusts frequently

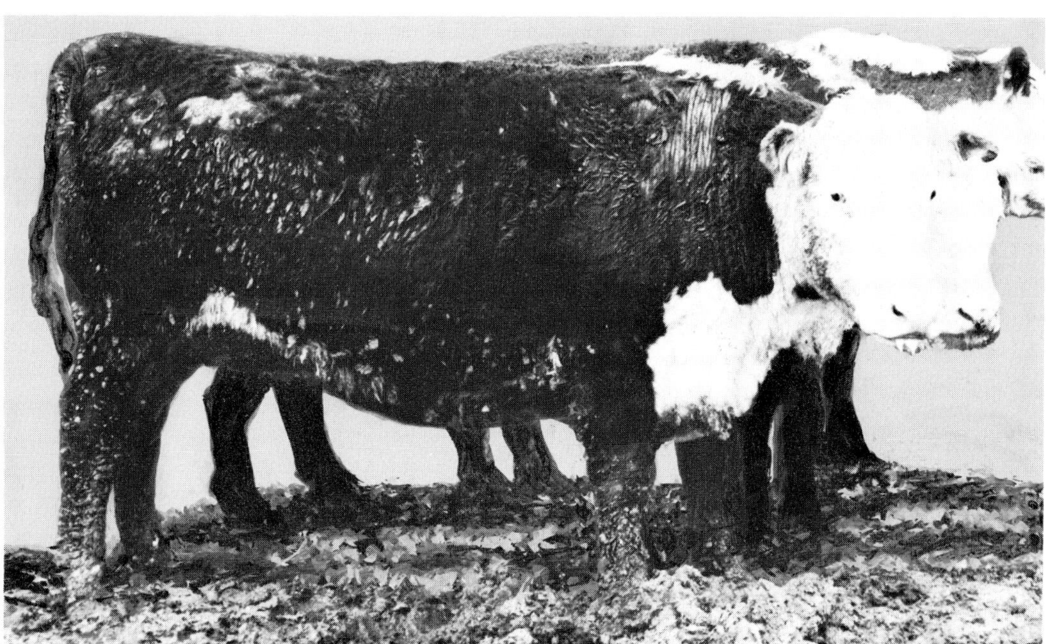

FIG. 49. Steers with psoroptic mange. (From Jensen, R., and Mackey, D. R.: *Diseases of Feedlot Cattle.* Ed. 2, Philadelphia, Lea & Febiger, 1971.)

stained with blood. In the early stages the scab may be about the size of a pea, but as the mites seek the healthy skin around the edges of the wound the crust gradually increases in size.

Some mites migrate to other parts of the body and start new lesions, which extend until they cover large areas. As the disease advances, increasingly large areas become denuded of hair and covered with thick, adherent crusts or scabs. The skin becomes tumefied, corrugated, and greatly thickened. The itching is severe and the animal is constantly irritated. In its efforts to relieve the itching and irritation the animal spends so much time licking, rubbing, and scratching that it has very little time for grazing. Consequently, it loses flesh, becomes weak and emaciated, and unless relieved finally dies.

Psoroptes ovis, the cause of sheep scab, has been known for two thousand years to exist wherever sheep are raised.

A little more than a half century ago, sheep scab was the greatest handicap to the sheep industry in the western states, and it also caused heavy losses in the corn-belt states. In fact, sheep scabies was so widespread that many ranchers were deterred from engaging in the sheep business, and farmers refused to buy undipped sheep for feeding purposes. So prevalent was the disease that in 1896 England prohibited the importation of sheep from the United States.

Economic losses are caused by mortality rates to 80 percent of massively infested susceptible flocks, destruction of fleece, and stress to survivors causing loss of condition and lowered production.

The female mite lays ova upon the thickly-wooled areas of the skin where they hatch in

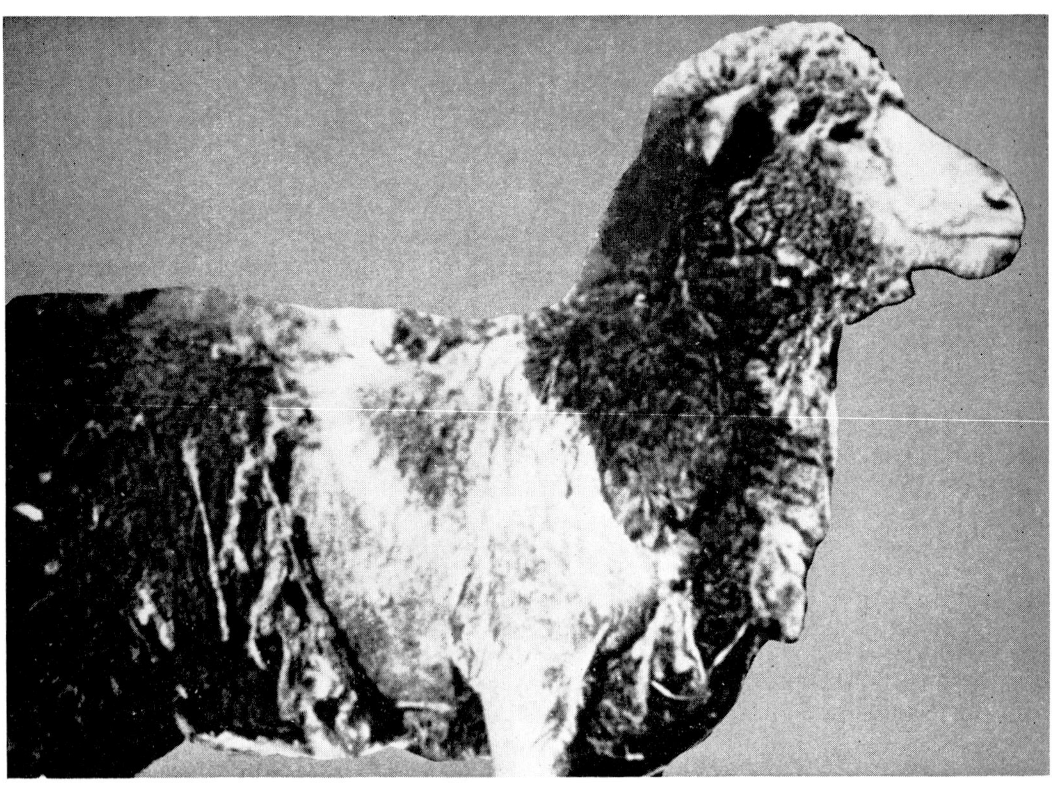

FIG. 50. Psoroptic mange. Note denuding of wool and scabbing of skin. (From Gibbons, W. J.: *Clinical Diagnosis of Diseases of Large Animals.* Philadelphia, Lea & Febiger, 1966.)

1 to 3 days, feed for 2 or 3 days, molt and become nymphs. The nymphs feed for 3 to 4 days and become adults. Thus, a few invading adults may have millions of descendants on a single host in a relatively short time.

These mites do not burrow under the skin, but the adults pierce the skin with their mouth parts and suck blood and tissue fluid. The skin wounds develop pustules which rupture and coalesce, leaking exudate which hardens to form crusts under which developing mites may be found.

Intense itching is usually the first symptom noted. The peak of the symptoms usually occurs about three months after initial infection, when the affected animals have developed anemia, a gradual loss of weight and loss of appetite. The wool becomes loose and is pulled out or rubbed off by the efforts of the sheep to obtain relief from itching. In heavy infestations the mites invade the ear canals, leading to rubbing of the head and further restlessness. Many sheep will die of sheep scabies unless treated.

Psoroptic sheep scabies is considered by the United States Department of Agriculture to be of such economic importance to livestock producers that the disease is reportable in all states and infested flocks are subject to quarantine until the mites are eliminated.

Chorioptic Mange Mites

Chorioptes bovis causes the most common type of mange found in cattle. Chorioptic mange mites do not usually produce such severe and conspicuous lesions as do either the psoroptic or sarcoptic mites. Furthermore, they do not spread as rapidly as do the psoroptic mites. After they have pierced the skin a small papule is formed. As the mites multiply, the papules merge with other adjoining ones and gradually build up a sizable inflamed area on the skin. Each papule exudes a small quantity of serum, which dries and leaves a thin crust. Under the crust the skin may be raw and inflamed. As the disease progresses, the skin becomes thickened and wrinkled, has a roughened corrugated appearance, is largely devoid of hair, and is covered with a thin, dried crust.

The chorioptic mites live in colonies on the skin, pierce the epidermis with their mouth parts and ingest lymph. The life cycle is similar to that of psoroptic mites, although it requires 19 to 23 days for completion. As a result, the spread of skin lesions is slow but inexorable.

The lesions of chorioptic mange are most commonly found on the escutcheon. From this region the mites spread upward to the base of the tail or downward to the inside of the thighs and forward to the flanks. In the more advanced cases, lesions extend to both the inside and outside of the hocks. Lesions, however, may be found almost anywhere on the body. They are less frequent around the coronary bands of the feet, but may appear above the knees and on the brisket.

Chorioptic mites cause considerable itching, although apparently not so severe as that produced by either psoroptic or sarcoptic mites. Infested animals kick and bite themselves, scratch themselves with their hind feet, rub against adjoining cattle, stamp their feet, switch their tails in the absence of flies, and strike their bodies with their hind feet. They commonly rub against stanchions, posts, trees, or any solid object.

The lesions develop rapidly in the winter, especially when the cattle are stabled, and it is during this period that the animals suffer most. As the weather warms in the spring, the lesions gradually recede. During the hot part of the summer, especially when the cattle are out in the open, the disease virtually disappears. However, symptoms appear on the same animals in the fall, and mange develops again during the winter.

Demodectic Mange Mites

A minute mite called *Demodex folliculorum* causes demodectic mange in domestic animals. There is lack of agreement as to the

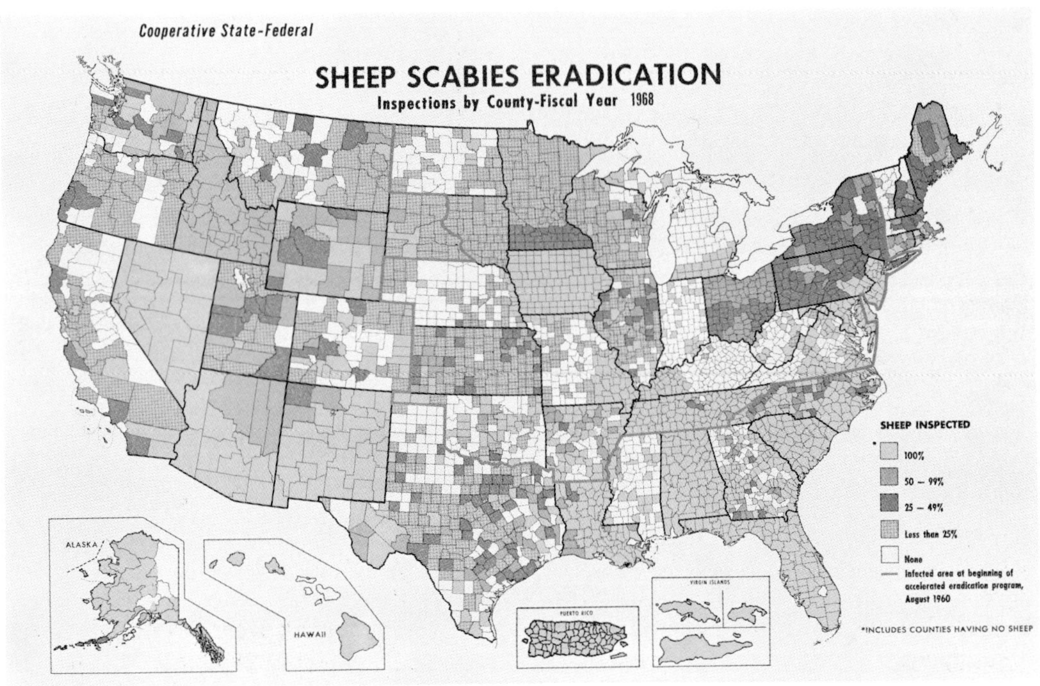

FIG. 51. Sheep scabies eradication.

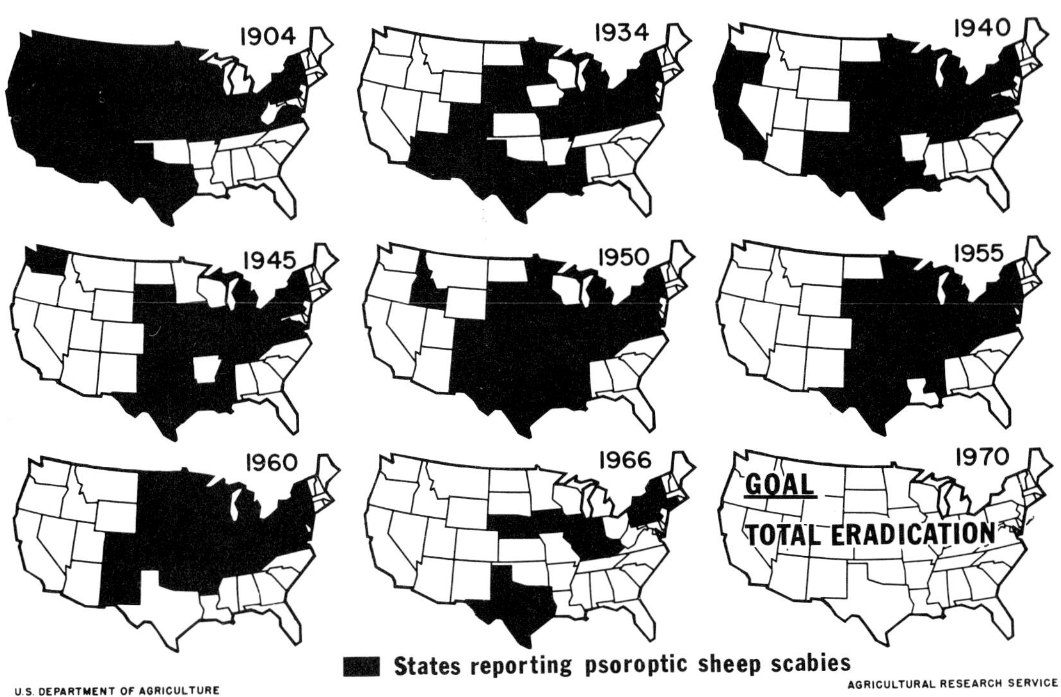

FIG. 52. Story of sheep scabies eradication.

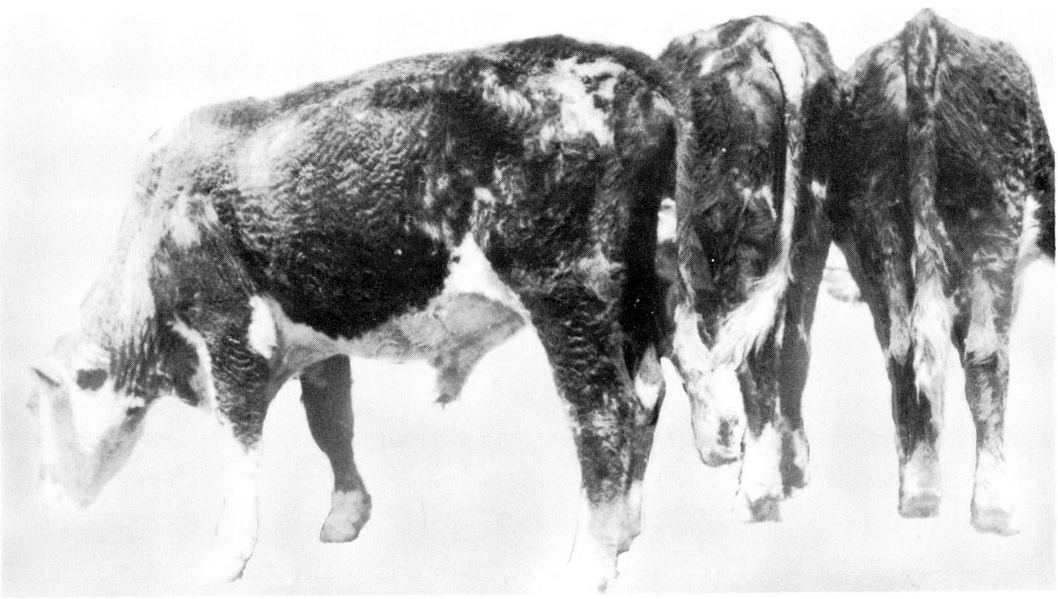

FIG. 53. Cattle with chorioptic scabies. (From Jensen, R., and Mackey, D. R.: *Diseases of Feedlot Cattle.* Ed. 2, Philadelphia, Lea & Febiger, 1971.)

host specificity of this mite. Many scientists believe there is only one form, but others believe that each host has its specific variety. Likewise, the life cycle is not fully known.

The mites live in the hair follicles and in the sebaceous glands, the tissues being injured mechanically or by the toxins produced. In cattle, demodectic mange is diagnosed most often in animals between 4 and 8 years of age. The course of the disease is mild and recovery is often spontaneous. In swine, sheep, and goats the clinical signs are similar to those found in cattle, although in goats the infestation occasionally progresses into a stubborn skin condition with serious damage to the hides.

The lesions of demodectic mange usually appear as nodules, most often in the skin of the neck, shoulders, breast, dewlap, and sometimes other parts. The nodules vary from the size of a pinhead to that of a hazelnut or larger. Except in advanced cases there are no marked changes in the hair coat, and, ordinarily, the lesions are not visible until the hair is parted. The nodules can be detected by passing the hand over the body with the fingers pressed firmly against the skin.

The nodules are usually firm, but in advanced cases several may unite to form a small abscess. When these larger lesions rupture and discharge their contents over the surrounding hair and skin, the condition resembles scabies. Ordinarily, the nodules contain a creamy-white material of cheesy consistency, and usually it is necessary to lance the nodule to obtain material for examination.

Psorergatic Mites

Psorergates ovis and *Psorergates bovis* are recently discovered mites infecting sheep and cattle, although they may also be found on mice and voles.

The psorergatic mites are about one third as big as the other mange mites. They cause a mild irritation and itchiness similar to that caused by lice. Sheep bite and scratch the parts most easily reached, such as the sides, flank and rump. Tags of wool are pulled out and the fleece has a ragged, tangled appearance.

The mite burrows into the skin, causing thickening, roughening, and scaling of the affected parts. The scabs are usually loose, dry and crumbly. Moist spots sometimes exist in the lesion.

The small size and the burrowing of the mites make them hard to find. Deep skin scrapings must be made with a scalpel or pocketknife and the material examined in light mineral oil under a microscope. The infection spreads slowly and may take 3 to 4 years to become generalized on sheep, and possibly longer on cattle.

Diagnosis

A positive diagnosis of mange depends upon finding the mites which cause the symptoms. To find them, scrape the outer edges of an infected area with a blunt-edged knife, transfer the scraping to a smooth, dark surface or a glass slide. If the scrapings are spread in the warm sun or near artificial heat, the mites become active and can be seen as minute, gray bodies moving against the background. They are plainly visible under a powered hand lens. By parting the hair of infested animals and removing the small scabs, the mites can sometimes be seen on the underlying moist, red skin and removed upon the point of a knife blade for examination. When the mites are causing irritation and the surface of the skin around the edges of the lesion, or under the small scabs, is red and moist, the parasites are usually present in large numbers. If the lesions and surrounding skin are dry and dull in appearance, the mites are probably inactive and will be difficult to find.

Control

If mites are found in a herd or flock, the grounds, pens, barns, corrals, and other premises frequented by infested livestock should be thoroughly cleaned and disinfected.

Remove and burn all litter, manure, and bedding to which mites may cling. Spray all exposed surfaces of buildings with one of the permitted dips or disinfectants. Mite-free livestock may safely occupy properly disinfected premises or buildings.

The control of scabies and mange of livestock requires the external application of chemicals capable of destroying the parasites without harming the animals. Dipping and spraying are the two methods of treatment commonly used. Dipping is the only method recognized by the U.S. Department of Agriculture for the official treatment of scabies in livestock. It is the most practical and effective method known, for the entire surface of the body receives a thorough wetting. Dipping vats are usually arranged so that cattle enter at one end, swim through the solution, and leave at the opposite end.

Spraying to control parasitic mites is done in many places because dipping vats are scarce. Spraying is less effective than dipping, since it may not thoroughly wet the hair coat and skin on all parts of the body. Scabies and mange can be cured, however, if generous amounts of liquid are used and the work is done carefully. Two sprayings with recommended pesticides, 10 to 12 days apart, are recommended. High-pressure power operated equipment is usually necessary, as a pressure of 200 to 400 pounds per square inch should be maintained.

Infestations of psoroptic, chorioptic, and sarcoptic mites are considered contagious and are reportable diseases in all states. Infested herds and individual animals are subject to quarantine and treatment under governmental supervision until the mites are eliminated. Livestock inspectors are stationed at public stockyards, sales yards, shipping terminals, and strategic inspection stations to prevent animals with contagious diseases from entering interstate commerce and to discover infested animals and their herds or flocks of origin.

58

Insects

INSECT pests in livestock are the cause of more loss to ranchers and farmers than any other single entity. In addition to damaging animals directly, they break down their resistance and make them susceptible to other microorganisms. They are often the transmitting agents of pathogenic microorganisms.

Hypoderma

Cattle grubs and heel flies are among the most destructive pests attacking cattle. Nearly all cattlemen know the conspicuous swellings which appear in the backs of cattle in winter; these swellings contain grubs, which are the maggot stage of heel flies.

Cattle grubs are larvae of two species of botflies, *Hypoderma bovis* and *Hypoderma lineatus.* In the United States, the first species is called the northern cattle grub and the second is called the common cattle grub. The disease caused by both species is called hypodermiasis.

The characteristic reaction (running about excitedly) of the cattle to the egg-laying activities of the flies is often referred to as gadding. Some people mistakenly think that the frightened running of the cattle is caused by the fly trying to sting or bite the animals, or trying to insert its eggs into the skin of the animal.

The larvae of *Hypoderma* are termed ox warbles, and the adults are referred to as warble flies. Warble also is a term applied to the inflammatory process resulting from the presence of second- and third-stage larvae in the subcutis of the animal's back.

These insects are obligatory parasites of cattle, and, to a limited extent, of a few other animals. Only one generation is produced each year, and the larvae spend their entire development period inside the body of the host.

Although the cattle grub has been present for thousands of years, only within the last hundred years has any serious attempt been made to assess the damage caused by larvae of *Hypoderma* species or to eliminate the loss.

Life Cycle

The life cycle of the two species of cattle grubs is quite similar, differing only in oviposition habits, migration routes, and seasonal occurrence.

Adult flies emerge from pupae early in the morning. They are sexually mature and have been observed to mate as soon as one hour after emergence. Mating is brief, and the females are capable of laying fertile eggs 20 minutes later.

The flies do not have functional mouth parts, and therefore do not feed. They are very active, and exhaust themselves rapidly if weather conditions are favorable for egg laying. They may live only 2 to 3 days if the weather is warm, but during periods of cool weather they are less active and have been known to live as long as 25 days.

The best information available indicates that heel flies range less than a mile from the emergence site if cattle are available, but are capable of much longer flights if necessary to find cattle for oviposition.

Heel flies are active during different months in different parts of the world, but typically appear during the first warm, sunny days of spring. The adults of *Hypoderma bovis* are determined and persistent in their attacks on cattle. They deposit their eggs one at a time in quick succession, and terrorize the cattle far more than does *H. lineatus.* The heel or lower leg is the preferred place for the eggs of *H. bovis,* but, as the flies deposit eggs while pursuing the running animals, many eggs are deposited higher on the legs, especially on the thighs and on the rump.

In contrast, the adults of the common cattle grub are often unnoticed by the cattle. They may cause some gadding, but frequently they approach the animals while they are lying down and attach their eggs to the hairs on the udder, the escutcheon, or the side near the ground. The eggs are attached in rows of 2 or 3 to 25 or 30 along a single hair. Each female may lay from 400 to 800 eggs, the average number being approximately 500. The eggs hatch in 2 to 6 days depending on the temperature. With the common cattle grub, the eggs nearest the body hatch sooner than those located farther out on the hair, apparently because of the influence of body heat.

The larva of both species of *Hypoderma* emerges from the distal end of the egg and crawls along the hair to the skin. It usually penetrates the skin through or near the hair follicle by use of its mouth parts and movement of its body, with assistance from the action of enzymatic secretion. Several hours are required for the larva to penetrate the skin. When several larvae enter the skin near one place, a rash occurs from which clear serum is secreted. The rash is readily apparent shortly after penetration and remains visible for a week or more, when a dry scab forms and the rash disappears.

After penetration of the animal's skin, the larva enters the connective tissue through which it migrates for a period of approximately 8 months before reaching the back of the animal. The two species differ in that larvae of the northern cattle grub migrate to the vertebral canal while those of the common cattle grub go to the esophagus. They spend several months in these areas before moving to an area immediately under the skin on the animal's back. When the larva reaches the back it cuts a small hole, usually called a breathing hole. After a 3- to 4-day period of rest, the larva molts to the second stage.

Growth of the second-stage larva is rapid, but there is a gradual change from the second to the third stage. The second stage is milky white but, as the third stage forms, the color becomes first tan and then progressively darker until at the time of emergence it is quite dark and in some instances completely black.

The time spent in the larval stages varies with species and geographic location. In Texas, the larval period in the animal's back may be as short as 35 days for *H. lineatus,* while in Montana a period of 99 days has been observed for *H. bovis*. The average period appears to be about 50 days for *H. lineatus* and 65 for *H. bovis*.

The larva is larger in diameter than the exit hole, but it forces itself out segment by segment; it usually takes 2 to 3 minutes for this process. The larva then drops to the ground and crawls to the nearest shelter, often no more than debris or leaves. There it becomes inactive and in 2 or 3 days turns into a pupa. The length of the pupal period depends on the temperature of the area. The adults of *H. lineatus* may emerge in less than 3 weeks in Texas, while in Canada the time may be as long as 60 days. The time spent in the pupal stage by *H. bovis* may be shorter in the northern states since it emerges from one to two months later, in the spring when the weather is warmer.

Distribution of Species

In North America *Hypoderma bovis* is abundant in southern Canada and extends as far south as an imaginary line through the northern part of South Carolina, Tennessee, Oklahoma, Arizona, and the southern part of California. Although many *H. bovis*-infested cattle are shipped south of this line, the species does not ordinarily perpetuate itself in states farther south, such as Texas.

Hypoderma lineatus is found in all states except Alaska, and in Canada. Heel fly activity may occur at various times of the year, depending on the locality and the temperature. In west Texas, it is not uncommon to see heel fly activity from September to January. In this area, larvae of *H. lineatus* may be found in animals' backs as early as July; however, most larvae appear in September and October. Thus, treatment of cattle in or from western Texas with systemic grubicides can be dangerous after July 1, since many larvae are congregated in the esophageal region at that time. In some areas of the southwest, grubs are never present in the esophageal region in sufficient numbers to cause trouble, even though systemic grubicide treatments are applied at the time the larvae are in the esophagus.

Host-parasite Relationship

Both species of *Hypoderma* larvae are dependent upon the host for the entirety of their parasitic existence, which spans several months. Other than the reaction shown toward adult flies during oviposition and some slight irritation at the time of larval penetration into the skin, the host shows no visible signs of incompatibility as long as the natural movement of the larva is not disturbed. However, when many larvae have accumulated in the esophagus or vertebral canal and are killed by the administration of a systemic organophosphate, the reactions are sometimes quite severe; the degree of reaction is directly dependent upon the number and size of the larvae. When many larvae are present in the esophagus at the time of treatment, enough foreign protein is released by the disintegrating larvae to cause swelling to the extent that the animal may bloat. If many larvae are present in the vertebral canal, the resulting swelling may produce partial to complete paralysis of the hindquarters. These signs are frequently mistaken for toxic symptoms caused by the systemic grubicide. Such signs are generally transitory, and subside in 48 to 72 hours or less.

Control

The transportation of cattle from various areas to feedlots often creates problems when grub-control treatments are applied. The location of the larvae in these animals usually does not correspond to the larval development in native cattle. It is, therefore, extremely important to know the origin of cattle before systemic grub treatments are applied. A concerted effort should be made to treat animals as soon as possible after the adult heel fly has ceased egg-laying activity. Treatment at this period will avoid the host-parasite reactions noted above, and at the same time will not result in unsightly swellings on the backs of infected cattle at a later date, as the minute larvae will be killed in situ.

Profit losses from grubs and heel flies are estimated at up to 400 million each year. These losses occur through: (1) injury and weight loss caused by running to escape the adult heel flies during the egg-laying season; (2) slower weight gains and even loss of weight or milk flow in heavily-infested herds; (3) injury to the hide by perforation of grubs, thus lowering hide values; (4) injury to meat by the grubs, causing extra trimming of damaged flesh.

It is easy to detect animals being attacked by the heel fly. The animals run and kick up their heels, with their tails in the air, when attempting to evade the flies. They commonly injure themselves in attempts to escape the attacks of the flies. Cattle constantly attacked by heel flies do not graze and feed properly and will thus lose weight.

To control cattle grubs, it is necessary to have a knowledge of the particular cycle in the area in which the cattle are raised. The most recent method of control is by systemic insecticides or grubicides which are absorbed through the skin. The circulatory system carries the insecticide to the site where the grubs localize. Only one application is necessary, but it should be made as soon as possible after heel fly activity has stopped for the year.

Face Fly

In recent years a new pest of livestock called *Musca autumnalis,* or face fly, has moved into the United States and is causing concern among livestock producers. At first this pest affected cattle only in the extreme northeastern part of the nation. By 1960, however, it had spread to every state east of the Mississippi River north of and including Kentucky and North Carolina, and to some states west of the Mississippi—Iowa, Kansas, Minnesota, Nebraska, North Dakota, Missouri, Wyoming and California. In many areas face flies are so profuse that they have seriously decreased milk production, prevented proper gains in beef cattle, and created difficulties in handling horses. For example, infestations of 200 flies per head of cattle were reported in New York, over 100 flies per head in Vermont and 75 flies per head in New Jersey. It is apparent that in some states the face fly has become the single most important insect affecting livestock. This pest is continuing to spread to other areas, particularly along main transportation routes, and it probably will be only a matter of time before the whole nation is infested.

The pest probably came from Europe, where cattle have been bothered by it for years. The face fly came to North America in 1952, first reported in Nova Scotia. It was discovered in the United States in 1953, on Long Island, New York. The worldwide distribution of the face fly now includes parts of Canada and the United States, Europe (and the British Isles), Israel, Kashmir, and China.

The egg of the face fly is stalked, and the mature larva has a characteristic yellow color. The adult resembles an oversized housefly except that it is somewhat darker. The male face fly has eyes set very close together, practically meeting. His abdomen is orange-yellow with a black median stripe. The cheeks are white and the thorax is bluish gray. The female's eyes are set wider apart, the abdomen is light gray, the cheeks are gray and the thorax is slate gray with four broad black stripes.

Life Cycle

Male flies and hibernating females seem content to live on a diet of nectar and pollen and pose no particular threat to livestock. The active female causes the damage. She apparently needs animal secretions for producing eggs. Up to 30 eggs are laid singly in fresh feces by one female; several hundred, however, may be laid in a single dung pat. Most eggs are deposited by the time the feces are 20 minutes old, as the droppings lose their attractiveness within an hour through drying and crusting. The eggs incubate in 10 to 23 hours, and emerging larvae live in and feed upon the fresh manure. Larvae complete their development in 3 to 4 days. Pupation then occurs in the feces and the adult emerges about two weeks after oviposition.

Face flies hibernate in large numbers in buildings, barns, unheated attics, and other protected places during the winter. With the coming of warm weather the infestation begins and increases until late fall. Female insects accumulate primarily on the faces of animals, under and around the eyes, where they cause irritation and profuse lacrimation, and around the lips and nostrils. The face fly feeds on secretions from these areas and also on blood from wounds, injuries, and horsefly and other insect bites. Face-fly populations increase when biting flies are present, because blood from the bites provides additional food. Odor is probably the attractant.

Symptoms

The animals serving as primary hosts for the face fly are cattle, open-faced sheep, and horses. Flies attacking the moisture around the eyes, nose, and mouth during the warmer months interfere with normal grazing. Swarms of face flies cause nervousness in herds of cattle, and milk production decreases in lactating animals. Because these animals are trying to get rid of the flies, they neglect to graze; they therefore undergo weight loss and their weakened condition invites infestation from other disease vectors. The face fly has been incriminated as a mechanical spreader of *Moraxella bovis,* the cause of pinkeye, and of other diseases, and it is an intermediate host of mammalian eyeworm.

Control

Research has made little progress in developing effective materials and methods for control of the face fly; for one thing, it is difficult to rear these flies in the laboratory. Three methods of approach to control now under investigation involve the use of pesticide sprays, poison baits and feed additives. Sprays have given only temporary relief, and more than one application per day are necessary; work is being done to determine the required number. Poison baits have been more effective. Baits containing malathion, DDVP or Deptrix have been tested with favorable results. A 2 percent DDVP solution in syrup applied to the forehead worked well; it made the cattle unsightly, however, and they licked the syrup from each other's heads. Feed additives, or insecticides in range blocks, involve chemicals that will pass unchanged with feces, are harmless to the host, but will kill larvae developing in the feces. Feed additives are not designed to be systemic controls. With range cattle, insecticides can be applied with back-rubbers, or automatic spray devices on mineral and salt feeders. Proper placement of equipment or blocks is essential to encourage their use; otherwise, cattle will seek shade to avoid the flies.

In the years that the face fly has been in the United States, it has spread over wide areas and become a serious problem. It serves as an excellent example of the constant threat posed by exotic diseases and parasites to our economy and health. Although research is constantly ongoing to eliminate such diseases, they can get out of hand before appreciable control is developed. Further, control measures are limited by restrictions on the use of insecticides with cattle intended for slaughter and especially with dairy cattle. If face flies are detected in any area where they have not been seen before, swift control measures should be initiated to prevent their spread, aimed at restricting their breeding as well as killing them in their hibernating sites.

Screwworm

Myiasis is the term used to indicate any disease caused by the presence of larvae of flies on or in the living tissues and organs of man or animals. Screwworm myiasis is caused by the larvae of a dipterous fly which attacks all warm-blooded animals and deposits its ova in all kinds of fresh wounds. When the ova hatch, a cutaneous myiasis is initiated. The mature larval body tapers from a large posterior diameter and possesses clusters of spines which surround the body at each segment; thus the larva morphologically resembles a wood screw, from which it gets its name. It is bluish or blue-green and about twice the size of the housefly.

The screwworm, *Cochliomyia hominivorax,* is an obligatory parasite of warm-blooded animals. It has caused animal suffering and serious livestock losses for more than 125 years. Present annual livestock losses in the southwest are estimated to range to 100 million dollars. Wildlife losses are also known to be great, but estimates of total losses are not available.

Losses may occur as a result of death, crippling weight losses, or increased susceptibility to diseases. Labor that must be provided for animal inspections and treatment, and money spent for material for prevention or treatment of screwworm injury, also represent losses to livestock producers.

Screwworms have been known in Texas since 1842. During the summer months infestations spread to adjoining states, but subsequent cold, winter weather usually killed all but those in the Mexican border region. Screwworms were unknown in the southeast until the summer of 1933, when the first infestations were noted in Georgia. The flies spread rapidly and in a few years were found all over the southeast, although cold weather usually killed those which had migrated from the southern Florida reservoir.

By 1959, persistent efforts by cooperating federal and state agencies had eradicated screwworm flies from the southeastern part of the country, but they are still a menace in the southwest. The flies overwinter in the mild areas of Texas, New Mexico, Arizona, California and Mexico, and move northward in the summer months.

The adult fly is attracted by any fresh wound, such as a wire cut, scratch, castration, dehorning, branding, tick bite, fly bite, and the navel of a newly born animal. The extent of the infestation, the tissues involved, and the depth of penetration of the larvae depend on the number of active larvae and on whether or not the infestation is treated.

Life Cycle

The female lays eggs in batches of about 250 along the edges of open wounds. One female can lay about 4,000 eggs during her lifetime. While the fly lays her eggs in all types of wounds, she prefers fresh abrasions.

Within hours, the eggs hatch into tiny larvae or maggots that burrow deeply into the wound. At this stage, the larvae are barely visible and almost impossible to detect in a fly or tick bite, even on close inspection. Larvae do not crawl over the wound. With their rasping mouth parts, they tear at the wound and feed on the exudate for 5 to 6 days, growing to about one-half inch in length. They feed with their heads down; the tail, or blunt end, is exposed for breathing. An infested wound attracts additional female screwworm flies which lay eggs, and the toxemia and continuous destruction of these multiple infestations usually cause death of the host animal unless treated. The newly hatched larvae crowd together, lie into and rapidly destroy the host tissue by their feeding.

When fully developed, larvae drop from the wound and burrow into the soil to form brown, tough-shelled pupae. After about a week, screwworm flies emerge from the pupal shells. The life cycle of the screwworm averages about three weeks, but can be as long as 65 days during cold weather.

Symptoms

The clinical signs associated with screwworm myiasis are acute pain, apprehension, nervousness, and malodorous wounds. One of the most convenient aids for recognizing screwworm myiasis in range animals is the change in their behavior. Infested animals will separate from the rest of the herd or flock, seek shade, and bite and scratch at the infested wound. Even a small wound produces an odor that attracts not only screwworm flies but secondary blowflies as well. If wounds are untreated, the area of infestation increases through the addition of new larvae, and the secondary fly larvae attack necrotic tissue. In the terminal stages of an extensive infestation, the host is depressed, disoriented, and often prostrated. Death may occur after about ten days.

Control

Treatment of screwworm infestations is accomplished by the proper and timely application of insecticides which are not toxic to the infested host. An old remedy is the application of benzol to kill the larvae, but this will not prevent reinfestation. About 1940, a formulation known as Smear 62 was developed by the Bureau of Entomology and Plant Quarantine of the United States Department of Agriculture and was found highly effective in controlling screwworm infestation. This medication will protect wounds for about three days; it is, however, inferior to EQ-335, developed about 1950. The latter contains lindane, is less volatile than Smear 62 (which contains benzol), and is more effective in that screwworm flies returning to a treated wound will be killed through the residual action of the lindane. Reapplication of both of these formulations may be necessary until wound healing has occurred.

Prevention of screwworm infestations depends to a great extent on good management practices and the use of effective and approved insecticidal formulations. Fences, corrals, and equipment should be kept in good repair so that animals do not suffer cuts, minor wounds, scratches, and abrasions. Cuts from the milk teeth of suckling pigs and lacerations from rough handling may attract adult screwworm flies. Procedures such as castration and ear-tagging should be performed during the cooler months of the year when the screwworm menace is at a minimum.

If such recommendations cannot be met, all wounds should be treated with an approved screwworm remedy and the wounded animals placed in close confinement where they can be examined daily and treated until the wounds heal.

In response to strong interest on the part of livestock producers and others, the Secretary of Agriculture on February 13, 1962 announced the beginning of a cooperative program to eradicate screwworms from large areas of the southwest. Screwworm flies have already been completely eliminated by this method in the southeast, particularly in Florida.

This program seeks to eradicate the worms by releasing laboratory-raised flies made sterile by exposing the pupae to gamma rays from radioactive cobalt. These sterile male flies mate with normal screwworm females and they are unable to produce offspring (the flies mate only once in a lifetime). A plant for producing sterile screwworm flies located near Mission, Texas, can produce millions of such flies per week.

Although the eradication program may take a long time, progress is being made and the next few years could see the screwworm pest problem eliminated within the United States. The livestock producer may aid in this program by following very closely the nine steps outlined by the U.S. Department of Agriculture:

1. Examine animals regularly for open wounds.
2. Manage livestock as to prevent injury.
3. Collect maggots or eggs in wounds, put them in alcohol or water and send them to the U.S.D.A. for positive identification.

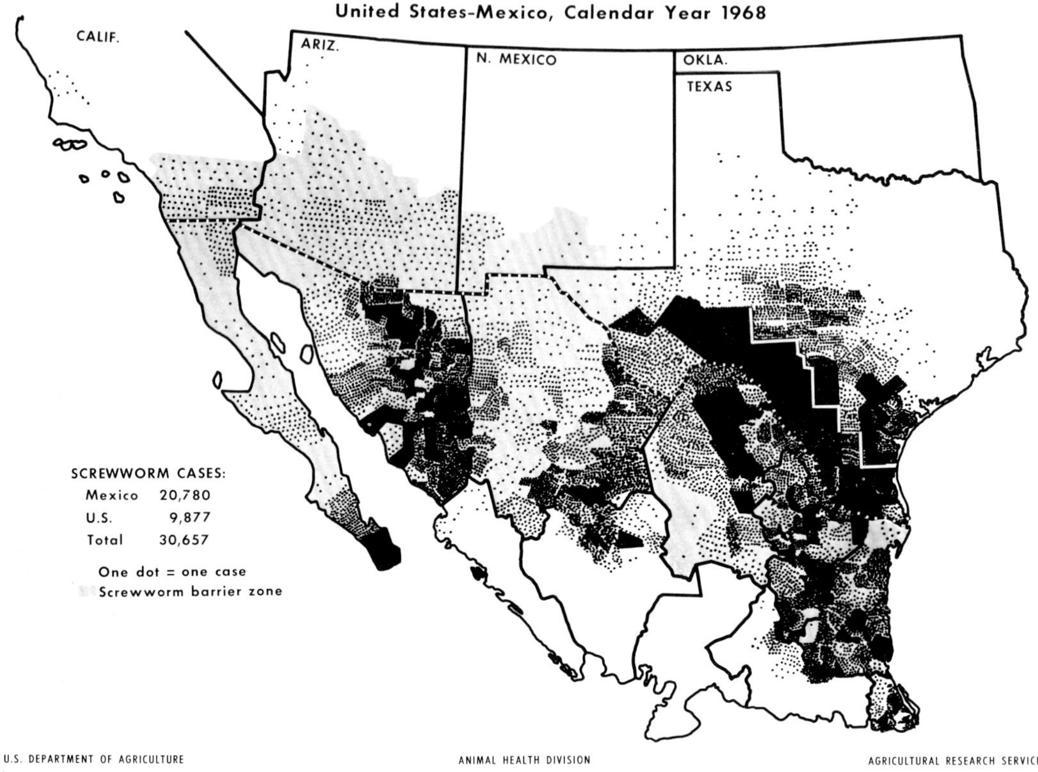

FIG. 54. Concentration of laboratory-confirmed screwworm cases, 1968.

4. Treat wounds with proper medication.
5. Apply approved preventive sprays.
6. Observe closely restrictions on animals and animal shipments.
7. Check purchased animals to be sure they are free of screwworms at point of origin.
8. Cooperate with neighbors and the U.S. Department of Agriculture.
9. Maintain constant vigilance for screwworms.

Horn Flies, Stable Flies, Deer Flies

Horn Flies

These are small black flies that appear in large numbers on cattle during the summer. Horn flies resemble houseflies, but are more slender and only about half as big. Like most other cattle flies, they are bloodsuckers.

The scientific name of the horn fly is *Haematobium irritans,* and it is primarily a pest of cattle. The horn fly entered this country from Europe in the 19th century. Thus far, it has not been incriminated as a vector of any cattle diseases; however, it causes stress and thus makes the animal more susceptible to a variety of diseases.

Fighting the flies drains an animal's energy and interferes with feeding and resting. The animal may lose half a pound a day during fly season; studies show that during the grazing season cattle treated for horn flies may gain 15 to 50 pounds more than untreated cattle. Milk production may also be reduced as much as 20 percent by horn fly attacks.

Horn flies are present from spring until fall, although they sometimes decrease in number during hot, dry weather.

They usually attack the backs of cattle, out of reach of the tail and the swing of the head. To avoid the sun or rain, they sometimes congregate on the underparts of the animal's body. When the air is cool, they often rest on the horns, hence the name.

The adult flies remain on the host except when depositing their eggs on fresh cattle droppings. Oviposition lasts only a few minutes, after which the flies return to the host.

The horn fly ova are oblong and reddish-brown. In warm weather, the ova hatch into larvae in less than a day. The larvae, upon hatching, enter the fresh manure, where they feed and mature in about five days. When full-grown the larvae change into the pupal, or resting, stage, either in the droppings in which they developed or on the soil beneath. The pupae develop into adults in about seven days, and begin to lay eggs in another two days.

The complete life cycle, from egg to adult, takes only about two weeks. One adult female fly can lay as many as 400 eggs, so numbers can grow very rapidly during favorable weather.

With the coming of cold weather, the adult flies die and the pupae overwinter in the soil to reappear the following spring as adult horn flies.

Stable Flies

The stable fly is a serious pest of livestock. It usually annoys cattle on the lower parts of the legs; the pain of the biting flies causes them to stamp their feet incessantly. The stable fly looks somewhat like a robust housefly, but can be distinguished easily by the proboscis, which is held forward bayonet-like when the fly is at rest, and by the seven dorsal spots on the abdomen. It is common in the central section of the United States and lives around barns and stables rather than on the open range.

Horse and Deer Flies

Horse flies and deer flies are among the most annoying of livestock pests. Over 300 species have been recorded in North America. They are the vectors of many diseases, and they are vicious biters. They cut a small slit in the hide of animals with their lance-like mouth parts and suck large amounts of blood daily.

Control

There are four methods of controlling flies: (1) sprays, (2) dusts, (3) rubbing devices, and (4) dipping. Spraying with an approved insecticide is the best means of control.

59
Protozoa

PROTOZOOLOGY is that division of parasitology dealing with diseases caused by unicellular animals, or protozoa.

There are many species of protozoa and they vary markedly in their morphological and biological characteristics. Many simple species are morphologically primitive, but others are complex in their organization.

The ability of protozoan parasites to exist under various ecological and environmental conditions is illustrated by their varied localization in the body of the host. Protozoa can become parasitic in the blood, in the epithelial cells of the intestines, in the liver, kidneys, and urogenital tract, and in the lumen of the stomach and intestines.

The biological differences in protozoan parasites are complex and varied. Some develop in the body of only one host, often in a specific area within the host which they invade directly from the outside by way of feed, water and fomites. Others require one or more hosts, one definitive and one intermediate, in which the most drastic pathological changes are noted.

Reproduction in protozoa is sexual or asexual, but always by means of fission. In sexual reproduction, a reorganization takes place in the nucleus accompanied by a rejuvenation of nuclear matter. Fertilization is by copulation, conjugation, or autogamy, by fusing two nuclei apparently of different sexes. Asexual reproduction results from fission of the cell into two formations, each of which receives an equal part of the nucleus and cytoplasm.

Some protozoa reproduce only asexually, others only sexually, while a third group reproduces by alternation of both methods, in which case the sexual stage takes place in the definitive host if there is more than one host.

Often, pathogenic protozoa that have caused disease do not disappear from the body of the animal after it has recovered but persist for a long period, creating the carrier state. The carrier animal then serves as a focus of infection from which the disease may be transmitted to susceptible livestock. Carriers must be discovered before eradication can be successful.

Trichomoniasis

Trichomoniasis is a contagious venereal disease of cattle caused by a protozoan parasite, *Trichomonas foetus.* It is characterized by sterility, pyometra, early abortion in cows and inflammation of the genital tract in bulls. The first cases of the disease reported in the United States were in the east in 1932; subsequently, the disease has been discovered in all parts of this country. Trichomoniasis is distributed worldwide, wherever cattle are raised.

Etiology

Trichomonas foetus, a pyriform, pleomorphic protozoan, is the causative agent. It is distinguishable by 4 to 6 polar flagella, an undulation membrane extending the length of the organism, and an axostyle. It is generally ovoid, and 15 x 5 μ in size.

The organism is found in the genital tract of both sexes and is a strict parasite. *T. foetus* is spread by coitus, contaminated instruments, and infected semen used in artificial insemination. The infection rate is high. An infected bull may infect 90 percent of the heifers and cows in a herd, and will remain a carrier for an indefinite period unless treated. The parasite is insidious, and when first introduced into a herd the infection rate is high. In time, however, cows develop an apparent resistance to the point that the protozoan can be present but easily overlooked.

Symptoms

The invasion of the parasite may cause a low-grade vaginitis and endometritis with uterine, cervical, and vaginal catarrh.

External signs of the disease are slight reddening and swelling of the vulva and vaginal walls and an increased quantity of watery, mucous vaginal discharge in the cow, and inflammation of the penis and prepuce in the bull. One or two days after infection in bulls, pain and edema in the prepuce are noted, accompanied by a putrid discharge. The mucous membranes of the penis and prepuce are covered with small wheals, and small necrotic ulcers appear at the external edge of the prepuce. After two weeks the disease regresses, but bulls remain infective until cured by persistent treatment.

Infertility in the cow or heifer is a cardinal sign of the disease. It is indicated by repeat breedings, long, irregular estrus cycles, early embryonic mortality, or abortion by the fifth month of gestation. Conception may occur but, because of the uterine infection, abortion may follow. Abortion may take place at any time during gestation but usually occurs 2 to 16 weeks following infection. Late abortions are rare, and under certain conditions normal gestation and calving may occur, although the calf is usually weak. A vaginal discharge may be seen several days prior to abortion, and persist until the subsequent heat period; it is milky in color and heavily charged with parasites.

Postcoital pyometra occurs in some infected females. This results from death and maceration of the fetus. There is usually a slight discharge into the vagina when pyometra is present. In cases where the corpus luteum and the cervical seal persist, no pus will be discharged into the vagina. When pyometra persists, estrus may not occur for several months, although cows tend to rid themselves of the infection even without treatment and begin to cycle about 90 days after aborting.

Abortion is rapid and there may be little or no evidence of it. It is usually complete, without retention of the placenta and with little discharge. The discharges in trichomoniasis are always odorless and thus markedly different from those associated with other pathogenic infections.

Pathogenesis

T. foetus can be isolated in vaginal discharges, fetal membranes, mouth cavity and stomach contents of the fetus, fetal fluids, and exudate from the uterus of aborted cows. Investigations have shown that the duration of infection and fluctuations of numbers of parasites in the reproductive tract are related to the physiological state, the estrus cycle, and the development of specific antibodies. Thus, it would appear that (1) the true locus of infection is the uterus; (2) the presence of parasites in the vagina prior to estrus is due to extrusion from the uterus; (3) the development of antibodies in the vaginal secretions overcomes the parasites in the vagina, but that infection in the uterus is more resistant in animals with pyometra.

In the nonpregnant cow, the parasites appear periodically in the vagina, remain in the uterus, and will cause endometritis for one to several months in duration.

The bull carries the organism without ill effects except the possible swelling of the external genitalia. The organism may be isolated from the glans penis or the prepuce by the use of a preputial pipette with a rubber bulb and preinjection of a saline solution, or by the use of swabs. For positive diagnosis, weekly tests of this nature must be undertaken until the infective protozoa are isolated.

Diagnosis

Aids to diagnosis such as breeding history and external symptoms are helpful but not conclusive. A positive diagnosis depends upon identification of *Trichomonas foetus* in vaginal and uterine exudate, aborted fetuses, or preputial secretions. Motile parasites can be demonstrated by microscopical examination.

Control

The bull will remain permanently infected if not treated, and even then treatment is not completely effective. Infected cows or heifers will usually return to normal after a 90-day sexual rest.

The prevention of the entry of *T. foetus* into a disease-free herd is the primary method of control. This may be accomplished by checking the breeding records of newly acquired stock, medical examination of these animals, and quarantine upon their arrival. If the parasite has been introduced into the herd, the first step is separation of infected from noninfected cattle. Do not breed the infected females for 90 days, and then only after thorough examination. Breed noninfected females to a noninfected bull. Isolate and treat infected bulls, or dispose of them if the infection persists. Artificial insemination may be employed at this point on the noninfected animals, and after 90 days on the infected ones.

Coccidiosis

Coccidiosis is usually an enzootic disease occurring in young animals, although older animals may be affected. The disease is caused by microscopic one-celled parasites (protozoa) known as coccidia. These parasites affect the lining of the intestines by invading and destroying the epithelial cells, thus giving rise to hemorrhagic intestinal evacuations. All coccidia pathogenic to domestic animals belong to either the genus *Eimeria* or the genus *Isospora.*

Some authors believe that coccidia cause greater economic loss among domesticated animals of the temperate zone than any other group of protozoa. In some parts of the world they unquestionably are of major importance among pathogenic microorganisms attacking poultry, rabbits, cattle, sheep and swine. There is ample evidence to incriminate coccidia as parasitic to calves, sheep, goats, dogs, cats, and laboratory animals. Horses and related species seem to be relatively free of these parasites, although there are a few reports of their existence in these animals.

The life history of *Eimera cavae,* a parasite of the guinea pig, is described to illustrate the development of coccidiosis, since it is representative of those species causing coccidiosis in domestic animals. It is parasitic in the epithelial cells of the colon of the guinea pig, and may destroy many or most of the cells of this part of the alimentary canal, but, although the destruction of cells may be extensive, the health of the guinea pig is not seriously affected.

The infective stages of *Eimeria cavae* are the sporozoites. They enter the epithelial cells of the colon and become trophozoites, which feed and grow inside these cells and destroy them. The full-grown trophozoite is an oval cell with broad ends, and practically fills the cell destroyed by its growth. It ceases to grow and undergoes a process of multiple division called schizogony; it is therefore called a schizont. The divisions occur in the long axis of the schizont; 12 to 32 cigar-shaped individuals are produced, each of which is 6 to 16 μ long. They resemble the sporozoites in shape but are called merozoites. They are produced by asexual multiple division, not by the multiple division that follows the union of male and female gametes producing the sporozoites and called sporogony.

The merozoites leave the remains of the cells in which they were formed and infect other cells, inside which they develop into tropozoites. The trophozoites become schizonts, which repeat the process of schizogony.

In this manner, several generations of asexually-produced merozoites and schizonts may be formed and large numbers of the cells they parasitize may be destroyed. The destruction of the epithelium of the colon in this manner does not affect the health of the guinea pig, but the similar destruction of the epithelial and other cells by other species of *sporozoa,* in other animals, may cause serious complications and death. It is usually this asexual schizogonous phase of the life history that causes the disease of domesticated animals known as coccidiosis.

After several generations have been produced by schizogony, asexual multiplication ceases and sexual reproduction begins. The trophozoites mature and become, not schizonts, but gametocytes, which form gametes. The gametocytes are sexually differentiated into male and female, although this fact is not, in this species, evident until gamete formation has begun.

The male gametocytes of *Eimeria cavae* divide to form a large number of minute, comma-shaped, active male gametes, each provided with two flagella. They are exactly comparable to the spermatozoa of higher animals. The female gametocyte does not divide and is not active. Its nucleus undergoes a process of maturation similar to, but more primitive than, the maturation of the ova of higher animals, and the cytoplasm stores up reserves of feed. The female gametocyte is then a female gamete ready to be fertilized by the male gamete. The gametes are thus, like those of higher animals, anisogametes, and active male gametes leave the cells in which they were formed and seek out and fertilize the passive female gametes. The resulting zygote is thus exactly comparable to the fertilized ovum of higher animals.

The zygote, while still inside the cell in which it is parasitic, forms a resistant envelope around itself and is then called an oocyst. The oocyst is liberated by bursting the host cell, and is passed out in the host's excreta.

Outside the host the zygote divides inside the oocyst into two sporoblasts. These again divide into two, so that four sporoblasts are formed. Each of these four sporoblasts secretes a resistant wall around itself which is called a sporocyst. In this manner, each sporoblast becomes a spore. Each oocyst of *Eimeria sp.* thus contains four spores. The contents of each spore then divides to form two sporozoites. The production of four spores, each containing two sporozoites, so that there are eight sporozoites in each oocyst, is characteristic of all species of the genus *Eimeria.* The species of the genus *Isospora,* also found in some domestic animals, form only two spores, each of which contains four sporozoites. Species of these two genera may be differentiated by this feature. Other species of *Coccidia* produce variable numbers of spores.

The process by which spores and sporozoites are formed is called sporulation. This term must be carefully distinguished from the term sporogony, the name given to the whole sexual cycle producing the sporozoites to distinguish it from the asexual multiple division producing merozoites and called schizogony.

Sporulation—the division of the zygote to form sporoblasts and the division of these to form sporozoites enclosed in spores—always occurs outside the host, although occasionally the feces of constipated animals, retained for abnormal periods of time in the rectum, may contain oocysts in which sporulation is in progress or has been completed. When sporulation is complete, the oocyst can, if swallowed by another host of the same species, cause infection. However, it is not infective until the sporozoites have been fully formed. Thus, the infectivity of oocysts is governed by the time required for their sporulation. The oocysts of most species of *Eimeria* complete this process in 2 or 3 days, provided temperature, moisture, and other environmental factors influencing the rate of sporulation are adequate. The life histories of most of the species of the genus *Eimeria* are direct, that is, schizogony and sporogony occur in the same host. All of the *Coccidia* which affect domestic animals have direct life histories.

Transmission

The sporulated oocyst is the infective stage of coccidial parasites. As already stated, the sporulation process requires a lapse of time after the immature oocyst leaves the host, plus optimum temperature and moisture. Once the oocyst is mature it is infective, unless unfavorable environmental conditions destroy its viability.

Under ordinary farm conditions there is ample opportunity for the direct transmission of infective oocysts from host to host through contamination of feed and water, or by young animals licking themselves or the walls of pens, or sucking other contaminated animals or objects.

Mechanical transmission is also possible, as the infective oocysts can be carried from place to place on the feet and clothing of attendants, on the feet of rodents and birds, on the hooves of adult livestock, and by running surface water. Insects may play a similar role in the mechanical transfer of parasites, and may carry them in their intestines and deposit them in droppings where they are available for ingestion by susceptible hosts. It has been noted that birds and mammals may at times convey from place to place coccidial oocysts to which they are not susceptible.

Coccidia are normal inhabitants of the intestines of young cattle maintained in confinement, and clinical coccidiosis develops as the result of lowering the resistance of host to parasite. Carrier animals are able to initiate an outbreak of coccidiosis when mixed with susceptible animals under bad management conditions, such as crowding, overstocking of lush areas where the oocysts may sporulate, and poor hygiene. It has been shown that contaminated pens in feeder sheep barns carry the infection from year to year, and that bedding is usually the source of viable oocysts for young lambs.

Prevention

It is easier to prevent clinical coccidiosis than to cure it, especially in large animals. Strict attention to hygiene is necessary at all times with any class of livestock, although, unless pastures are overstocked, the problem is not as pressing with beef cattle.

It is recommended that sanitary precautions and management practices be designed to prevent young animals from swallowing large numbers of infective sporulated oocysts.

Young animals should never be introduced into a group of animals of various ages. They will pick up a few stray oocysts, develop nonclinical infections, and then pass large numbers of oocysts. Other young animals will ingest the oocysts and clinical cases will occur.

If it is possible to isolate animals or keep the pens cleaned daily, segregation of young animals into separate pens according to age groups will help. Animals fed outside on wet ground around feed sheds, watering troughs or haystacks are a problem. All puddles and wet spots should be drained and filled. Manure should be removed often. Rotation of feeding places is valuable.

Immunity

Critically conducted experiments have shown that susceptible animals may be made to develop a more or less complete immunity to reinfection by the repeated administration of sublethal doses of viable sporulated oocysts. However, reports indicate that, in certain types of swine coccidiosis, a protracted period of frequent reinfection is necessary to establish even a temporary immunity.

Little is known concerning the effects of age upon susceptibility to infection. It often appears that older animals are more resistant than younger animals, but this apparent age immunity may well be illusory, as the animals may have at some time in the past picked up enough sporulated oocysts to acquire what scientists call "a partial immunity constituting protection against symptoms of the disease although not against reinfection."

It is definitely known that immunity in coccidiosis is specific; an animal immunized against one species does not become resistant to other species for which it is also the host.

Host Specificity

At one time it was believed that coccidia were nonspecific insofar as the host was concerned. Experimental work has shown that a degree of host specificity exists with the various species. The coccidia of the genus *Eimeria* are host specific, even organ specific, while the coccidia of the genus *Isospora* are not so particular and in general less pathogenic. Certain species of the *Eimeria,* which are responsible for the most serious infections of domesticated animals, may occasionally be found in closely related species of animals, such as sheep and goats, but this is the exception rather than the rule.

Coccidiosis of Cattle

Thirteen species of *Eimeria* may infect cattle, although some are more pathogenic than others. The species most commonly responsible for the production of clinical coccidiosis in cattle are *Eimeria zurnii* and *Eimeria bovis.*

Symptoms

The symptoms of coccidiosis may include rough coat, weakness, listlessness, nervousness, poor appetite, diarrhea, and loss of or poor gains in weight. The general weakness may cause calves to defecate without rising, thus soiling the tail, hindquarters, and lower part of the body. When standing, the calf may attempt to defecate and is unable to; the intense straining results in an arched back, raised tail, and a "pumping" of the sides. The diarrhea may be watery or only slightly liquid, being quite unlike the "white scours" of calves less than 3 weeks old. Diarrhea caused by coccidiosis may contain strands of gelatinous mucus and streaks of blood. In infections with *Eimeria zurnii* and *Eimeria bovis,* feces may be extremely bloody and may even contain shreds of intestinal tissue or occasionally short lengths of the tubular lining of the damaged intestine.

Gross lesions observed on postmortem include: erosion and necrosis of areas of the mucosa, thickening of the intestinal wall and circumscribed or diffuse hemorrhage. The mucosa may be irregularly thickened and the surface pitted or rough and granular in appearance. In severe cases, a diphtheritic membrane may be found on the surface of the cecum or colon. Most of the lesions occur in the lower small intestine, the cecum and colon. In infections with *Eimeria bovis,* minute white dots may be seen microscopically in the villi of the lower small intestine. These

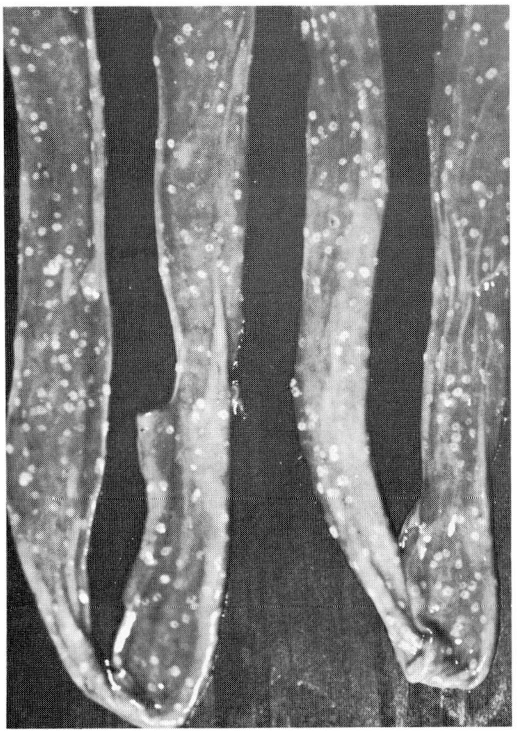

FIG. 55. Infection with *Eimeria arlongi.* The white dots are schizonts in the mucosa of the small intestine.

are large schizonts developing in the endothelial cells beneath the epithelial lining.

Calves between the ages of 3 weeks and 6 months are most commonly affected. Symptoms usually begin about two weeks after infection and diarrhea is the most characteristic symptom.

Coccidiosis of Sheep

There are ten species of *Eimera* affecting sheep and goats, although clinical coccidiosis is usually due to mixed infections with two or more species; *Eimeria arlongi, Eimeria faurei,* and *Eimeria ansata* are considered the most common.

Coccidiosis has long been recognized in Europe and the United States as a disease of some importance in sheep. It is well known that coccidia are usually present in large numbers in apparently healthy young sheep and in smaller numbers in older animals. There is, however, a syndrome attributed to coccidiosis, although published descriptions of the disease vary somewhat in detail.

Life History

The infection arises from the ingestion of sporulated oocysts, from which the sporozoites are liberated in the digestive tract of the host. The sporozoites invade the epithelial cells of the gut where asexual and, later, sexual reproduction takes place with consequent damage to the host tissue. The end-product of the sexual phase is the oocyst, which passes to the exterior in the feces.

The oocyst is fairly resistant and, under suitable conditions of moisture, warmth, and oxygen tension, it will develop further and in 1 to 4 days will be found to contain 4 sporocysts, each with 2 sporozoites.

Conditions favoring sporulation have been studied in the field. It was found that, in shallow water at temperatures near freezing, sporulation occurred slowly; at room temperature, it was rapid, but at higher temperatures (103 F) sporulation did not occur and the cysts died in about 3 days. This failure was attributed to lack of oxygen due to putrefaction. About 20 percent of the unsporulated oocysts were still viable after 10 months at temperatures near freezing. It was concluded that in the field oocysts could accumulate and survive in wet situations over the colder months of the year. Inside moistened pellets, sporulation proceeded normally at room temperature, but drying was lethal to the oocysts within several days.

Symptoms

The disease has usually been described in lambs between the ages of 4 to 6 months. The affected animals show signs of abdominal pain, anemia, loss of weight, and diarrhea. The feces are foul smelling, brownish to yellow-green, and often blood streaked. There is a marked enteritis and yellowish-white

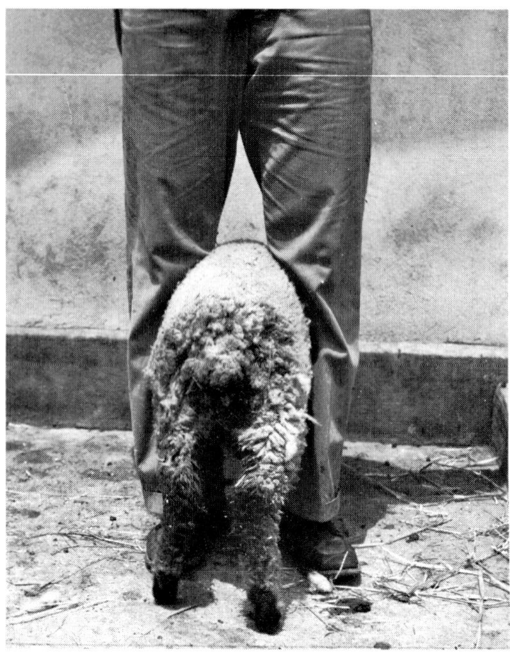

FIG. 56. Coccidiosis in the sheep. Note the soiling of the rump and rear of legs from diarrhea.

spots can be seen from the serosal surface; they vary from 0.5 to 6.0 mm in diameter. These areas are filled with macrogametocytes and oocysts. In some cases the lesions take the form of papilliform growths, the interior of which is filled with parasites. There is frequently inflammation of the large intestine as well. The disease occurs in lambs before and after weaning. Anemia is often present and occasionally lambs are paralyzed. There has been little work done with artificial infections and still less with pure strains, but there appears to be a general opinion that *E. arlongi* is one of the organisms most pathogenic for sheep.

Coccidiosis in Swine

There are five species of coccidia reported for swine in North America. Four of these species belong to the genus *Eimeria* and one to *Isospora*. Coccidiosis is a less important disease in swine than in sheep and cattle, and is usually self limiting. The disease lasts about two weeks, but a few oocysts may be shed for a long period of time by partially immune animals. *Eimeria debliecki* is the most pathogenic species, but *Eimeria scabra* and *Isospora suis* are most often encountered.

This disease is transmitted by ingestion of sporulated oocysts as contaminants in food or water. Cross transmission of coccidia between swine and other domestic animals has not been conclusively demonstrated.

Symptoms

Coccidiosis is a disease primarily of the young, as adult animals have usually experienced the infection and are partially immune, and clinical signs are not shown. The first sign of the infection is diarrhea which may be followed by constipation. This diarrhea, in contrast to that of coccidiosis in cattle, is rarely bloody upon close examination. In addition, however, dehydration and anorexia may occur. The morbidity varies widely in different outbreaks while the mortality remains low. Recovered animals are frequently stunted in growth and appear unthrifty. Lesions are found in the large intestine consisting of congestion, edema and catarrhal and hemorrhagic inflammation of the large intestine, but the small intestine may also be involved. In experimental infections, the coccidia are confined to the surface epithelium, causing destruction and loss of cells in addition to a mild cellular reaction which results in a slight thickening of the gut.

Diagnosis

Coccidiosis is diagnosed by fecal examination. A direct smear in water or saline should suffice, although concentration by salt or heavy sugar solution will not destroy the oocysts. Species identification is difficult and usually not necessary.

Treatment and Control

The most effective therapeutic agents are the sulfonamides; however, in most cases, the animals showing clinical signs are past the stage for optimum benefit. Symptomatic treatment of the diarrhea and the prevention of secondary infections are indicated. Control measures should include adequate clean water from fountains or troughs, and adequate racks or troughs for food. Space should be provided to avoid overcrowding. Pasture rotation to reduce the amount of contamination is helpful, but this measure alone is not sufficient; it has been shown that coccidia remain viable in soil for 15 months with the surface temperature ranging from 103 F to 20 F, and withstand freezing for at least a month.

Prophylaxis of clinical coccidiosis is based upon controlling the intake of sporulated oocysts by young animals so that the infection becomes established in immunizing proportions without causing the frank disease. Good feeding, proper sanitation, and modern management practices accomplish this goal.

PART 7
Selected References and Additional Reading

Anthony, D. J., and Lewis, E. F.: *Diseases of the Pig,* 5th ed. Bailliere, Tindall & Cox, London, 1961.

Blood, D. C., and Henderson, J. A.: *Veterinary Medicine.* Williams & Wilkins, Baltimore, 1960.

Brandly, C. A., and Jungherr, E. L. (Eds.): *Advances in Veterinary Science.* Academic Press, New York, 1953 to date.

British Veterinary Association: Handbook on Tropical Diseases. London, 1962.

Gibbons, W. J. (Ed.): *Diseases of Cattle.* American Veterinary Publications, Santa Barbara, 1963.

Hagan, W. A., and Bruner, D. W.: *The Infectious Diseases of Domestic Animals,* 4th ed. Comstock Publishing Associates, Ithaca, 1961.

Henning, M. H.: *Animal Diseases in South Africa,* 2nd ed. Central News Agency, Johannesburg, 1949.

Horton-Smith, C. (Ed.): *Biological Aspects of the Transmission of Disease,* 1st ed. Oliver & Boyd, London, 1957.

Hull, T. G.: *Diseases Transmitted from Animals to Man,* 5th ed. Charles C Thomas, Springfield, 1963.

Hutyra, F., Marek, J., and Manninger, R.: *Special Pathology and Therapeutics of the Diseases of Domestic Animals.* Alexander Eger, Chicago, 1949.

Lovell, R.: *The Aetiology of Infective Diseases: With Special Reference to the Subsidiary and Important Nonspecific Factors.* Michigan State Univ. Press, East Lansing, 1959.

Marsh, H.: *Newsom's Sheep Diseases,* 2nd ed. Williams & Wilkins, Baltimore, 1958.

Miller, A. R.: *Meat Hygiene,* 2nd ed. Lea & Febiger, Philadelphia, 1958.

Pool, W. A. (Ed.): *Veterinary Annual.* Williams & Wilkins, Baltimore, 1959 to date.

Radeleff, R. D.: *Veterinary Toxicology.* Lea & Febiger, Philadelphia, 1970.

Riley, W. F., Jr., Smith, K. W., and Flynn, R. J. (Eds.): *Year Book of Veterinary Medicine.* Year Book Medical Publishers, Chicago, 1963.

Siegmund, O. H., McLean, J. W., Armistead,

W. W., Hagan, W. A., Hutchings, L. M., and Schnelle, G. B. (Eds.): *Merck Veterinary Manual,* 2nd ed. Merck & Co., Rahway, 1961.

Smith, H. A., and Jones, T. C.: *Veterinary Pathology.* Lea & Febiger, Philadelphia, 1961.

Smith, L. D. S.: *Introduction to Pathogenic Anaerobes.* Univ. of Chicago Press, Chicago, 1954.

Stableforth, A. W., and Galloway, I. A. (Eds.): *Infectious Diseases of Animals: Diseases Due to Bacteria,* Vols. 1 and 2. Academic Press, New York, 1959.

Udall, D. H.: *The Practice of Veterinary Medicine,* 6th ed. Ithaca, 1954. Printed by Geo. Banta Publishing Co., Menesha, Wisconsin.

United States Department of Agriculture: *Keeping Livestock Healthy.* The Yearbook of Agriculture, 1942.

United States Department of Agriculture: *Animal Diseases.* The Yearbook of Agriculture, 1956.

Index